Pocket Guide
to
Low Sodium
Foods

Pocket Guide
to
Low Sodium
Foods

Bobbie Mostyn

**Second Edition
Revised**

InData Group, Inc.

Pocket Guide to Low-Sodium Foods. Copyright 2003, 2006 by Bobbie Mostyn. All rights reserved. This book, or parts thereof, may not be reproduced in any form without permission from the publisher, exceptions are made for brief excerpts used in published reviews. Published by InData Group, Inc., P.O. Box 11908, Olympia, WA 98508-1908.

Printed in the United States of America

Cover design: Gray Ponytail Studio - www.grayponytail.com

Pocket Guide to Low-Sodium Foods Web site:

www.LowSaltFoods.com

Library of Congress Cataloging-in-Publication Data

Mostyn, Bobbie
  Pocket guide to low sodium foods / Bobbie Mostyn. -- 2006 ed., completely rev.
    p.cm.
    Includes index.
    LCCN 2002117596
    ISBN 0-9673969-6-4

  1. Food--Sodium content--Tables.   I. Title.
TX553.S65M67 2006   613.2'85

CONTENTS

DEDICATED TO:

*My husband, Mike – without your continued support and help
this whole project would not be possible –
you are the light of my life!*

*All my friends and family – thanks for your understanding
and patience for all the calls and emails
that went unanswered.*

*Food manufacturers and restaurants who are
reducing the sodium in their product offerings –
thanks for your interest in our well-being –
we, in turn, will support your products.*

*Those who are watching their sodium intake –
hopefully this guide makes your food
choices a little bit easier.*

Salt is contributing to a U.S. health crisis and the medical community is sounding the alarm. According to estimates, Americans consume 4,000-6,000 milligrams (mg) of sodium per day – two to three times more than the National Institutes of Health recommended level of 2,400mg (or about 1 teaspoon salt).

There is reason for concern. Excessive sodium has been linked to the development of high blood pressure (or hypertension). Once developed an individual's risk for heart attack, stroke, kidney and other problems increases significantly.

More than 50 million Americans (one in four adults) have high blood pressure and that number is expected to increase as our population ages. In fact, fifty percent of people over the age of 60 develop hypertension.

Nevertheless, there is good news. Studies show that a substantial decrease in the amount of sodium consumed can lower blood pressure and may even help prevent hypertension. Medical experts are now recommending sodium reduction for everyone, not just hypertensive patients. *NOTE: At this writing, the National Academy of Sciences' Institute of Medicine is recommending that sodium guidelines be reduced to 1,500mg per day (less for older people).*

USE LESS SALT

Reducing one's intake of salt is not easy. Nearly everything we eat contains some natural sodium, even small amounts occur naturally in fruits and vegetables, but the vast majority comes off the grocery shelves and from restaurant meals. Surprisingly, less than 15% of the salt we consume comes from the saltshaker.

Thanks in part to our busy lifestyles, we have become accustomed to salty snacks and foods. Because we have less time to plan meals, we rely more on convenience and fast foods, which are loaded with salt. Unfortunately, the more salt we consume, the more we crave. It's a vicious cycle, but it can be modified.

Although lifestyle changes may be difficult, particularly when it comes to eating, you can retrain your tastebuds to enjoy less salt in about 6-8 weeks. If you start gradually, using a little less salt each day, not only will your use of sodium decrease, but also your craving. In fact, many foods that used to taste good will now taste salty.

Tips to Reducing Salt

Eliminate the saltshaker. Don't salt before you taste. Break the habit of automatically reaching for the saltshaker.

Choose lower sodium foods. Eat more fruits and vegetables and use less prepared foods (the less processing, the less sodium). Look for foods labeled *sodium free, low sodium, reduced sodium, unsalted* and *no salt added*. (See Nutritional Content Claims, page xv, for more information.)

Read the label. Know how much sodium is in each serving. Be alert to "salty" terms, like *brine, cured, marinated, pickled* and *smoked*. Notice serving sizes. What is listed may be smaller than what you will actually eat.

Use less salt in cooking. In most recipes salt can be reduced or, in many cases, omitted without compromising the flavor. Use more herbs and spices, particularly onion and garlic powder. Also, low-sodium bouillon can add extra flavor, as can wine, vinegar, lemon or lime juice.

Prepare low-salt recipes. Get a good low-sodium cookbook. Many are available at your local bookstore. Also, search the Internet where there is an abundance of low-salt recipes.

Order low-sodium foods at restaurants. Ask how foods are prepared and whenever possible request that no salt be added to your entree. Find restaurants that feature "heart-healthy" meals or will accommodate your dietary restrictions. (NOTE: "Heart-healthy" usually indicates a menu item is low fat or low cholesterol and may not always be low sodium.)

BECOME SODIUM CONSCIOUS

Although experts have been warning us for years to cut back on salt, most consumers are not listening. The problem is most of us are unaware of how much sodium we actually take in. Many people mistakenly think the amount they are consuming is okay, because they do not use it at the table or in their cooking. Although the saltshaker contributes about 15% of the salt we consume, the majority of it comes off the grocery shelves. The bottom line, if you don't know how much salt is in a product, you cannot take control of your diet.

As you become more aware of the amount of sodium in grocery items, you will discover two things: (1) nearly every food has a low-salt alternative and (2) there is a large disparity among brands. For instance, some pasta sauces contain as much as 850mg sodium per serving, others have around 200mg, and no-salt-added sauces have less than 50mg. Another example is teriyaki marinade—some brands have up to 3,050mg sodium per tablespoon. As a substitute, try one of the many grilling sauces with less than 140mg. Use the *Pocket Guide to Low-Sodium Foods* to find low-salt substitutes for the following high-sodium products.

Foods High in Sodium

Bakery items – bagels, breads, donuts, and pastries
Canned foods – soups, meats, fish, sauerkraut, beans, and vegetables
Convenience foods – frozen dinners, pizza, cereals, and packaged mixes , such as pancakes, food "helpers," stuffing, and rice dishes
Dairy products – cheese and cottage cheese
Deli items – bacon, luncheon meats, corned beef, smoked meats or fish, anchovies, and mayonnaise-based salads, like cole slaw and potato salad
Snack foods – crackers, chips, and dips
Condiments – mustard, ketchup, mayonnaise, salad dressings, pickles, olives, capers, salsas, and packaged seasoning mixes
Sauces – gravy, steak, pasta, teriyaki or soy sauce
Baking needs – self-rising flour, baking and biscuit mixes, bouillon cubes, batter and coating mixes, breadcrumbs, corn syrup, cooking wines, meat tenderizers, monosodium glutamate (MSG), baking powder and baking soda
Beverages – tomato and vegetable juices, Bloody Mary and chocolate drink mixes

---

HIDDEN SOURCES OF SODIUM

You may not be aware of the numerous sources of hidden sodium that are in over-the-counter health aids. For example, certain dentifrices, aspirin, and medications that contain ibuprofen (such as *Advil* and *Nuprin*) contain sodium, as do antacids, like *Rolaids* and *Alka-Seltzer* (some have as much as 761mg). Check labels for low-sodium alternatives or ask your pharmacist or healthcare provider for suggestions.

Also, many households have water-softening systems that contain sodium chloride. To remedy this, potassium chloride (where potassium replaces the salt) can be used. Of course, if it is still a concern you can always drink bottled water.

NOTE TO THE HYPERTENSIVE

"High blood pressure is a time bomb in your blood vessels, just waiting to explode in a stroke or heart attack," says Pat Kendall, Ph.D., R.D., a nutrition specialist at Colorado State University Cooperative Extension. "It just keeps ticking away, speeding the artery-clogging process until the blood vessels finally burst."

THE DASH DIET

Scary stuff, but there is new research that has determined diet can have a positive effect on blood pressure. Funded by the National Heart, Lung and Blood Institute (NHLBI), the Dietary Approaches to Stop Hypertension (DASH) clinical study shows that the DASH diet not only lowers blood pressure, but may also help prevent and control hypertension.

According wo the DASH study, sodium reduction lowers blood pressure regardless of race or sex and has the greatest effect on hypertensive individuals. Subsequent research indicates the lower the salt intake, the better the results.

The DASH diet, based on 2,000 calories a day, is low in fats and cholesterol. It is also high in fiber and plentiful in fruits, vegetables, and low-fat dairy products. What's more, following the DASH diet may also reduce your risk of cancer, osteoporosis, and diabetes.

NOTE: Diet is only one part of the prevention and treatment of hypertension and other maladies. Other factors include exercise, maintaining a healthy weight, quitting smoking, and increasing your intake of calcium and magnesium. Before making any major changes in salt consumption or beginning an exercise program, be sure to talk with your healthcare provider.

SALT SUBSTITUTES

If you are taking certain diuretics and other prescription drugs for the treatment of hypertension, be cautious of salt substitutes. Many contain potassium which may adversely affect your medication. Additionally, many foods that are low in sodium also have added potassium. Check with your healthcare provider before using salt substitutes or consuming potassium-enhanced foods.

— Other Culprits That Raise Blood Pressure —

Caffeine (including coffee, tea, soft drinks, chocolate, and some medications) – may temporarily increase blood pressure

Licorice – consumed in large amounts

Phenylalanine (used in sugar-free foods that contain aspartame, such as *Nutra-Sweet* and *Equal*) – may elevate blood pressure in sensitive individuals

Alcohol – more than 1 glass of wine or 24 ounces of beer is considered excessive and may cause a rise in blood pressure

Cold and cough remedies – decongestants (such as, pseudoephedrine, phenylpropanolamine, dextromethorphan) found in many cough and cold medications may elevate blood pressure

Appetite suppressants – ingredients (like diethylpropion) found in many weight reducing agents may raise blood pressure

---

The Food and Drug Administration (FDA) regulates food labeling to assure consumers that the information they receive is accurate and not misleading. Labels contain a lot of useful information to help you compare products and make healthy food choices.

WHAT THE LABEL TELLS YOU

Serving Size – Identified in familiar units (such as cups or tablespoons) followed by the metric equivalent (i.e. grams) and is determined by the amount typically eaten.

Amount per Serving – Nutritional information is based on one serving. In the example below, the serving size is 1 cup. If you eat 2 cups you need to double the calories, nutrients, and *% Daily Value*.

Nutrition Facts

Serving Size 1 cup (55g)
Servings Per Container about 8

Amount Per Serving

Calories 170   Calories from Fat 10

	% Daily Value*
Total Fat 1 g	
Saturated Fat 0g	**2 %**
Trans Fat 0g	**0 %**
Cholesterol 0mg	**0 %**
Sodium 85mg	**0 %**
Total Carbohydrate 41g	**4 %**
Dietary Fiber 7g	**14 %**
Sugars 21g	**28 %**
Protein 6g	

Vitamin A 0%	▪	Vitamin C 0%
Calcium 0%	▪	Iron 6%

*Percent Daily Values are based on a 2,000 calorie diet. Your daily values may be higher or lower depending on your calorie needs.

		Calories	2,000	2,500
Total Fat	Less than		65g	80g
Sat Fat	Less than		20g	25g
Cholesterol	Less than		300mg	300mg
Sodium	Less than		2,400mg	2,400mg
Total Carbohydrate			300m	375mg
Dietary Fiber			25g	30 g

Calories from Fat – This is the amount of fat multiplied by 9 (number of calories per gram of fat). Dietary guidelines suggest no more than 30% of daily calories come from fat. To calculate percentage, divide *Calories from Fat* by *Calories* (in this example, $10 \div 170 = 6\%$).

Nutrients – Values are listed in grams except for *Cholesterol* and *Sodium* which are in milligrams. Use these figures to compare fat, sodium, etc. between products. If a nutrient is not shown, there is no significant amount in the product.

% Daily Value – This shows how much of the *Recommended Daily Values* (RDVs) each nutrient provides and is another way to compare similar products. Calculations are based on 2,000 calories. In this example, the total RDV for sodium (2,400mg) is divided by the amount of sodium per serving (85g), which means this serving equals 4% of your RDV for sodium.

Ingredients – Listed in order from most to least amount. Generally, if sodium is one of the first 3 ingredients, there is probably too much salt for a low-salt diet.

NUTRITIONAL CONTENT CLAIMS

Label content claims describe the level of a nutrient or dietary substance in the product, using terms, such as *free*, *high*, and *low*. They can also compare the nutrient amount in a particular food to that of another food using terms, such as *more*, *reduced*, and *lite*. The following claims are used on nutritional labels and are based on one serving.

	FREE	LOW	REDUCED/ LESS	LIGHT/ LITE
Cal	< 5 calories	40 calories or less	25% less than normal	50% less than normal
Fat	< 0.5g fat	3g or less fat	25% less than normal	50% less than normal
Sat Fat	< 0.5g sat fat & < 0.5g trans fatty acids	1g or less saturated fat	25% less than normal	50% less than normal
Chol	< 2mg chol & 2g or less sat fat	< 20mg chol & 2g or less sat fat	25% less than normal	50% less than normal
Sug	< 0.5g sugar		25% less than normal	50% less than normal

	FREE	VERY LOW	LOW	UNSALTED/NSA
Sod	< 5mg sod	< 35mg sod	<140mg sod	No salt added to normally salted food

NOTE: *Low-fat* and *non-fat* do not mean low sodium or low sugar; manufacturers often replace the fat with added salt and sugar.

CALORIES AND NUTRIENTS

CALORIES

Calories measure the amount of energy contained in foods and are calculated based on the amount of carbohydrates, fat, and protein within the food. (Alcohol also provides calories.)

Once consumed and digested, food is converted to glucose which fuels everything the body does, like walking, talking, breathing. The amount of calories needed is different for every individual. For example, the more active an individual, the greater the caloric need. However, when the body takes in more calories than it requires, the extra energy is stored as body fat.

CHOLESTEROL AND FATS

Cholesterol and fats are essential to the human body, however, too much of either can be detrimental to your health.

CHOLESTEROL

Cholesterol is a waxy, fat-like substance produced naturally in the body and is necessary for many bodily functions. The body manufactures all the cholesterol it needs and circulates it via the bloodstream, which separates it into "good" and "bad" lipoproteins.

The bad, or low-density lipoproteins (LDL), stick to the blood vessel walls contributing to clogged arteries and hypertension, and is the leading cause for heart disease. The good, or high-density lipoproteins (HDL), unstick LDLs and help move them through the bloodstream and out of the body. This is why the ratio of HDL to LDL is important.

Over time the LDL deposits (along with fat) build up, causing the arteries to clog. As the arteries narrow, the flow of blood decreases and blood pressure increases. This build-up of fatty deposits is also a major factor in coronary disease and strokes.

Research indicates that saturated fats and trans-fatty acids have a greater impact in raising cholesterol than from eating dietary cholesterol. It should be noted, that most foods high in cholesterol are also high in saturated fats, and vice versa.

Cholesterol is found mainly in animal foods (meat, poultry, fish, egg yolks, and dairy products), it is not found in plant foods. The daily recommendation for cholesterol is less than 300mg.

FAT

Not all fats are harmful and have been classified as either good or bad. Saturated fat is considered bad, as too much of it raises LDL cholesterol levels. Monounsaturated and polyunsaturated fats help lower cholesterol and are considered good. (Although too much of any fat raises blood cholesterol levels, all fats should be used in moderation.)

Trans fatty acids, considered saturated and classified as bad, not only raise LDLs, but also decrease HDLs. Many experts believe trans fats are as bad as, if not worse than, saturated fats.

Types of Fat

Saturated — Usually solid at room temperature (comes mainly from animal products, such as butter, cheese, meat products, egg yolks, and whole milk dairy products).

Monounsaturated — Liquid at room temperature, but solidifies in the refrigerator (found in plant foods, such as olive oil, canola oil, avocados, and nuts).

Polyunsaturated — Liquid at room temperature and also in the refrigerator (examples are vegetable oils, including corn oil, safflower oil, and sunflower oil).

Trans fatty acids — Result of hydrogenation and used for shelf stability or solidifying a fat product (found in margarine, crackers, cookies, potato chips, and fast foods, such as french fries).

If a product lists *hydrogenated* or *partially hydrogenated* in the ingredients, it has trans-fatty acids. Be aware that many low-fat, low-cholesterol products may have trans fats.

The American Heart Association (AHA) suggests no more than 30% of total calories come from fat and no more than 10% from saturated fat (7% if you have heart disease, diabetes, or high LDL cholesterol). As a general rule, any food that has 5% or less fat is considered low in fat; 20% or more, is high. Choose fats with 2g or less saturated fat per serving.

CARBOHYDRATES, FIBER AND SUGAR

Carbohydrates are the body's supplier of energy. Once consumed carbohydrates convert into two basic forms: simple carbohydrates (found in sugars) and complex carbohydrates (comprised of starches and fibers). Except for fiber, which is not digestible, all carbohydrates turn directly into sugar (glucose) in the bloodstream and affect blood glucose in different ways.

Carbohydrates

Simple carbohydrates – generally have no nutritive value and produce a rapid rise in blood glucose followed by a rapid fall.
Complex carbohydrates – are more nutritious and produce a slower, more sustained blood glucose response.

Foods high in complex carbohydrates are usually low in calories, saturated fat, and cholesterol. They are found primarily in plant foods, such as fruits, vegetables, whole grains, beans, and legumes. They also are present in dairy products.

Daily caloric intake of carbohydrates should be between 55-60% (or 25-35 grams) with an emphasis on complex carbohydrates.

FIBER

Fiber is the part of food that is not digested. There are two types of fiber – soluble and insoluble.

Soluble fiber – dissolves in fluids of the large intestine. Soluble fiber is found in oats, barley, rye, nuts, fruits, vegetables, psyllium seeds (used in fiber laxatives), beans, and legumes. Consumed in large amounts, soluble fiber can decrease blood cholesterol, improve blood glucose levels, and appears to reduce hypertension. It also may help with weight loss by increasing the feeling of fullness.

Insoluble fiber – instead of dissolving, it passes straight through the intestines and helps maintain regularity. It is found in whole grains, seeds, bran, fruit, and vegetable skins. It also is associated with reduced risk of colon cancer.

The amount of fiber also affects blood glucose. The more fiber in a food, the slower the digestion and absorption of sugars. To help understand fiber's influence on blood glucose, the glycemic index (GI) was developed. Using glucose (the highest rated GI) as a standard, a food is ranked by how fast it is digested and how much it causes blood glucose to rise. We will not get into GI rankings in this book, but suffice to say, this new information is changing the way nutritionists and the medical society are looking at carbohydrates.

The recommended level of total soluble and insoluble fiber is 20-35 grams per day. Look for a minimum of 3 grams of fiber, but 5 grams or more is better.

SUGAR

Sugar consumption has been on the increase and experts believe diets high in sugar are contributing to many of today's health problems, including hypertension and heart disease.

Current research indicates long-term consumption of a diet high in refined (simple) carbohydrates produces higher insulin levels. As insulin levels elevate, adrenaline production is stimulated, which can cause blood vessel constriction and increased sodium retention. Additionally, high carbohydrate intake has been linked to increased LDL and decreased HDL cholesterol.

Even though the RDVs have no sugar guidelines, the US Department of Agriculture (USDA) advises limiting sugar to 10 teaspoons (47g) a day (based on a 2,000-calorie diet).

SODIUM

Sodium is essential to the body. About 500mg a day is needed to help regulate fluids and maintain normal functioning of nerves and muscles. If excess sodium is not used, fluid builds up (water retention) increasing the work of the heart and kidneys.

Select foods that contain less than 5 percent of the daily value for sodium (or about 100mg per serving). Experts suggest limiting any food that has more than 480mg sodium per serving.

DINING OUT

The most difficult time to control salt consumption is when dining out. Making good nutritional choices can be difficult, especially when we do not know what has been added to the foods we order. For example, a healthy garden salad with lowfat dressing oftentimes has more sodium than a hamburger and french fries. Hard to believe, but depending on how it is prepared, what we think is healthy may not be low sodium.

Another fast food misconception is chicken or fish sandwiches being a better choice than beef. There may be less fat, but not salt. In most instances added seasonings, coatings, deep frying, and other preparations create a much higher sodium meal.

Perhaps one day, with enough public pressure, nutritional data will be available at all restaurants. In the meantime, follow the suggestions below in selecting healthier, low-sodium menu items.

Watch the Salt

- **Order low-sodium foods.** Ask how foods are prepared; choose steamed, broiled, grilled, or roasted entrees without sauces.
- **Avoid fried foods.** Most batters are salted, plus additional saturated or trans-fats are in the frying liquid.
- **Stay away from soups and creamed sauces.** Most have way too much sodium to be included in a low-salt diet.
- **Go easy on the bread.** One small piece maay have several hundred milligrams of sodium, and that's before you add the margarine or butter.
- **Use oil and vinegar on salads.** Watch out for the salad bar, many items are mayonnaise-based or pickled, which adds too much salt.
- **Order the smallest portion.** Eat half or save the rest for the next day.
- **Request condiments served on the side.** Then you control amount used.
- **Ask that salt not be added to your meal.** Most restaurants can accommodate you, however, fast food eateries often premake many items and may not be able to handle special requests.

PLAN AHEAD

If you know you will be dining out, eat a low-salt breakfast and lunch. If you have too much salt at one meal, keep your sodium intake low for the next couple of meals.

You can also place low-sodium condiments, like ketchup, mustard, mayonnaise and salad dressing, in small plastic containers and take them with you. The important thing is you do not have to deprive yourself. Just use moderation. Remember, low salt does not mean no salt.

FAST FOODS QUICK REFERENCE

Wondering where to get a hamburger and french fries with the lowest sodium? Which pizza won't put you over the top in your daily salt consumption? For your convenience a *Restaurant Quick Reference* has been included (see page 231-244). Use this to find the best places to get lower sodium favorites and stay within low-sodium guidelines.

USING THIS GUIDE

With our increasingly busy lifestyles, making healthy, low-sodium food choices at the supermarket and when dining out is challenging. Most of us do not have time to compare the labels of thousands of grocery items. We also have no idea of what's in the restaurant foods we are consuming.

This is where the *Pocket Guide to Low Sodium Foods* can help. It includes common products found in most grocery stores and menu items from 64 national restaurant chains. It's small enough to put in a purse or coat pocket and can be used as a quick reference when grocery shopping or eating out.

Only low-salt foods within acceptable Nutritive Criteria (see pg xxv) are listed. Calories, fat, saturated fat, trans fat, cholesterol, carbohydrates, fiber, sugar, and sodium are shown for each food product. These are the most important nutrients to consider for healthy eating.

The book is broken down into two parts: *Grocery Products* and *Quick-Serve Restaurant Chains*.

GROCERY PRODUCTS

All foods are listed alphabetically within the following 16 categories and approximates the aisles of your supermarket.

Baking and Cooking Needs
Beverages
Breads, Rolls and Bread Products
Breakfast Products
Condiments and Sauces
Dairy Products and Alternatives
Desserts and Sweets
Dinners, Entrees and Side Dishes

Ethnic Foods
Fish and Seafood
Fruits
Meat, Poultry and Substitutes
Pasta, Noodles, Rice and Grains
Snack Foods
Soups, Stews and Chilis
Vegetables, Beans and Legumes

Generic nutrient analysis is shown for each food type (listed by amount of sodium in ascending order) and represents the average or typical values for that particular food. This is followed by brand named products in alphabetical order and, when applicable, are divided into subcategories, such as *Canned*, *Frozen/Refrigerated*, and *Shelf-Stable*. Only low-salt foods within the Nutritive Criteria are listed. (NOTE: Products exceeding these guidelines may be shown if substantially less than the non-brand product.)

QUICK-SERVE RESTAURANT CHAINS

This section includes national fast-food and quick-serve restaurant chains listed in alphabetical order. Although fast foods are loaded with fat and sodium and are not necessarily the best choice for healthy, low-sodium diets, they are a fact of life. Use the *Pocket Guide to Low-Sodium Foods* to help you make the wisest selections.

Restaurant menu selections are broken down into categories, such as *Sandwiches, Salads, Side Dishes*, and *Desserts*. Only low-salt foods within the Nutritive Criteria are listed. However, if all choices within a category exceed sodium guidelines, the menu item with the least amount of salt may be listed as a reference. Additionally, some lower fat items (i.e. chicken and fish), may be shown even though salt content is higher than the nutritive guidelines.

Unfortunately, not all restaurant chains were willing or responsive to requests to reprint nutritional data. In order to give readers some idea of sodium content for these eateries, menu items with the least salt are listed. Foods are grouped by amount of sodium in 50mg increments (i.e., 0-50mg, 50-100mg, etc.).

NOTE: Although a majority of quick-serve food is excessive in sodium, when you do consume these foods, you may want to eat a smaller portion to keep within daily guidelines.

NUTRITIVE CRITERIA

The amount of sodium per serving determines which foods are listed in the guide. However, the criteria is different for fast foods— if we used the same criteria, there would be very few selections, consequently sodium amounts are greater than for grocery store items.

	Maximum Sodium	
	Grocery	Fast Food
Main dishes (i.e. frozen dinners, sandwiches)	> 550g	> 600g
Sides (i.e. baked goods, desserts, vegetable dishes)	> 250g	> 300g
Condiments and individual foods	> 200g	> 250g

All information contained in the *Pocket Guide to Low-Sodium Foods* is based on nutritional data provided by the US Department of Agriculture, food manufacturers, restaurant chains, and author calculations.

Data is for informational purposes only and is subject to change. No endorsement is intended of companies and their products, nor is any adverse judgment implied for companies and products not mentioned.

Availability of products, menu items and variations in serving sizes or product ingredients may occur dependent upon geographical region, local suppliers, season of the year and production changes. Read manufacturer's product labels or contact individual restaurants for the most up-to-date analysis of food items. Data was collected during 2006.

AUTHOR'S NOTE:

Although several organizations, including the American Public Health Association, are urging the food industry to reduce sodium by 50% by 2010, food manufacturers are opposed to these changes. They contend that low-sodium products often do not fare well in the marketplace. Taste is the main reason people buy a particular product and when salt is removed, consumers react negatively to the loss of flavor.

Unfortunately, food manufacturers cannot be forced to produce low-salt items. It is much easier for them to stop manufacturing a product than it is to create a new item, particularly one that probably will not be embraced by consumers.

While gathering data for this second edition of the *Pocket Guide to Low Sodium Foods*, it became evident that many food manufacturers and quick-serve restaurants are not lowering the sodium in their products, instead they are adding more sodium! Additionally, many smaller manufacturers that previously produced low-salt products are either out-of-business or no longer producing them. A sad state for those of us who are concerned about the salt in our diets.

Consequently, read labels and continue to re-read them. You may be surprised to discover a favorite low-sodium food suddenly having more salt listed than the last time you used it. And continue to support manufacturers and products that are lower in sodium; we need them to survive.

ABBREVIATIONS AND SYMBOLS

all	all varieties/flavors	NSA	no salt added
approx	approximately	orig	original
avg	average	oz	ounce
cal	calories	pc	piece(s)
carb	carbohydrate	pkg	package
choc	chocolate	pkt	packet
chol	cholesterol	prep	prepared to product
cinn	cinnamon		directions
envl	envelop	refrg	refrigerated
FF	fat free	reg	regular
fl oz	fluid ounce	sat	saturated fat
g	gram	serv	serving
lb	pound	sl	slice
LF	low fat	sm	small
mayo	mayonnaise	sod	sodium
med	medium-sized	sq	square
mg	milligram(s)	tbsp	tablespoon
micro	microwave	tsp	teaspoon
misc	miscellaneous	veg	vegetable
most	most varieties	w/	with
NF	nonfat	w/o	without

-	nutritional data unavailable
<	less than

FOOD MEASUREMENTS AND EQUIVALENTS

1 1/2 tsp	=	1/2 tbsp	=	0.25 oz	=	7 grams
3 tsp	=	1 tbsp	=	0.5 oz	=	14 grams
2 tbsp	=	1/8 cup	=	1 oz	=	28 grams
4 tbsp	=	1/4 cup	=	2 oz	=	55 grams
8 tbsp	=	1/2 cup	=	4 oz	=	115 grams
16 tbsp	=	1 cup	=	8 oz	=	225 grams

LIQUID

1/2 fl oz	=	15 ml	=	1 tbsp
1 fl oz	=	30 ml	=	1/8 cup
2 fl oz	=	60 ml	=	1/4 cup
4 fl oz	=	120 mil	=	1/2 cup
8 fl oz	=	240 ml	=	1 cup
16 fl oz	=	480 ml	=	1 pint

2 cups	=	1 pint	=	1/2 quart
4 cups	=	2 pints	=	1 quart
4 pints	=	2 quarts	=	1/2 gallon
8 pints	=	4 quarts	=	1 gallon

READING THE NUTRITIVE VALUES

Food	Cal	Fat	Sat	TFat	Chol	Carb	Fib	Sug	Sod
FROSTING									
Vanilla, ready-to-spread, 2 tbsp	140	5	2	0	0	23	0	20	70
Cream cheese, ready-to-spread, 2 tbsp .	140	5	2	0	0	23	0	20	80
Chocolate, ready-to-spread, 2 tbsp	130	5	2	0	0	21	0	18	90
BRANDS . . .									
MIX									
Calorie Control Lemon, Vanilla, Choc, or Cream Cheese (typ), 2 tbsp	93	3	1	0	0	8	0	1	27
Estee, all, prep, 2 tbsp	67	1	0	0	0	13	0	-	0
READY-TO-SPREAD									
Betty Crocker Soft Whipped									
Fluffy White, 2 tbsp	100	5	2	0	0	15	0	14	25
Vanilla, 2 tbsp	100	5	2	0	0	15	0	14	25

Generic foods are listed first, followed by brand-name products. Values are an average for all foods of this type.

Nutritional information unavailable.

All nutrient values are rounded off to the nearest whole number. If the nutrient value on a food label is:

    <5 (less than 5mg or 5g), the Pocket Guide uses: 5
    <1 (less than 1mg or 5g), the Pocket Guide uses: 1
    tr (trace amount present), the Pocket Guide uses: 0

If the nutrient value is not listed, there is no significant amount present; the Pocket Guide uses 0.

PART 1

GROCERY PRODUCTS

Food	Cal	Fat	Sat	TFat	Chol	Carb	Fib	Sug	Sod

BAKING AND COOKING NEEDS

ALMOND PASTE

(also see Pie/Pastry Fillings, pg 10)

Food	Cal	Fat	Sat	TFat	Chol	Carb	Fib	Sug	Sod
Almond paste, 2 tbsp	180	11	1	0	0	19	1	17	0

BRANDS ...

Most brands are within the generic range.

BAKING CHOCOLATE AND MORSELS

Food	Cal	Fat	Sat	TFat	Chol	Carb	Fib	Sug	Sod
Cocoa powder, unsweetened, 2 tbsp	25	1	1	0	0	6	4	0	2
Baking chocolate:									
Semi-sweet, 1 oz	136	9	5	0	0	18	2	15	3
Sweet, 1 cz	143	10	6	0	0	17	2	15	5
Unsweetened, 1 oz	140	15	9	0	0	8	5	0	7
White, 1 oz	151	9	5	0	4	17	0	17	25
Morsels:									
Choc, semi-sweet, 1 oz	134	8	5	0	0	18	2	15	3
Carob, grain sweetened, 1 oz	70	4	3	0	0	11	0	5	4
Butterscotch, 1 oz	160	8	7	0	0	18	0	18	30
White, 1 oz	160	8	7	0	0	18	0	18	40
Carob, unsweetened, 1 oz	70	4	3	0	0	8	2	7	50
Carob, sweetened, 1 oz	70	3	3	0	0	8	0	5	65
Peanut butter, 1 oz	160	8	8	0	0	14	0	12	70

BRANDS ...
Most brands are within the generic range.

BAKING MIXES

(also see mixes for specific items, i.e. Biscuits, Brownies, Cakes, Cookies, etc.)

Food	Cal	Fat	Sat	TFat	Chol	Carb	Fib	Sug	Sod
All-purpose baking mix, 1/4 cup	129	5	1	1	0	19	1	1	368
BRANDS ... *(1/4 CUP UNLESS NOTED)*									
Authenic Foods Pancake & Baking Mix	130	2	0	0	0	24	2	1	170
Bob's Red Mill Low Carb Baking Mix	100	2	0	0	0	11	5	0	115
Carbquick Biscuit & Baking Mix	50	4	0	0	0	9	7	0	110
Ener-G Brown Rice Mix	148	4	0	0	0	25	3	2	35
Potato Mix	133	0	0	0	0	34	1	1	110
Kingsmill Unimix All-purpose	100	2	0	0	0	20	0	0	0

Food	Cal	Fat	Sat	TFat	Chol	Carb	Fib	Sug	Sod

BAKING POWDER AND BAKING SODA

(see Leavening Agents, pg 7)

BATTER, SEASONING AND COATING MIXES

(also see Breadcrumbs, Cracker and Other Crumbs below)

Food	Cal	Fat	Sat	TFat	Chol	Carb	Fib	Sug	Sod
Tempura batter mix, 1/4 cup	100	0	0	0	0	23	0	0	175
Batter mix, 1/4 cup	100	0	0	0	0	22	1	0	690
Seasoning & coating mix, 1/4 pkg	80	4	0	0	0	10	0	1	800

BRANDS . . . *(1/4 CUP UNLESS NOTED)*

Food	Cal	Fat	Sat	TFat	Chol	Carb	Fib	Sug	Sod
Aunt Candice Breading Mix, 1.5 oz	159	4	0	0	0	30	2	0	157
Chef's Delight Predust, NSA	9	1	0	0	1	31	1	1	6
Fry Crisp SF Batter or Coating Mix	100	1	0	0	0	22	1	1	5
Golden Dipt Sharables	36	0	0	0	0	9	0	1	23
Ka-Me Tempura	200	0	0	0	0	44	0	0	10
Louisiana Fish Fry Fish Fry, 2 tsp	20	0	0	0	0	5	0	0	5
Seasoned Fish Fry, 2 tsp	20	0	0	0	0	5	0	0	135
Shake 'N Bake Hot & Spicy, 2 tsp	40	1	0	0	0	7	0	1	170
Garlic & Herb, 2 tsp	35	1	0	0	0	7	0	1	180
Sun Luck Tempura	100	0	0	0	0	23	1	1	50
Tony Chachere's Fish Fry Creole	120	0	0	0	0	26	1	2	35
Zatarain's Fish Fry, SF, 1.5 tbsp	45	0	0	0	0	10	0	0	0
Wonderful Fish Fry, 1 tbsp	45	0	0	0	0	0	0	0	0

NOTE: Although some of the above coating mixes exceed sodium guidelines, they are substantially less than the generic.

BREADCRUMBS, CRACKER AND OTHER CRUMBS

Food	Cal	Fat	Sat	TFat	Chol	Carb	Fib	Sug	Sod
Matzoh meal, 1/4 cup	145	1	0	0	0	31	1	1	3
Cracker meal, 1/4 cup	110	0	0	0	0	23	1	0	8
Panko Breading, 1/4 cup	44	0	0	0	0	9	0	1	38
Cookie crumbs, 1/4 cup	140	6	2	-	10	26	0	14	110
Breadcrumbs, plain, 1/4 cup	107	1	0	0	0	19	1	2	198
Graham cracker crumbs, 1/4 cup	107	3	1	-	0	17	1	3	200
Breadcrumbs, seasoned, 1/4 cup	115	2	0	0	0	21	2	2	528

BRANDS . . . *(1/4 CUP UNLESS NOTED)*

BREADCRUMBS

Food	Cal	Fat	Sat	TFat	Chol	Carb	Fib	Sug	Sod
4C Plain, SF, 1 oz	110	1	0	0	0	23	2	2	5
Edward & Sons Lightly Salted, 1/3 cup	110	1	0	0	0	21	1	2	110
Ener-G	90	5	0	0	0	13	2	1	95
Golden Dipt Light N' Crunchy	44	0	0	0	0	9	0	1	39

Food	Cal	Fat	Sat	TFat	Chol	Carb	Fib	Sug	Sod
BREADCRUMBS (CONT'D)									
Hol-Grain Brown Rice, SF	40	0	0	0	0	9	0	0	0
Jaclyns Plain, 1/3 cup	120	1	0	0	0	23	3	2	5
Nu-World Foods Amaranth	122	2	0	0	0	22	3	0	2
Southern Homestyle									
Tortilla Crumbs, 2 tbsp	40	0	0	0	0	9	0	1	50

CRACKER AND OTHER CRUMBS

Most brands are within the generic range.

COCONUT

Raw, 1 oz	35	3	3	0	0	2	1	1	2
Coconut milk, 1/4 cup	111	12	11	0	0	2	0	2	7
Shredded, unsweetened, 1 oz	187	18	16	0	0	7	5	0	10
Sweetened, 1 oz	58	4	4	0	0	6	1	5	30
Flaked, sweetened, 1 oz	134	9	8	0	0	13	1	12	73

BRANDS . . . *(1 OZ UNLESS NOTED)*
Most brands are within the generic range.

CORNMEAL

Degermed, white or yellow, 1/4 cup	126	1	0	0	0	27	3	0	1
Blue, 1/4 cup	137	2	0	0	0	27	3	1	2
Whole-grain, white or yellow, 1/4 cup	110	0	0	0	0	23	2	0	11
Self-rising, white or yellow, 1/4 cup	122	1	0	0	0	26	2	0	465

BRANDS . . .
Most brands are within the generic range.

CORNSTARCH

Cornstarch, 1 tbsp	30	0	0	0	0	7	0	0	1

BRANDS . . .
Most brands are within the generic range.

EGGS – DRIED/POWDERED

Egg whites, powdered, 1 tbsp	53	0	0	0	0	1	0	1	173
BRANDS . . . *(1 TBSP UNLESS NOTED)*									
Bob's Red Mill Egg Replacer	30	1	0	-	0	2	1	1	20
Deb El Just Whites, 2 tsp	12	0	0	0	0	0	0	0	51
Whole Eggs, 2 tsp	80	6	2	0	245	1	0	1	75
Ener-G Egg Replacer, 1 1/2 tsp	15	0	0	0	0	4	0	0	5
Kingsmill									
Egg Replacer, powder, 1 tsp	10	0	0	0	0	3	0	0	15

BAKING AND COOKING NEEDS
Fats, Oils and Cooking Sprays

Food	Cal	Fat	Sat	TFat	Chol	Carb	Fib	Sug	Sod

FATS, OILS AND COOKING SPRAYS

Food	Cal	Fat	Sat	TFat	Chol	Carb	Fib	Sug	Sod
Cooking spray, 1/3 sec spray	0	0	0	0	0	0	0	0	0
Lard or shortening, 1 tbsp	115	13	5	4	12	0	0	0	0
Oil, all varieties, 1 tbsp (avg)	119	14	2	0	0	0	0	0	0

BRANDS . . .
Most brands are within the generic range.

FAT SUBSTITUTES

BRANDS . . . *(1 TBSP UNLESS NOTED)*

Food	Cal	Fat	Sat	TFat	Chol	Carb	Fib	Sug	Sod
Mrs. Bateman's ButterLike	36	1	0	-	5	8	0	0	20
Rokeach Neutral Nyafat	99	11	-	-	0	0	0	0	0

FLAVORINGS AND EXTRACTS

Food	Cal	Fat	Sat	TFat	Chol	Carb	Fib	Sug	Sod
Flavorings & extracts, 1 tsp (avg)	10	0	0	0	0	0	0	0	0

BRANDS . . .
Most brands are within the generic range.

FLOUR

Food	Cal	Fat	Sat	TFat	Chol	Carb	Fib	Sug	Sod
Rice flour, white, 1 cup	578	2	1	0	0	127	4	0	0
Cake flour, 1 cup	496	1	0	0	0	107	2	0	0
Rye flour, dark, 1 cup	415	3	0	0	0	88	29	4	1
Light, 1 cup	374	1	0	0	0	82	15	0	2
All-purpose flour, 1 cup	495	2	0	0	0	99	3	0	3
Wheat flour, whole-grain, 1 cup	407	2	0	0	0	87	15	3	6
Soy flour, 1 cup	366	17	3	0	0	30	8	0	11
Rice flour, brown, 1 cup	574	4	1	0	0	121	7	0	13
Potato flour, 1 cup	571	1	0	0	0	133	9	0	88
Self-rising flour, 1 cup	443	1	0	0	0	93	3	0	1588

BRANDS . . .
Most brands are within the generic range.

FROSTING, ICING AND DECORATIONS

Food	Cal	Fat	Sat	TFat	Chol	Carb	Fib	Sug	Sod
Ready-to-spread, vanilla frosting, 2 tbsp	138	5	1	2	0	22	0	21	61
Ready-to-spread, cream cheese, 2 tbsp	137	6	2	2	0	22	0	21	63
Ready-to-spread, choc, 2 tbsp	163	7	2	2	0	26	0	24	75
Mix, choc, 1/4 pkg	150	4	2	1	0	28	1	26	130

BRANDS . . . .
There are many low-sodium frostings, the following have less than 70mg per serving.

Food	Cal	Fat	Sat	TFat	Chol	Carb	Fib	Sug	Sod
FROSTING, ICING AND DECORATIONS (CONT'D)									
MIX *(2 TBSP UNLESS NOTED)*									
Calorie Control Lemon	93	3	1	0	0	8	0	1	27
Vanilla, Choc, or Cream Cheese	67	3	1	0	0	8	0	1	27
Oetker Simple Organics									
Choc or Vanilla	110	0	0	0	0	26	0	24	65
Sweet N'Low Choc	60	4	2	0	0	7	1	0	20
White	60	3	2	0	0	10	0	0	20
READY-TO-SPREAD *(2 TBSP UNLESS NOTED)*									
Betty Crocker									
Whipped:									
Fluffy White or Strawberry Mist	110	5	2	2	0	15	0	13	25
Lemon, Vanilla, or Butter Cream	110	5	2	2	0	15	0	13	25
Whipped Cream	100	5	2	2	0	15	0	13	25
Cream Cheese	110	5	2	2	0	15	0	13	45
Milk Choc	100	5	2	1	0	14	0	12	50
Choc or Choc Mousse (avg)	100	5	2	1	0	14	1	12	55
Rich & Creamy, Coconut Pecan	140	7	3	2	0	18	1	16	55
Duncan Hines									
Home-Style, Vanilla or French Vanilla	140	5	2	2	0	22	0	21	60
Home-Style, Cream Cheese	140	5	2	2	0	22	0	21	60
Wild Cherry Vanilla	140	5	2	2	0	22	0	21	60
Home-Style, Lemon Supreme	140	5	2	0	0	21	0	21	65
Fun Frosters M&Ms	140	6	2	2	0	23	0	22	65
Pillsbury Whipped, Cream Cheese	100	5	2	2	0	14	0	13	20
Whipped Supreme	100	5	1	2	0	14	0	13	50
Creamy Supreme, Milk Choc	140	6	2	2	0	21	1	19	55
Creamy Supreme, Coconut Pecan	160	10	4	2	0	17	1	16	60

ICING AND DECORATIONS

Sprinkles, 1 tsp	20	1	1	0	0	3	0	3	0
Decorating icing, 1 tsp	25	1	1	0	0	4	0	4	10

BRANDS . . .
Most brands are within the generic range.

LEAVENING AGENTS

Yeast, baker's, dry, 1 tbsp	35	1	0	0	0	5	3	0	0
Cream of tartar, 1 tsp	8	0	0	0	0	2	0	0	2
Baking powder, 1 tsp	2	0	0	0	0	1	0	0	488
Baking soda, 1 tsp	0	0	0	0	0	0	0	0	1259

Food	Cal	Fat	Sat	TFat	Chol	Carb	Fib	Sug	Sod

LEAVENING AGENTS (CONT'D)

BRANDS . . . *(1 TSP UNLESS NOTED)*

Food	Cal	Fat	Sat	TFat	Chol	Carb	Fib	Sug	Sod
Ener-G Baking Powder, SF	0	0	0	0	0	0	0	0	0
Baking Soda, SF	0	0	0	0	0	0	0	0	0
Hain Featherweight Baking Powder, SF	0	0	0	0	0	0	0	0	0

MARSHMALLOWS

Food	Cal	Fat	Sat	TFat	Chol	Carb	Fib	Sug	Sod
Marshmallow creme, 2 tbsp	91	0	0	0	0	22	0	16	14
Marshmallows, miniatures, 1 oz	90	0	0	0	0	23	0	17	30

BRANDS . . .
Most brands are within the generic range.

MILK AND MILK SUBSTITUTES – CANNED AND POWDERED

Food	Cal	Fat	Sat	TFat	Chol	Carb	Fib	Sug	Sod
Milk, powdered, NF, 1 tbsp	15	0	0	0	0	2	0	2	23
Buttermilk, powdered, 1 tbsp	20	0	0	0	1	3	0	3	41
Goat milk, powdered, 1 tbsp	70	4	2	0	13	6	0	6	58
Canned, 1/2 cup	140	8	6	0	20	12	0	12	120
Evaporated milk, canned, 1/2 cup	169	10	6	0	37	13	0	13	133
Skim, canned, 1/2 cup	100	0	0	0	5	15	0	15	147
Condensed milk, sweetened, canned, 1/2 cup	491	13	8	0	52	83	0	83	194

BRANDS . . .

Food	Cal	Fat	Sat	TFat	Chol	Carb	Fib	Sug	Sod
Meyenberg Condensed, 1/2 cup	71	4	2	0	13	6	0	6	58
Ener-G Soy Quik, powdered, 1/8 cup	50	2	0	0	0	4	2	2	0

NUTS – BAKING

(see Nuts and Seeds, pg 146)

PASTRY DOUGH/SHELLS

(also see Pie Crusts, pg 9; Crepes, pg 27)

Food	Cal	Fat	Sat	TFat	Chol	Carb	Fib	Sug	Sod
Phyllo (fillo) dough, 1 sheet	57	1	0	0	0	10	0	0	92
Puff pastry, 1/6 sheet (1.4 oz)	170	11	3	4	0	14	1	1	200
Puff pastry shell, 1 shell	190	13	4	4	0	16	1	0	230

BRANDS . . .

FROZEN/REFRIGERATED

Apollo or *Athens*

Food	Cal	Fat	Sat	TFat	Chol	Carb	Fib	Sug	Sod
Mini Fillo Shells, 2 shells	35	2	0	0	0	4	0	0	25
Shredded Fillo Dough (Kataifi), 2 oz	120	2	0	0	0	22	1	1	115
Fillo Factory Mini Shells, 3 shells	45	1	0	0	0	7	0	0	30
Large shells, 1 shell	80	2	0	0	0	13	0	0	55

Food	Cal	Fat	Sat	TFat	Chol	Carb	Fib	Sug	Sod
PASTRY DOUGH/SHELLS (FILLO FACTORY CONT'D)									
Kataifi, 2 oz	180	2	0	0	0	35	4	1	140
Fillo Dough, 2 sheets, 1.6 oz	130	1	0	0	0	28	1	0	160
Kineret Puff Pastry, 2 oz sq	250	18	5	-	0	20	1	0	140
Oronoque Orchards									
Tart Shell, 3" shell	140	9	2	-	0	12	0	0	140

(PASTRY/PIE FILLINGS)

(see Pie/Pastry Fillings, pg 10)

(PIE CRUSTS)

Food	Cal	Fat	Sat	TFat	Chol	Carb	Fib	Sug	Sod
Cookie crumb crust, shelf-stable									
Vanilla, 1/6	140	7	2	0	5	18	1	10	65
Choc, 1/8	110	5	1	0	0	14	1	7	100
Flour crust, frozen, 1/8	73	5	1	1	0	7	0	0	92
Mix, prep, 1/8	100	6	2	0	0	10	0	0	146
Graham cracker crust, shelf-stable, 1/8	140	7	2	0	0	10	0	9	125

BRANDS . . .

FROZEN/REFRIGERATED *(1/8 OF 9" SHELL UNLESS NOTED)*

Food	Cal	Fat	Sat	TFat	Chol	Carb	Fib	Sug	Sod
Countrys Delight	80	5	1	-	0	8	0	1	75
Great Value	100	7	2	-	0	9	0	0	40
Deep Dish	100	7	2	-	0	9	0	0	50
Oronoque Orchards, regular	80	6	2	-	0	7	0	0	90
Pet-Ritz	80	4	2	0	0	9	0	1	70
Deep Dish, All Vegetable	90	5	1	2	0	11	0	1	85
Deep Dish	90	5	2	0	0	11	0	1	85

MIX *(1/8 SHELL UNLESS NOTED)*

Food	Cal	Fat	Sat	TFat	Chol	Carb	Fib	Sug	Sod
Arrowhead Mills Graham Mix	100	5	2	-	0	12	0	6	55
Gluten Free Pantry Perfect Pie, 1/6	60	0	0	0	0	15	1	0	70
Krusteaz	100	6	2	2	0	10	1	1	90

SHELF-STABLE *(1/8 SHELL UNLESS NOTED)*

Food	Cal	Fat	Sat	TFat	Chol	Carb	Fib	Sug	Sod
Fifty50									
Sugar Free Graham Cracker	100	5	2	-	0	11	0	0	50
Keebler									
Shortbread	100	5	1	0	0	15	1	6	95
Graham Cracker, Reduced Fat	100	4	1	0	0	15	0	6	100
Graham Cracker, 4 oz single shell	120	5	3	2	0	16	1	6	125
Kemach Graham Cracker	100	4	1	-	0	14	1	5	50
Mother's Own Graham Cracker	110	6	2	-	0	12	1	5	115
Nabisco Nilla	140	7	2	-	5	18	1	10	65

Food	Cal	Fat	Sat	TFat	Chol	Carb	Fib	Sug	Sod

PIE/PASTRY FILLINGS

(also see Puddings and Gelatins, pg 84)

Pastry Filling:

Food	Cal	Fat	Sat	TFat	Chol	Carb	Fib	Sug	Sod
Almond paste, 2 tbsp	180	11	1	0	0	19	1	17	0
Marzipan, 1 oz	116	4	1	0	0	18	1	16	5
Date filling, 1 oz	100	0	0	0	0	22	3	16	40

Pie Filling:

Food	Cal	Fat	Sat	TFat	Chol	Carb	Fib	Sug	Sod
Peach pie filling, 3 oz	80	0	0	0	0	21	0	17	30
Cherry pie filling, 3 oz	100	0	0	0	0	24	0	15	40
Apple pie filling, 3 oz	90	0	0	0	0	22	2	17	40
Blueberry pie filling, 3 oz	90	0	0	0	0	22	1	12	50
Lemon pie filling, 3 oz	120	0	0	0	15	29	0	25	220
Mincemeat pie filling, 4 oz	200	2	0	0	0	48	0	44	250
Pumpkin pie mix, 4 oz	141	0	0	0	0	36	11	24	281

BRANDS . . .

PASTRY FILLINGS

Most brands are within the generic range.

PIE FILLINGS *(4 OZ UNLESS NOTED)*

Most brands are within the generic range; the following have less than the generic.

Food	Cal	Fat	Sat	TFat	Chol	Carb	Fib	Sug	Sod
Comstock Lemon pie filling, 3.25 oz	130	2	0	0	0	28	0	20	120
Libby									
100% Pumpkin, no added ingredients	40	1	0	0	0	9	5	4	5
Pumpkin Pie, premixed	100	0	0	0	0	25	2	22	150

SALT AND SEASONINGS

SALT AND SALT SUBSTITUTES

Food	Cal	Fat	Sat	TFat	Chol	Carb	Fib	Sug	Sod
Salt substitute, 1 tsp	2	0	0	0	0	0	0	0	0
Lite salt, 1 tsp	0	0	0	0	0	0	0	0	1160
Seasoned salt, 1 tsp	0	0	0	0	0	0	0	0	1280
Table salt, 1 tsp	0	0	0	0	0	0	0	0	2325

BRANDS . . . *(1 TSP UNLESS NOTED)*

Most brands are within the generic range.

HERBS, SPICES AND SEASONINGS

Food	Cal	Fat	Sat	TFat	Chol	Carb	Fib	Sug	Sod
Chili powder, 1 tbsp	24	1	0	0	0	4	2	1	76
Liquid aminos, all purpose, 1/2 tsp	2	0	0	0	0	0	0	0	110
MSG, 1 tbsp	0	0	0	0	0	0	0	0	150
Old Bay Seasoning, 1/4 tsp	0	0	0	0	0	0	0	0	160
Meat tenderizer, 1/4 tsp	0	0	0	0	0	0	0	0	240

Food	Cal	Fat	Sat	TFat	Chol	Carb	Fib	Sug	Sod
HERBS, SPICES AND SEASONINGS (CONT'D)									
All-purpose seasoning, 1/2 tsp	5	0	0	0	0	0	0	0	300

NOTE: Individual herbs and spices have little or no sodium, however, herb and spice blends may contain added salt. Check labels for sodium content or list of ingredients if nutrient values are not listed.

BRANDS . . . *(1 TSP UNLESS NOTED)*

Food	Cal	Fat	Sat	TFat	Chol	Carb	Fib	Sug	Sod
Accent Flavor Enhancer, 1/8 tsp	0	0	0	0	0	0	0	0	80
Bell's SF Seasoning	0	0	0	0	0	0	0	0	0
Blazing Blends	0	0	0	0	0	0	0	0	0
Blue Crab Seafood or Salmon Seasoning	0	0	0	0	0	0	0	0	0
Chef Paul Prudhomme, all Magic SF Seasonings, Pizza & Pasta Magic	0	0	0	0	0	0	0	0	0
Eden Dulce Flakes	3	0	0	0	0	0	0	0	15
Eden Shake (Furikake), 1/2 tsp	5	0	0	0	0	1	1	0	25
Gomasio (sesame salt), all varieties	15	2	0	0	0	1	0	0	80
Fortner's SF, all	0	0	0	0	0	0	0	0	0
Frontier, SF, all	0	0	0	0	0	0	0	0	0
Kernal Season's Popcorn Seasoning									
Apple Cinnamon, 1/4 tsp	4	0	0	0	0	0	0	0	0
Choc Marshmallow, 1/4 tsp	0	0	0	0	0	0	0	0	1
BBQ, 1/4 tsp	3	0	0	0	0	1	0	1	5
Lawry's SF 17	0	0	0	0	0	0	0	0	0
Longhorn Grill Mesquite, 1/4 tsp	0	0	0	0	0	0	0	0	5
McCormick Salt Free, all	5	0	0	0	0	0	0	0	0
Mickey & T Gourmet, all	0	0	0	0	0	0	0	0	0
Mrs. Dash SF, all	8	0	0	0	0	0	0	0	4
Nantucket Off-Shore, all	0	0	0	0	0	0	0	0	0
Simply Organic All-Purpose Blend	0	0	0	0	0	0	0	0	0
Italian Blend	0	0	0	0	0	0	0	0	0
Spice Hunter SF, all	0	0	0	0	0	0	0	0	0
Spice Island SF, all	0	0	0	0	0	1	0	0	0
Spike SF Seasoning	0	0	0	0	0	0	0	0	0
Sylvia's SF Secret Seasoning	0	0	0	0	0	0	0	0	0
Tony Chachere Salt Free Seasoning	0	0	0	0	0	0	0	0	0
Wassi's Own Sausage Seasoning, all	0	0	0	0	0	0	0	0	0
Wayzata Bay Spice Co, all	0	0	0	0	0	0	0	0	0
Zatarain's Shrimp and Crab Boil	0	0	0	0	0	0	0	0	0

SWEETENERS

Food	Cal	Fat	Sat	TFat	Chol	Carb	Fib	Sug	Sod
Sugar, powdered, 1/4 cup	117	0	0	0	0	30	0	29	0
Granulated sugar, 1/4 cup	194	0	0	0	0	50	0	50	0

BAKING AND COOKING NEEDS
Wheat Germ

Food	Cal	Fat	Sat	TFat	Chol	Carb	Fib	Sug	Sod
SWEETENERS (CONT'D)									
Brown sugar, packed, 1/4 cup	207	0	0	0	0	54	0	53	21
Honey, 1/4 cup	258	0	0	0	0	70	0	70	3
Rice syrup, brown, 1/4 cup	170	0	0	0	0	42	0	19	5
Fruit sweetener, 1/4 cup	120	0	0	0	0	30	2	28	10
Molasses, 1/4 cup	244	0	0	0	0	63	0	47	31
Blackstrap, 1/4 cup	193	0	0	0	0	50	0	35	45
Corn syrup, light, 1/4 cup	241	0	0	0	0	65	0	22	53
Dark, 1/4 cup	235	0	0	0	0	64	0	22	127

BRANDS . . .
Most brands are within the generic range.

SUGAR SUBSTITUTES

Food	Cal	Fat	Sat	TFat	Chol	Carb	Fib	Sug	Sod
Fructose, 1 tsp	15	0	0	0	0	4	0	4	0
Sweetener w/aspartame, 1 tsp	8	0	0	0	0	1	0	0	0
Sweetener w/saccharin, 1 tsp	4	0	0	0	0	1	0	0	0
Sucralose, 1 tsp	0	0	0	0	0	0	0	0	0

BRANDS . . .
Most brands are within the generic range.

(WHEAT GERM)

Food	Cal	Fat	Sat	TFat	Chol	Carb	Fib	Sug	Sod
Wheat germ, 2 tbsp	50	1	0	0	0	6	2	1	0

BRANDS . . .
Most brands are within the generic range.

12

Food	Cal	Fat	Sat	TFat	Chol	Carb	Fib	Sug	Sod

BEVERAGES

ALCOHOLIC BEVERAGES

BEER AND ALE

Food	Cal	Fat	Sat	TFat	Chol	Carb	Fib	Sug	Sod
Beer, regular, 12 fl oz	153	0	0	0	0	13	0	0	14
Non-alcoholic, 12 fl oz	70	0	0	0	0	15	0	3	10
Light, 12 fl oz	103	0	0	0	0	0	0	0	14

BRANDS . . .
Most brands are within the generic range.

LIQUOR AND SPIRITS

Food	Cal	Fat	Sat	TFat	Chol	Carb	Fib	Sug	Sod
Distilled, all (i.e. gin, rum, whiskey), 1 fl oz	64	0	0	0	0	0	0	0	0
Creme de menthe, 1 fl oz	125	0	0	0	0	14	0	14	2
Coffee liqueur, 1 fl oz	107	0	0	0	0	11	0	11	3
Coffee liqueur w/cream, 1 fl oz	102	5	3	0	5	7	0	7	29
Daiquiri, canned, 6.8 fl oz	258	0	0	0	0	32	0	-	83
Whiskey sour, canned, 6.8 fl oz	249	0	0	0	0	38	0	-	92
Whiskey sour, mix, 1 pkt	65	0	0	0	0	17	0	17	47
Pina colada, canned, 6.8 fl oz	526	17	15	0	0	61	0	-	158

BRANDS . . .
Most brands are within the generic range.

WINE AND CHAMPAGNE

Food	Cal	Fat	Sat	TFat	Chol	Carb	Fib	Sug	Sod
Sake, 3.5 fl oz	136	0	0	0	0	5	0	0	2
Red wine, 3.5 fl oz (avg)	87	0	0	0	0	3	0	1	4
White wine and champagne, 3.5 fl oz (avg)	85	0	0	0	0	3	0	1	5
Dessert wines, dry, 3.5 fl oz	157	0	0	0	0	12	0	1	9
Dessert wines, sweet, 3.5 fl oz	165	0	0	0	0	14	0	8	9
Cooking wines, 1 fl oz	14	0	0	0	0	2	0	0	182

NOTE: Instead of cooking wines, use madeira, marsala, sherry, vermouth, etc. from the wine department, which have little or no sodium.

BRANDS . . .
Most brands are within the generic range.

COCKTAIL MIXERS

(also see Water, Tonic and Seltzers, pg 20)

Food	Cal	Fat	Sat	TFat	Chol	Carb	Fib	Sug	Sod
Daiquiri mix, 8 fl oz	140	0	0	0	0	35	0	33	0
Margarita mix, 8 fl oz	100	0	0	0	0	25	0	23	0
Cream of coconut, 1 fl oz	85	2	2	0	0	18	1	17	45

BEVERAGES
Cocoa/Hot Chocolate

Food	Cal	Fat	Sat	TFat	Chol	Carb	Fib	Sug	Sod
COCKTAIL MIXERS (CONT'D)									
Collins mix, 8 fl oz	110	0	0	0	0	25	0	25	55
Whiskey sour mix, 8 fl oz	217	0	0	0	0	55	0	54	85
Pina colada mix, 8 fl oz	360	0	0	0	0	86	0	80	130
Sweet & sour mix, 8 fl oz	276	0	0	0	0	70	0	61	131
Bloody Mary mix, 8 fl oz	56	0	0	0	0	12	1	6	1174
BRANDS . . .									
FROZEN/REFRIGERATED *(8 FL OZ PREP UNLESS NOTED)*									
Bacardi Real Fruit Mixers, Pina Colada	170	4	3	0	0	35	0	35	20
READY-TO-DRINK *(8 FL OZ UNLESS NOTED)*									
Baja Bob's Sugar Free Drink Mixes, all ...	0	0	0	0	0	0	0	0	90
Finest Call Tom Collins Mix	280	0	0	0	0	68	0	66	20
Pina Colada Mix	340	1	0	0	0	78	0	72	40
Major Peters Pina Colada Mix	400	3	0	0	0	99	0	93	63
Mr. & Mrs. T Sweet & Sour	200	0	0	0	0	46	0	42	100

COCOA/HOT CHOCOLATE

(also see Drink Mixers and Additives, pg 16)

Food	Cal	Fat	Sat	TFat	Chol	Carb	Fib	Sug	Sod
Cocoa powder, 1 envl	113	1	1	0	2	24	1	21	146
Cocoa powder, sugar-free, 1 envl	56	0	0	0	0	10	1	7	171
Gourmet hot choc, 1 serv	160	0	0	0	0	28	0	22	240
BRANDS . . . *(1 SERVING UNLESS NOTED)*									
Caffe D'Amore Bellagio White Hot Choc	150	4	3	0	0	28	0	17	40
Bellagio Hot Choc	140	4	3	0	0	28	0	17	85
Carnation Hot Cocoa Mix, FF	25	0	0	0	0	5	1	4	120
Droste Cocoa	15	1	1	0	0	2	1	1	35
Equal Exchange Hot Cocoa Mix	70	0	0	0	0	13	1	-	60
Giradelli Hot Choc Mix, most (avg)	80	2	1	0	0	19	1	16	0
Double Choc	80	2	1	0	0	19	1	17	30
Nestlé Carnation Rich Choc	110	1	0	0	0	24	0	21	100
Swiss Miss Milk Choc	120	3	1	0	0	22	1	17	130

COFFEE/COFFEE-FLAVORED DRINKS

Food	Cal	Fat	Sat	TFat	Chol	Carb	Fib	Sug	Sod
Coffee, brewed, 6 fl oz	2	0	0	0	0	0	0	0	4
Instant, 6 fl os	4	0	0	0	0	1	0	0	4
Espresso, 6 fl oz	4	0	0	0	0	0	0	0	25
Cappuccino-flavor, instant mix, 8 fl oz	88	1	1	0	0	19	0	15	39
Mocha-flavor, instant mix, 8 fl oz	60	2	1	0	0	10	0	8	41
Coffee drink, ready-to-drink, 9.5 oz	190	3	2	0	12	39	0	30	110
French-flavor, instant mix, 8 fl oz	97	5	1	0	0	13	0	8	111

14

Food	Cal	Fat	Sat	TFat	Chol	Carb	Fib	Sug	Sod

COFFEE/COFFEE-FLAVORED DRINKS (CONT'D)

BRANDS ...

COFFEE

Most brands are within the generic range.

COFFEE-FLAVORED DRINKS

MIX *(8 FL OZ PREP UNLESS NOTED)*

CAPPUCCINO

Most cappuccino-flavored drink mixes are within the generic range.

OTHER FLAVORS

Food	Cal	Fat	Sat	TFat	Chol	Carb	Fib	Sug	Sod
Caffe D'Vita French Vanilla	60	3	3	0	0	10	0	7	30
Caffe D'Amore Bellagio Caffe, most	110	3	2	0	0	23	0	14	15
Bellagio Caffe Biano	110	3	2	0	0	22	0	14	50
Folgers Cafe Latte, most (avg)	100	5	2	0	5	14	0	7	80
General Foods International Hazelnut or French Vanilla *Cappuccino Coolers*	60	0	0	0	0	15	0	15	0
Choc *Cappuccino Coolers*	60	0	0	0	0	16	1	16	0
Viennese Choc Cafe	50	2	2	0	0	11	0	9	25
Swiss White Choc	70	3	3	0	0	12	0	9	30
Suisse Mocha, Sugar Free	30	2	2	0	0	2	0	0	30
Suisse Mocha	60	2	2	0	0	10	0	8	40
French Vanilla Cafe, Sugar Free	30	3	2	0	0	2	0	0	50
Creme Caramel	60	2	2	0	0	12	0	10	50
French Vanilla Cafe	60	3	1	0	0	10	0	8	55
French Vanilla Nut	60	3	3	0	0	10	0	8	55
Hazelnut Belgian Cafe	70	2	2	0	0	12	0	9	55
Cafe Vienna, Sugar Free	30	2	2	0	0	2	0	0	60

READY-TO-DRINK *(12.5 FL OZ UNLESS NOTED)*

Food	Cal	Fat	Sat	TFat	Chol	Carb	Fib	Sug	Sod
Arizona Iced Coffee, Latte Supreme or Mocha Latte, 15.5 fl oz (avg)	110	0	0	0	0	21	1	17	96
Blue Luna Cafe Latte	130	2	1	0	7	24	0	18	90
Mocha	70	2	1	0	7	10	0	9	90
Folgers Jakada Coffee Latte, 10.5 fl oz	170	4	2	0	10	31	0	30	70
Kogee Cafe Organic, 9.5 fl oz	200	0	0	0	0	39	0	39	100
Starbucks Doubleshot, 6.5 fl oz	140	6	4	0	20	18	0	17	70
Frappuccino Mocha Lite, 9.5 fl oz	100	3	2	1	30	12	3	11	80

COFFEE CREAMERS AND FLAVORINGS

Food	Cal	Fat	Sat	TFat	Chol	Carb	Fib	Sug	Sod
Non-dairy soy creamer, 1 tbsp	20	2	0	0	0	2	0	1	0
Cream substitute, powder, 1 tsp	11	1	1	0	0	1	0	1	4
Liquid, 1 tbsp	20	2	0	0	0	2	0	2	12

Food	Cal	Fat	Sat	TFat	Chol	Carb	Fib	Sug	Sod
COFFEE CREAMERS AND FLAVORINGS (CONT'D)									
Flavored creamer, 1 tbsp	45	2	0	0	0	7	0	5	5
Cream, liquid, 1 tbsp	29	3	2	0	10	1	0	0	6
Syrup flavoring, all, 1 oz	85	0	0	0	0	21	0	20	8

BRANDS . . .
Most brands are within the generic range.

COFFEE SUBSTITUTES

Cereal grain, prep w/water, 6 fl oz	11	0	0	0	0	2	1	0	2
Cereal grain, prep w/milk, 6 fl oz	120	6	4	-	24	10	0	8	91

BRANDS . . .
Most brands are within the generic range.

DIET AND NUTRITIONAL DRINKS

(also see Sports and Energy Drinks, pg 19)

Diet, mix for 8 fl oz	110	4	1	0	5	18	4	11	140
Nutritional, ready-to-drink, 8 fl oz	250	6	1	0	5	40	0	23	200
Diet, ready-to-drink, 11 fl oz	190	5	2	0	10	24	5	13	220

BRANDS . . .

MIX

Alba Dairy Shakes (avg)	70	0	0	0	5	12	2	7	140
Slim Fast Optima, all (avg)	110	4	1	0	0	18	4	10	130

READY-TO-DRINK *(8 FL OZ UNLESS NOTED)*

Boost Breeze	160	0	0	0	0	31	0	31	50
Vanilla Drink	240	4	1	0	5	41	0	23	130
High Protein Drink	240	6	1	0	10	33	0	16	170
Calorie Shed Shake, all (avg)	90	2	2	0	10	18	1	4	60
Grainaissance Amazake Most (avg)	180	2	0	0	0	35	4	30	20
Gimme Green Rice Shake	190	3	1	0	0	37	4	29	35
Amazing Mango	170	2	0	0	0	35	4	30	40
Rice Nog	190	2	0	0	0	39	4	34	65
RW Knudsen Recharge, all	70	0	0	0	0	18	0	17	25
Simply Nutritious (avg)	120	0	0	0	0	31	0	27	25

DRINK MIXERS AND ADDITIVES

(also see Cocoa/Hot Chocolate, pg. 14)

Strawberry syrup, 2 tbsp	100	0	0	0	0	28	0	26	5
Strawberry, mix, 1 serv	86	0	0	0	0	22	0	21	8
Carob flavor, powder, 1 tbsp	45	1	0	0	0	11	1	9	12

Food	Cal	Fat	Sat	TFat	Chol	Carb	Fib	Sug	Sod
DRINK MIXERS AND ADDITIVES (CONT'D)									
Choc syrup, 2 tbsp	109	0	0	0	0	25	1	19	28
Choc, mix, 1 serv	88	1	1	0	0	20	1	18	30
Malted milk, choc, powder, 1 tbsp	86	1	1	0	0	18	1	15	40
Malted milk, natural, powder, 1 tbsp	90	2	1	0	5	15	0	10	85

BRANDS . . . *(1 SERV UNLESS NOTED)*

Most syrup additives and drink mixers are within the generic range; the following have less than the generic.

Gosh That's Good! Choc Mix									
Classic, Sugar Free, 2 tbsp	35	2	0	0	0	4	0	1	0
White Velvet, Sugar Free, 2 tbsp	35	2	2	0	0	5	0	12	5
Classic, 2 tbsp	100	2	0	0	0	21	0	16	10
Ovaltine Classic Malt Mix	80	0	0	0	0	18	0	14	5

(EGGNOG)

Eggnog, ready-to-drink, 8 fl oz	343	19	11	0	150	34	0	21	137

BRANDS . . .

Most brands are within the generic range.

(ENERGY DRINKS)

(see Diet and Nutritional Drinks, pg 16; Sports and Energy Drinks, pg 19)

(FLAVORED DRINKS)

(see Sodas/Soft Drinks, pg 18)

(FRUIT JUICE AND FRUIT-FLAVORED DRINKS)

Fruit-flavored drink mix, 8 fl oz	60	0	0	0	0	16	0	16	0
Fruit juice, all citrus, 8 fl oz	112	0	0	0	0	27	0	21	2
Cranberry juice cocktail, 8 fl oz	137	0	0	0	0	34	0	30	5
Lemonade, frozen, prep, 8 fl oz	131	0	0	0	0	34	0	33	7
Mix, prep, 8 fl oz	60	0	0	0	0	16	0	16	25
Apricot nectar, 8 fl oz	141	0	0	0	0	36	2	31	8
Fruit punch, frozen, prep, 8 fl oz	114	0	0	0	0	29	0	29	10
Ready-to-drink, 8 fl oz	119	0	0	0	0	32	0	28	25
Apple juice, 8 fl oz	110	0	0	0	0	29	0	23	15
Grape drink, canned, 8 fl oz	153	0	0	0	0	40	0	33	40
Fruit & vegetable drink, 8 fl oz	110	0	0	0	0	29	0	26	50

BRANDS . . .

Most brands are within the generic range. NOTE: Some fruit blends with less than 25% juice may contain as much as 80mg sodium per serving.

Food	Cal	Fat	Sat	TFat	Chol	Carb	Fib	Sug	Sod

RICE AND SOY BEVERAGES

(see Milk Products and Non-Dairy Alternatives, pg 65)

SELTZER

(see Water, Tonic and Seltzers, pg 20)

SODAS/SOFT DRINKS

(also see Sports and Energy Drinks, pg 19)

Food	Cal	Fat	Sat	TFat	Chol	Carb	Fib	Sug	Sod
Cola, 12 fl oz	136	0	0	0	0	35	0	33	15
Diet, 12 fl oz	7	0	0	0	0	1	0	0	28
Ginger ale, 12 fl oz	124	0	0	0	0	32	0	32	26
Diet, 12 fl oz	0	0	0	0	0	0	0	0	60
Lemon-lime, 12 fl oz	151	0	0	0	0	38	0	38	37
Diet, 12 fl oz	0	0	0	0	0	0	0	0	30
Pepper-type, 12 fl oz	151	0	0	0	0	38	0	38	37
Orange, 12 fl oz	179	0	0	0	0	46	0	46	45
Diet, 12 fl oz	0	0	0	0	0	0	0	0	80
Cream soda, 12 fl oz	189	0	0	0	0	49	0	49	45
Diet, 12 fl oz	0	0	0	0	0	0	0	0	35
Root beer, 12 fl oz	152	0	0	0	0	39	0	39	48
Diet, 12 fl oz	0	0	0	0	0	0	0	0	45
Grape, 12 fl oz	160	0	0	0	0	42	0	42	56
Lemonade, 12 fl oz	150	0	0	0	0	42	0	40	120

BRANDS . . . *(12 FL OZ UNLESS NOTED)*
Most brands are within the generic range; the following have less than the generic.

Food	Cal	Fat	Sat	TFat	Chol	Carb	Fib	Sug	Sod
Blue Sky Natural or Organic, all (avg)	180	0	0	0	0	45	0	45	10
Canfield's Diet, all	0	0	0	0	0	0	0	0	0
Diet Riet, all	0	0	0	0	0	0	0	0	0
Green River	180	0	0	0	0	45	0	45	15
Jones Naturals, all	100	0	0	0	0	23	0	23	0
Soda, all	170	0	0	0	0	46	0	46	14
Minute Maid Diet Orange	2	0	0	0	0	0	0	0	0
Natural Brew Root Beer or Grapefruit	180	0	0	0	0	44	0	39	0
Vanilla Creme, Outrageous Ginger Ale, or Ginseng Cola	170	0	0	0	0	42	0	38	18
Polar, all (avg)	0	0	0	0	0	0	0	0	0
Santa Cruz Root Beer	140	0	0	0	0	36	0	32	0
Virgil's Root Beer	160	0	0	0	0	42	0	42	0

Food	Cal	Fat	Sat	TFat	Chol	Carb	Fib	Sug	Sod

SODAS/SOFT DRINKS (CONT'D)

ALTERNATIVE DRINKS/SODAS

There are many low-sodium alternative drinks, the following have less than 40mg per serving.

Food	Cal	Fat	Sat	TFat	Chol	Carb	Fib	Sug	Sod
Ginseng Up, most (avg)	160	0	0	0	0	41	0	41	10
Apple or Ginger Beer (avg)	160	0	0	0	0	41	0	41	30
Orangina	120	0	0	0	0	28	0	26	0

SOY BEVERAGES

(see Milk Products and Non-Dairy Alternatives, pg 65)

SPORTS AND ENERGY DRINKS

(also see Water, Tonic and Seltzers, pg 20)

Food	Cal	Fat	Sat	TFat	Chol	Carb	Fib	Sug	Sod
Sports drink, fruit flavored, 8 fl oz	66	0	0	0	0	14	0	13	73
Energy drink, 8 fl oz	115	0	0	0	0	28	0	26	214

BRANDS . . .

Food	Cal	Fat	Sat	TFat	Chol	Carb	Fib	Sug	Sod
Elements Energy Drinks (avg)	120	0	0	0	0	29	0	27	10
Hansen's Energy, 8.3 fl oz (avg)	120	0	0	0	0	31	0	29	25
Honest Ade, all	100	0	0	0	0	26	0	26	10
Powerade, all	70	0	0	0	0	19	0	15	55
Rockstar Energy Drink	110	0	0	0	0	29	0	27	35
SoBe Sports & Energy drinks (avg)	130	0	0	0	0	33	0	31	20

TEA AND CHAI

Food	Cal	Fat	Sat	TFat	Chol	Carb	Fib	Sug	Sod
Tea, instant, lemon-flavored, prep, 8 fl oz	39	0	0	0	0	9	0	1	6
Tea, regular, prep, 8 fl oz	2	0	0	0	0	1	0	0	7
Tea, ready-to-drink, flavored, 8 fl oz	88	0	0	0	0	22	0	22	51
Chai, mix, prep, 8 fl oz	120	2	0	5	0	21	0	19	180

BRANDS . . .

CHAI

MIX *(8 FL OZ PREP UNLESS NOTED)*

Food	Cal	Fat	Sat	TFat	Chol	Carb	Fib	Sug	Sod
Caffe D'Amore Chai Amore	150	4	3	0	0	29	0	17	25
General Foods Int'l Chai Latte, no sugar	30	3	2	0	0	0	0	0	35
Pacific Chai Decaf Vanilla	120	2	2	0	0	23	0	14	38
Spice or Vanilla	120	2	1	0	0	25	0	21	55

TEA

INSTANT AND REGULAR

Most brands are within the generic range.

BEVERAGES
Vegetable Juice

Food	Cal	Fat	Sat	TFat	Chol	Carb	Fib	Sug	Sod
TEA AND CHAI (TEA CONT'D)									
READY-TO-DRINK (8 FL OZ PREP UNLESS NOTED)									
Arizona	89	0	0	0	0	22	0	22	9

VEGETABLE JUICE

Food	Cal	Fat	Sat	TFat	Chol	Carb	Fib	Sug	Sod
Mixed vegetable and fruit, 8 fl oz	72	0	0	0	0	18	0	5	52
Carrot juice, 8 fl oz	94	0	0	0	0	22	2	9	68
Tomato juice, 8 fl oz	41	0	0	0	0	10	1	9	653
Vegetable juice cocktail, 8 fl oz	46	0	0	0	0	11	2	8	655
Clam/tomato juice, 8 fl oz	116	0	0	0	0	26	1	8	875
BRANDS . . . (8 FL OZ UNLESS NOTED)									
After The Fall 24 Karrot Orange	120	0	0	0	0	28	0	25	55
Kogome Autumn Reds	170	0	0	0	0	40	1	34	25
RW Knudsen Very Veggie, LS	50	1	0	0	0	11	2	6	35
SoBe Orange Carrot Elixir	90	0	0	0	0	24	0	23	20
V8 Vegetable, LS	50	0	0	0	0	10	2	8	140

WATER, TONIC AND SELTZERS

(also see Sports and Energy Drinks, pg 19)

Food	Cal	Fat	Sat	TFat	Chol	Carb	Fib	Sug	Sod
Water, bottled, 8 fl oz	0	0	0	0	0	0	0	0	5
Seltzer, includes fruit-flavored, 8 fl oz	0	0	0	0	0	0	0	0	10
Tonic, 8 fl oz	83	0	0	0	0	22	0	24	29
Diet, 8 fl oz	0	0	0	0	0	0	0	0	35
Club soda, 8 fl oz	0	0	0	0	0	0	0	0	50

NOTE: Some fruit-flavored seltzers may contain as much as 46mg sodium per serving.

BRANDS . . . (8 FL OZ UNLESS NOTED)
Most bottled seltzers are within the generic range, the following hae less than the generic.

Food	Cal	Fat	Sat	TFat	Chol	Carb	Fib	Sug	Sod
Canada Dry Club Soda, LS	0	0	0	0	0	0	0	0	35

Food	Cal	Fat	Sat	TFat	Chol	Carb	Fib	Sug	Sod

BREAD, ROLLS AND BREAD PRODUCTS

BAGELS

Food	Cal	Fat	Sat	TFat	Chol	Carb	Fib	Sug	Sod
Cinnamon raisin bagel, med, 2.5 oz	194	1	0	0	0	39	2	4	229
Plain bagel, med, 2.5 oz	182	1	0	0	0	36	2	4	318
Mini, 1 oz	69	0	0	0	0	13	1	1	116
Large, 3.9 oz	283	2	0	0	0	56	2	6	493
Egg bagel, med, 2.5 oz	197	1	0	0	13	38	2	4	359
Oat bran bagel, med, 2.5 oz	181	1	0	0	0	38	3	1	360

BRANDS . . .

MIX

Food	Cal	Fat	Sat	TFat	Chol	Carb	Fib	Sug	Sod
Gluten Free Pantry, 1 bagel	150	0	0	0	0	36	1	4	170

SHELF-STABLE *(3.3 oz unless noted)*

Food	Cal	Fat	Sat	TFat	Chol	Carb	Fib	Sug	Sod
French Meadow Spelt	210	2	0	0	0	48	6	0	225
Natural Ovens Raspberry, 3 oz	280	2	0	0	0	38	5	10	110
Whole Grain, 3 oz	170	3	0	0	0	35	6	6	200
Golden Crunch Lo-Carb, 3 oz	190	11	0	0	0	15	8	5	200
Blueberry, 3 oz	190	2	0	0	0	40	4	10	220
Cinnamon Raisin, 3 oz	180	1	0	0	0	40	5	9	240
Hearty Grains & Onion, 3 oz	190	4	1	0	0	37	7	6	250
Silver Hills Squirrelly	210	4	1	0	0	32	6	3	170
Flax	210	3	0	0	0	33	19	2	210
Multigrain	210	2	0	0	0	36	8	2	250

NOTE: Although many of the above bagels exceed sodium guidelines, they are less than the generic.

BISCUITS

Food	Cal	Fat	Sat	TFat	Chol	Carb	Fib	Sug	Sod
Mixed grain, refrg dough, 2 1/2" (1.6 oz)	116	2	1	0	0	21	0	3	295
Plain biscuit:									
Mix, prep, 2 1/2" (1.1 oz)	95	3	1	-	1	14	1	3	271
Refrg dough, 2 1/2" (1.1) oz	90	4	1	0	0	12	0	2	314
LF refrg dough, 2 1/2" (1.1 oz)	73	1	0	0	0	13	1	2	354
Ready-to-eat, 2 1/2" (1.3 oz)	128	6	1	0	0	17	1	1	368

BRANDS . . . *(1 oz biscuit unless noted)*

MIX

Food	Cal	Fat	Sat	TFat	Chol	Carb	Fib	Sug	Sod
Bernard, LS	170	4	2	0	0	30	0	0	10
Carbquick Biscuit & Baking Mix	50	4	0	0	0	9	7	0	110

Food	Cal	Fat	Sat	TFat	Chol	Carb	Fib	Sug	Sod
BREAD – DOUGH AND MIXES									
(also see Bread – Shelf-Stable, pg 23)									
Multigrain, mix, 1/4 cup	130	2	0	0	0	22	2	1	150
Whole wheat, mix, lowfat, 1/4 cup	120	2	0	0	0	22	3	1	160
White, mix, 1/4 cup	120	2	0	0	0	22	3	1	170
Banana, mix, prep, 2.1 oz slice	196	6	1	0	26	33	1	17	181
Rye, mix, 1/4 cup	120	2	0	0	0	22	3	1	190
Wheat, bread machine mix, 1/3 cup	150	2	0	0	0	28	1	5	260
White, bread machine mix, 1/3 cup	150	2	0	0	0	28	1	5	280
BRANDS . . .									
FROZEN/REFRIGERATED *(1 OZ UNLESS NOTED)*									
Kineret Challah	70	1	0	0	10	14	1	2	110
The Upper Crust Banana Bread, 2 oz	177	7	3	0	22	26	1	17	113
Corn Brean, 2 oz	180	5	2	0	25	33	1	16	170
MIX *(1 SLICE UNLESS NOTED)*									
Arrowhead Mills Multigrain, 2 oz	140	1	0	0	0	28	3	1	115
Pumpernickel, 2 oz	120	1	0	0	0	25	4	2	130
Whole Wheat, 2 oz	140	1	0	0	0	27	4	2	140
French, 2 oz	130	1	0	0	0	27	1	2	150
Bob's Red Mill Low-Carb Bread Mix	90	2	0	0	0	9	4	0	92
Glutano Bread & Cake Mix, 2 slices	70	0	0	0	0	34	0	6	120
Gluten Free Pantry French Bread & Pizza	110	0	0	0	0	25	1	0	115
Ketogenics White, Honey Wheat, or									
Pumpernickel Rye (avg)	80	1	1	0	0	7	5	1	60
McCann's Irish Brown, 1/14	90	1	0	0	0	17	2	0	100
Sylvan Border Farm Dark, White, or									
Wheat-Free, 2 oz	140	4	1	0	35	24	1	6	120
QUICK/SWEET BREADS									
MIX *(1 SLICE UNLESS NOTED)*									
Betty Crocker Cinnamon Streusel	160	4	1	1	0	28	0	15	150
Chébé Cinnamon Roll-ups, 0.8 oz	73	0	0	0	0	18	0	0	100
Gluten Free Pantry Lemon Poppyseed	120	0	0	0	0	28	1	12	75
Pumpkin	120	0	0	0	0	28	1	11	75
Banana	120	0	0	0	0	28	1	13	75
Lollipop Tree Summer Berry, 1.2 oz	130	2	2	0	0	26	1	15	85
Cherry w/Belgian Choc, 1.2 oz	130	2	1	0	0	27	1	18	105
Pear Spice, 1.2 oz	120	0	0	0	0	29	1	16	105
Caramel Apple, 1.2 oz	130	0	0	0	0	29	1	19	110
Lemon w/Lemon Peel, 1.2	120	0	0	0	0	28	1	16	115

Food	Cal	Fat	Sat	TFat	Chol	Carb	Fib	Sug	Sod

BREAD – SHELF-STABLE

(also see Bread – Dough and Mixes, pg 22)

Food	Cal	Fat	Sat	TFat	Chol	Carb	Fib	Sug	Sod
Raisin bread, 1.1 oz slice	82	1	0	0	0	16	1	2	117
Rice bran bread, 1 oz slice	66	1	0	0	0	12	1	1	119
Oat bran bread, 1.1 oz slice	71	1	0	0	0	12	1	2	122
Mixed grain bread, 1.1 oz slice	75	1	0	0	0	14	2	3	146
Wheat bread, 1.1 oz slice	74	1	0	0	0	13	1	2	150
Cracked wheat bread, 1.1 oz slice	78	1	0	0	0	15	2	1	161
Oatmeal bread, 1.1 oz slice	81	1	0	0	0	15	1	2	180
French or sourdough bread, 1.1 oz slice	88	1	0	0	0	17	1	0	195
Pumpernickel bread, 1.1 oz slice	75	1	0	0	0	14	2	0	201
White bread, 1.1 oz slice	80	1	0	0	0	15	1	1	204
Rye bread, 1.1 oz slice	83	1	0	0	0	15	2	1	211
Boston brown, canned, 1.6 oz slice	88	1	0	0	0	19	2	1	284
Focaccia bread, 1 oz slice	78	1	0	0	0	15	1	1	308

BRANDS . . . *(1 SLICE UNLESS NOTED)*

There are many low-sodium breads, the following have less than 100mg per slice.

Food	Cal	Fat	Sat	TFat	Chol	Carb	Fib	Sug	Sod
Alvarado St. Bakery Multi-Grain, SF	90	1	0	0	0	15	2	2	10
Arnold Golden Wheat Light	40	0	0	0	0	10	3	2	80
Raisin Cinnamon	80	2	0	0	0	15	1	7	95
The Baker Yoga	70	1	0	0	0	12	2	-	80
Honey Cinnamon Raisin	85	1	0	0	0	17	2	-	85
Seeded Whole Wheat	75	2	0	0	0	14	2	-	85
Whole Grain Bran or Whole Grain Flax	50	1	0	0	0	8	3	-	90
Barkat Cinnamon Raisin Rice	110	2	0	0	0	23	1	1	0
Flax Seed Rice	110	2	0	0	0	23	1	1	0
Breadsmith Vanilla Egg	77	0	0	0	9	16	0	-	39
Cranberry Orange Dessert	86	3	2	0	14	13	1	3	68
Panettone or Greek Olive (avg)	74	2	1	0	3	14	1	2	74
Gluten Free	74	3	0	0	11	10	0	1	78
Austrian Pumpernickel	53	1	0	0	0	13	2	3	84
Farmer's Wheat	70	1	0	0	0	13	1	3	92
Irish Soda Bread or Russian Rye (avg)	85	2	1	0	5	16	1	3	95
Country Buttertop, 1 oz	57	1	1	0	5	10	0	2	98
Ener-G Brown Rice	130	6	0	0	0	18	1	1	10
Rice Starch	160	5	0	0	0	29	4	5	10
Raisin	180	6	1	4	0	28	1	12	55
Hi-Fiber	100	3	0	0	0	20	2	2	60
Corn Loaf	40	3	0	0	0	8	4	1	60

BREAD, ROLLS AND BREAD PRODUCTS
Bread – Shelf-Stable

Food	Cal	Fat	Sat	TFat	Chol	Carb	Fib	Sug	Sod
BREAD – SHELF-STABLE (ENER-G CONT'D)									
Tapioca	70	8	0	0	0	10	1	0	65
Light White Rice	70	3	0	0	0	10	0	0	65
Tapioca, Thin Sliced, 2	90	5	0	0	0	12	2	0	90
Light Brown Rice	70	4	0	0	0	9	0	0	95
Food for Life Ezekiel LS	80	1	1	0	0	15	3	0	0
Genesis, Sprouted Grain & Seed	80	2	0	0	0	14	3	0	65
Cinnamon Raisin	80	0	0	0	0	18	2	5	65
Ezekiel, Low Carb	70	4	1	0	0	4	1	0	65
Ezekiel, Sprouted 7 Grain	80	1	0	0	0	15	3	1	80
French Meadow Rye, 100%, SF	103	1	0	0	0	22	3	0	0
Spelt	70	0	0	0	0	14	2	0	75
Flax & Sunflower Seed	92	2	0	0	0	18	3	0	90
Healthy Life 100% Whole Wheat	35	0	0	0	0	8	3	1	80
White	35	0	0	0	0	8	2	1	90
Irene's German Rye Lo-Carb	30	0	0	0	0	5	1	0	55
Loaves & Fishes Cinnamon Raisin, 4.2 oz	100	1	0	0	0	22	3	6	81
Sprouted Bread, 4.2 oz	100	1	0	0	0	17	4	0	94
Montana Mills Sunflower Millet	70	1	0	0	0	14	2	3	65
Cinnamon Raisin Walnut	70	1	0	0	0	14	2	1	70
Cranberry Orange or Woodstock (avg)	70	0	0	0	0	14	2	3	70
Multigrain	70	0	0	0	0	14	2	2	70
Raspberry Cheese Danish	60	1	0	0	0	12	1	2	70
Apple Raisin Challah	70	0	0	0	0	14	2	1	75
Blueberry Cobbler or King's Cake (avg)	70	1	0	0	5	15	1	5	75
Blueberry Cheese Danish	60	1	0	0	0	12	1	3	75
Blueberry Pancake or Sticky Bun (avg)	70	1	0	0	0	15	1	4	75
German Fruit & Nut Stollen	70	1	0	0	0	15	1	3	75
Maple Raisin Walnut	70	1	0	0	0	15	1	4	75
Red, White & Blue Cobbler	80	1	0	0	0	16	1	5	75
Honey Whole Wheat	70	0	0	0	0	14	2	2	80
Almond Bear Claw	80	2	0	0	0	14	1	2	85
Bavarian Rye	65	0	0	0	0	13	1	0	85
Cheese Danish or Choc Bobka (avg)	75	2	0	0	0	13	1	4	85
Cherry Choc or Raspberry Apricot	70	1	0	0	0	14	1	2	85
Hot Cross or Linzer Nut Tart (avg)	75	2	0	0	0	14	1	2	85
Venetian Pizza	60	1	0	0	0	13	1	1	85
Apple Raisin Cinnamon Swirl	70	0	0	0	0	15	1	3	90
Apricot Almond or Chessecake (avg)	70	0	0	0	0	15	1	3	90
Cherry Apple Strudel	70	1	0	0	0	10	1	3	90
Sesame Garlic Cheddar	70	2	0	0	0	12	1	1	90

Food	Cal	Fat	Sat	TFat	Chol	Carb	Fib	Sug	Sod
BREAD — SHELF-STABLE (MONTANA MILLS CONT'D)									
Blueberry Cheesecake	70	1	0	0	0	14	1	4	95
Blueberry White Choc	70	1	0	0	0	14	1	4	95
Cranberry Pecan Cornbread	80	2	0	0	0	14	1	4	95
Holiday Fruit or Stars 'n Stripes (avg)	65	0	0	0	0	14	1	2	95
Peaches 'n Creme	80	1	0	0	0	15	1	4	95
Natural Ovens Sunny Millet	70	2	0	0	0	13	4	1	60
Multi-Grain or Better White (avg)	70	1	0	0	0	16	3	1	75
Glorious or Happliness (avg)	75	1	0	0	0	16	2	4	80
Lo-Carb, Golden Crunch or Original (avg)	70	3	0	0	0	7	4	2	83
Nutty Natural	70	2	0	0	0	13	3	1	85
Right Wheat or Hunger Filler	60	1	0	0	0	13	4	1	85
100% Whole Grain	80	2	0	0	0	15	4	1	90
English Muffin Bread	80	1	0	0	0	16	1	2	95
Cracked Wheat	80	2	0	0	0	15	2	1	95
Nature's Path Manna Bread									
Millet Rice or Multigrain (avg)	130	0	0	0	0	28	5	9	3
Sun Seed	160	2	0	0	0	29	7	11	3
Carrot Raisin or Fruit & Nut (avg)	135	1	0	0	0	27	5	13	7
Whole Rye	150	0	0	0	0	32	5	7	10
Cinnamon Date	150	0	0	0	0	29	5	10	15
Pepperidge Farm Whole Wheat, Thin Sliced	70	1	0	0	0	11	2	1	95
Rudolph's SF Rye	124	1	0	0	0	26	4	0	2
Weissbrot	66	0	0	0	0	14	1	0	46
Ryelite	66	0	0	0	0	12	1	0	63
Sourdough or 5-Grain	77	1	0	0	0	16	1	0	76
Volkornbrot	55	0	0	0	0	13	2	0	87
Sara Lee Brown Sugar Cinnamon	100	3	2	0	0	15	2	8	95
Sunbeam Sandwich White	55	1	0	0	0	11	1	1	90
Weight Watcher's Whole Wheat	45	1	0	0	0	8	2	1	90
Wonder 100% Whole Wheat	55	1	0	0	0	9	2	1	90
BREAD BOWLS									
Lettieri's White Bread Bowl, 1.7 oz (1/3)	100	4	1	0	0	21	1	1	65
Seasoned Bread Bowl, 1.7 oz (1/3)	130	4	1	0	0	21	1	1	95

BREADSTICKS

Food	Cal	Fat	Sat	TFat	Chol	Carb	Fib	Sug	Sod
Plain, 0.5 oz	58	1	0	0	0	10	0	0	92
BRANDS . . . *(0.5 OZ UNLESS NOTED)*									
Glutino Pizza Flavored, 6	40	1	1	0	0	9	0	0	2
Sesame, 6	40	1	1	0	0	9	0	0	2

25

BREAD, ROLLS AND BREAD PRODUCTS
Buns, Croissants and Rolls

Food	Cal	Fat	Sat	TFat	Chol	Carb	Fib	Sug	Sod
BREADSTICKS (CONT'D)									
Stella D'oro SF, 0.4 oz	45	1	0	0	0	7	0	1	0
Original, 0.4 oz	40	1	0	0	0	7	0	0	40
Sesame, 0.4 oz	50	3	1	0	0	7	1	1	45
Mini, Original, 0.6 oz	70	2	0	0	0	12	1	1	65
Mini, Sesame, 0.6 oz	80	4	1	0	0	11	1	1	75
Toufayan Sesame or Whole Wheat	45	1	0	0	0	9	1	1	80

(BUNS, CROISSANTS AND ROLLS)

SANDWICH BUNS AND ROLLS

Food	Cal	Fat	Sat	TFat	Chol	Carb	Fib	Sug	Sod
Hot dog or hamburger, whole wheat	113	3	1	0	0	19	2	3	197
Hot dog or hamburger, plain	120	2	0	0	0	21	1	3	206
Reduced cal	84	1	0	0	0	18	3	3	190
Hoagie/submarine, small, 2.3 oz	173	3	1	0	0	33	5	6	311
BRANDS . . . *(1 BUN UNLESS NOTED)*									
Arnold Potato Hot Dog	140	2	1	0	0	24	1	5	170
Sesame Sandwich	140	4	1	0	0	25	1	4	200
The Baker Seeded Whole Wheat Rolls	100	2	0	0	0	18	3	-	115
Honey Cinnamon Raisin	150	2	0	0	0	29	3	-	140
7-Grain Sourdough Sandwich	110	1	0	0	0	22	4	-	190
Honey Whole Wheat Sandwich	120	1	0	0	0	24	4	-	190
Bread du Juor Italian Rolls	90	1	0	0	0	16	0	2	190
Brownberry Potato Hot Dog	120	2	0	0	0	22	1	4	160
Cybro's Rice Rolls (small)	60	1	0	0	0	14	1	0	160
Food for Life									
Hot Dog or Hamburger	150	3	0	0	0	28	5	2	140
Ezekiel Hamburger or Hot Dog	170	2	0	0	0	34	6	0	170
Ezekiel Sesame Hamburger	170	2	0	0	0	32	6	0	180
Francisco Int'l Sourdough	100	0	0	0	0	19	1	1	170
Harvest Pride Sandwich Rolls, 1.5 oz	150	2	1	0	0	29	1	3	200
Kings Hawaiian Deli Roll, 4.4 oz	90	2	1	0	10	15	0	4	85
Martin's Potato Rolls, Long or Sandwich	130	2	0	0	0	26	4	6	200
Mrs. Baird's Hot Dog	110	2	0	0	0	18	1	0	170
Natural Ovens Better Wheat Buns	140	2	0	0	0	30	5	4	120
Best Burger Buns	170	4	0	0	0	29	3	3	150
Nature Bake Sandwich, Multigrain	160	3	0	0	0	28	4	5	190
Nature's Own Wheat 'n Fiber Hamburger	80	2	0	0	0	28	5	2	160
Schmidts Potato Rolls, Long or Sandwich	140	1	0	0	0	28	2	5	190
Sunbeam Hamburger or Hot Dog	100	2	0	0	0	20	1	2	180
Village Hearth Light Wheat Hamburger	80	1	0	0	0	14	3	3	180

Food	Cal	Fat	Sat	TFat	Chol	Carb	Fib	Sug	Sod
CROISSANTS AND DINNER ROLLS									
Dinner roll, wheat, 1 oz	76	2	0	0	0	13	1	0	95
Whole wheat, 1 oz	74	1	0	0	0	14	2	2	134
Brown & serve, 1 oz	84	2	0	0	0	14	1	1	146
Rye, 1 oz	80	1	0	0	0	15	1	0	250
Hard roll (kaiser), 1 oz	83	1	0	0	0	15	1	1	154
French roll, 1 oz	79	1	0	0	0	14	1	0	173
Croissant, butter, 1 oz	115	6	3	0	19	13	1	3	211
BRANDS . . .									
FROZEN/REFRIGERATED *(1 ROLL UNLESS NOTED)*									
Pepperidge Farm Parker House Dinner ...	80	2	0	0	0	14	1	2	95
SHELF-STABLE *(1 ROLL UNLESS NOTED)*									
Breadsmith Hot Cross Buns, 1 oz	72	0	0	0	0	19	1	2	101
King's Hawaiian Honey Wheat Rolls	80	2	1	0	10	15	1	4	80
Sweet Rolls	90	2	1	0	10	15	0	4	85
Martin Potato Rolls	90	1	0	0	0	17	2	3	120
Potato Rolls, Sliced	100	2	0	0	0	15	1	3	140
Natural Ovens Dinner	70	1	0	0	0	15	4	3	70

SWEET ROLLS *(see Pastries and Coffeecakes, pg 37)*

COFFEECAKES

(see Pastries and Coffeecakes, pg 37)

CREPES

(also see Blintzes and Crepes, pg 89)

Food	Cal	Fat	Sat	TFat	Chol	Carb	Fib	Sug	Sod
Crepes, 1	37	1	1	0	5	5	0	3	60

BRANDS . . .
Most brands are within the generic range.

CROUTONS

(see Salad Toppings, pg 48)

ENGLISH MUFFINS

Food	Cal	Fat	Sat	TFat	Chol	Carb	Fib	Sug	Sod
Cinnamon-raisin, 2 oz	137	1	0	0	0	27	2	8	189
Wheat, 2 oz	127	1	0	0	0	26	3	1	218
Mixed-grain or granola, 2 oz	133	1	0	0	0	26	2	0	236
Plain or sourdough, 2 oz	129	1	0	0	0	25	2	2	242
Whole wheat, 2 oz	115	1	0	0	0	23	4	5	361

Food	Cal	Fat	Sat	TFat	Chol	Carb	Fib	Sug	Sod

ENGLISH MUFFINS (CONT'D)

BRANDS . . . *(1 MUFFIN UNLESS NOTED)*

CINNAMON/RAISIN MUFFINS

Food	Cal	Fat	Sat	TFat	Chol	Carb	Fib	Sug	Sod
Food for Life Ezekiel Cinnamon-Raisin ...	160	0	0	0	0	36	4	10	170
Thomas Cinnamon Raisin	140	1	0	0	0	30	1	8	180

OTHER MUFFIN VARIETIES

Food	Cal	Fat	Sat	TFat	Chol	Carb	Fib	Sug	Sod
Food for Life Genesis Whole Grain & Seed	180	4	0	0	0	30	6	0	140
Ezekiel 100% Whole Grain	160	1	0	0	0	30	6	0	160
Poi, 2.5 oz	150	0	0	0	0	32	1	3	210
Thomas Hearty Grain	130	1	0	0	0	27	2	4	180
Sourdough or Honey Wheat (avg)	115	1	0	0	0	25	1	2	190
Original Plain	120	1	0	0	0	25	1	1	200

(MUFFINS AND SCONES)

(also see English Muffins, pg 27; Snack Cakes, Pies and Sweet Snacks, pg 87)

MUFFINS

Food	Cal	Fat	Sat	TFat	Chol	Carb	Fib	Sug	Sod
Banana nut muffin, mix, 2 oz	150	5	1	0	5	23	0	11	205
Blueberry muffin, ready-to-eat, 2 oz	157	4	1	0	17	27	2	11	253
Mix, 2 oz	208	6	2	0	0	36	0	13	311
Corn muffin, ready-to-eat, 2 oz	173	5	1	0	15	29	2	4	295
Mix, prep, 2 oz	182	6	2	0	35	28	1	6	451

BRANDS . . .

MIX *(1 MUFFIN UNLESS NOTED)*

Food	Cal	Fat	Sat	TFat	Chol	Carb	Fib	Sug	Sod
Authentic Foods Choc Chip	150	5	0	0	0	29	3	18	140
Bernard Cornbread & Muffin, 2	150	2	1	0	0	31	1	0	20
Betty Crocker Twice the Blueberries	120	1	0	0	0	26	1	15	180
Lemon-Poppy Seed	140	2	1	1	0	29	1	19	190
Bob's Red Mill Raisin Bran	30	0	0	0	0	13	1	2	160
Oat Bran & Date Nut	120	2	0	0	0	22	2	1	160
Date Nut Bran	70	1	0	0	0	13	2	2	160
Spice Apple Bran	70	0	0	0	0	16	3	1	180
The Cravings Place Bread & Muffin	76	0	0	0	0	18	1	9	19
Cornbread Mix	110	2	0	0	0	23	2	0	31
Dixie Diner Corn	51	0	0	0	0	8	4	0	156
Apple Cinnamon, Cranberry Orange, or Blueberry Cream	31	0	0	0	0	7	3	2	179
Banana Nut	48	2	0	0	0	7	4	1	179
Firenza Corn Bread, 1 oz	100	0	0	0	0	23	1	9	100
Flax Z Snax Blueberrylicious	80	3	2	-	0	16	7	1	120

Food	Cal	Fat	Sat	TFat	Chol	Carb	Fib	Sug	Sod
MUFFINS AND SCONES (CONT'D)									
Gluten-Free Pantry Bran	130	1	0	0	0	27	4	8	30
Muffin & Scone	100	0	0	0	0	24	0	7	120
Hodgson Mill Apple Cinnamon	120	2	0	0	0	25	3	6	80
Bran	130	1	0	0	0	27	3	5	150
King Arthur Flour Blueberry	180	1	0	0	0	40	3	19	130
Cranberry-Orange	180	1	0	0	0	41	3	20	130
Krusteaz Cornbread w/Honey	110	3	1	0	0	20	1	6	190
Pantry Shelf Cinnamon Fudge, 1.5 oz	150	0	0	0	0	34	1	21	55
Gingerbread, 1.5 oz	200	0	0	0	0	48	1	28	95
SHELF-STABLE *(2 OZ UNLESS NOTED)*									
Awrey's Apple, 1.5 oz	140	7	2	0	30	18	0	8	120
Blueberry or Cranberry Nut, 1.5 oz (avg)	140	7	2	0	30	19	0	8	120
Corn, 1.5 oz	180	9	2	0	30	22	0	10	125
Banana Nut, 1.5 oz	170	9	2	0	30	20	0	10	135
Lemon Poppy Seed, 1.5 oz	190	11	2	0	30	20	0	10	140
Hostess Mini Muffins (avg)	160	8	2	-	0	16	0	8	110
Our Daily Muffin Choc	140	1	0	0	0	31	5	18	70
All others (avg)	120	0	0	0	0	31	9	16	140
SCONES									
Scone, mix, 1/4 cup	170	9	2	0	0	20	1	4	410
BRANDS . . .									
MIX *(1 SCONE UNLESS NOTED)*									
Bette's Diner Raisin	229	0	0	0	0	30	1	9	129
'Cause You're Special English	87	0	0	0	0	21	1	3	71
Gluten-Free Pantry Muffin & Scone	100	0	0	0	0	24	0	7	120
King Arthur Flour Cranberry Orange	180	1	0	0	0	38	1	14	105
Blueberry Sour Cream	180	2	1	0	5	37	1	14	140
Lollipop Tree Traditional English	140	0	0	0	0	30	1	6	85
Lemon Poppy Seed	140	1	0	0	30	0	1	8	135
Apricot Cranberry	130	0	0	0	0	30	1	10	140
Martha's Cranberry Orange	110	1	0	0	0	29	1	6	120
SHELF-STABLE *(1 SCONE UNLESS NOTED)*									
Breadsmith Cranberry	95	3	1	0	5	15	1	0	129
Health Valley Scones, all	180	0	0	0	0	43	5	18	190

PITA AND POCKET BREADS

Food	Cal	Fat	Sat	TFat	Chol	Carb	Fib	Sug	Sod
Whole Wheat pita, small 4" diam, 1	74	1	0	0	0	15	2	1	149
Large, 6.5" diam, 1	170	2	0	0	0	35	5	1	340

BREAD, ROLLS AND BREAD PRODUCTS
Wraps and Flatbreads

Food	Cal	Fat	Sat	TFat	Chol	Carb	Fib	Sug	Sod
PITA AND POCKET BREADS (CONT'D)									
White pita, small 4" diam, 1	77	0	0	0	0	16	1	0	150
Large, 6.5" diam, 1	165	1	0	0	0	33	1	1	322
BRANDS . . . *(1 PITA UNLESS NOTED)*									
The Baker White or Whole Wheat (avg)	140	0	0	0	0	28	2	0	115
Damascus Mini Pita, Plain, 1 oz	65	0	0	0	0	14	1	1	0
Mini Pita, Whole Wheat, 1 oz	65	0	0	0	0	14	2	1	75
Food for Life 7-Grain Pocket	90	1	0	0	0	19	3	1	110
Ezekiel Pocket	100	1	0	0	0	21	4	1	120
Garden of Eatin' Bible Bread, LS Pita	160	2	0	0	0	30	1	1	30
Bible Bread, LF Pita	160	2	0	0	0	31	2	1	115
Giant White Pita, Mini, SF, 2	150	0	0	0	0	32	1	2	0
Kangaroo Whole Grain Pockets	80	1	0	0	0	16	5	1	100
Salad Pockets or Pita Pockets (avg)	85	0	0	0	0	17	2	1	140
Pitaland Plain or Tandoor Pita, 1 oz	70	0	0	0	0	14	0	0	39
Sahara, Wheat, Mini, 1 oz	60	1	0	0	0	14	2	1	140

ROLLS

(see Buns, Croissants and Rolls, pg 26)

WRAPS AND FLATBREADS

(also see Tortillas and Taco Shells, pg 116)

Food	Cal	Fat	Sat	TFat	Chol	Carb	Fib	Sug	Sod
Flatbread, plain, 2 oz	260	0	0	0	0	58	2	2	300
BRANDS . . . *(1 WRAP UNLESS NOTED)*									
Lavash All Natural Roll-Ups	110	2	0	0	0	23	1	0	20
Nu-World Foods Amaranth Flatbread (avg)	161	4	1	0	0	30	5	0	12

Food	Cal	Fat	Sat	TFat	Chol	Carb	Fib	Sug	Sod

BREAKFAST PRODUCTS

BREAKFAST DRINKS/MEAL REPLACEMENTS

(also see Diet and Nutritional Drinks, pg 16)

Food	Cal	Fat	Sat	TFat	Chol	Carb	Fib	Sug	Sod
Choc mix, 1 envl	130	2	1	0	5	27	0	18	95
Vanilla mix, 1 envl	130	0	0	0	5	28	0	17	105
Meal replacement, mix, 3 tbsp	140	2	0	0	0	14	2	11	170
Vanilla, ready-to-drink, 8 fl oz	240	5	1	0	10	37	2	28	180
Choc, ready-to-drink, 8 fl oz	250	5	1	10	0	31	1	29	230

BRANDS . . .
Most brands are within the generic range.

CEREAL – COLD

Food	Cal	Fat	Sat	TFat	Chol	Carb	Fib	Sug	Sod
Puffed rice, 1 cup	56	0	0	0	0	13	0	0	0
Puffed wheat, 1 cup	44	0	0	0	0	10	1	0	0
Shredded wheat, 2 biscuits	155	1	0	0	0	36	6	0	3
Frosted corn flakes, 1 cup	152	0	0	0	0	37	1	16	198
Crispy rice, 1 cup	108	0	0	0	0	24	0	3	266
Corn flakes, 1 cup	101	0	0	0	0	24	1	2	266
Bran flakes, 1 cup	128	1	0	0	0	32	7	8	293
Wheat & barley, 1/2 cup	208	1	0	0	0	47	5	7	354
Bran & raisins, 1 cup	195	2	0	0	0	47	7	20	362

BRANDS . . . *(3/4 CUP UNLESS NOTED)*

PUFFED CEREALS OR SHREDDED WHEAT
Most brands are within the generic range.

OTHER CEREALS
There are many low-sodium cereals, the following have 50mg or less per serving.

Food	Cal	Fat	Sat	TFat	Chol	Carb	Fib	Sug	Sod
Alpen Original, 1.9 oz	200	3	0	0	0	44	4	11	30
No Sugar Added, 1.9 oz	200	3	0	0	0	40	4	7	30
Arrowhead Mills Amaranth Flakes	140	2	0	0	0	26	3	4	0
Nature-O's	130	2	1	0	0	25	2	1	0
Butte Creek Mill 10 Grain Hi Fiber, 1/4 cup	100	1	0	0	0	20	4	0	0
Ener-G Rice Bran, 1/2 cup	220	14	3	0	0	34	19	3	5
Erewhon Crispy Brown Rice, 1 cup	110	0	0	0	0	25	1	1	10
Rice Twice	120	0	0	0	0	26	0	8	60
Enjoy Life Very Berry Crunch, 1/2 cup	170	6	2	0	0	25	6	9	10
Cinnamon Crunch, 1/2 cup	160	5	0	0	0	26	5	5	10
Grainfields LS cereals (avg)	110	0	0	0	0	26	0	1	20

31

Food	Cal	Fat	Sat	TFat	Chol	Carb	Fib	Sug	Sod
CEREAL – COLD (CONT'D)									
Health Valley Blue Corn Flakes	100	0	0	0	0	24	3	5	10
Healthy Fiber Multigrain	100	0	0	0	0	23	4	3	15
Raspberry Rhapsody	200	3	0	0	0	41	4	11	30
Banana Gone Nuts or Cranberry Crunch	200	3	0	0	0	41	4	11	30
Kashi Heart to Heart or Honey Go Lean	120	1	0	0	0	28	10	7	35
Medley, 1/2 cup	100	1	0	0	0	20	2	5	50
Kellogg's Mini-Wheats, 2 oz (avg)	190	1	0	0	0	41	5	10	5
Honey Smacks	100	1	0	0	0	24	1	15	50
Nature's Path Synergy 8 Grain	100	1	0	0	0	24	5	4	0
Nu-World Foods Cereal Snaps, all (avg)	183	3	0	0	0	25	5	7	2
Amaranth O's, all (avg)	58	1	0	0	0	16	10	2	26
Post Golden Crisp	110	0	0	0	0	24	1	14	25
South Beach Diet									
Toasted Wheats, 1 1/4 cups	210	1	0	0	0	48	8	3	0
GRANOLA AND MUSELI									
Granola, 1/2 cup	299	15	3	0	0	32	5	12	101
BRANDS . . . *(1/2 CUP UNLESS NOTED)*									
Back to Nature Granola, Classic	180	3	0	0	0	36	4	5	5
Raisin	190	2	0	0	0	35	4	15	5
Apple Cinnamon	180	3	0	0	0	36	4	11	15
Apple Strawberry or Apple Blueberry (avg)	190	3	0	0	0	37	4	6	20
French Vanilla or Cranberry Pecan (avg)	220	6	2	0	0	35	4	12	50
The Baker Pecan Granola	130	8	0	0	0	12	2	-	0
Nut & Berry or Honey Crunch Muesli (avg)	255	8	0	0	0	37	6	-	0
Forest Berry Muesli	210	3	0	0	0	41	6	-	15
Bear Naked Granola, Fruit & Nut	210	9	2	0	0	28	4	12	0
Familia Museli, No Sugar	200	3	2	0	0	41	5	8	0
Breadshop Granola									
Super Natural or Crunchy Oat Bran (avg)	215	9	1	0	0	31	5	10	0
Blueberry or Raspberry 'n Cream	220	8	1	0	0	32	4	7	0
Triple Berry Crunch, 2/3 cup	220	7	0	0	0	36	4	9	35
Pralines 'n Cream or Mocha Almond Crunch	210	7	0	0	0	34	4	8	40
Cinnamon Raisin	220	6	1	0	0	37	4	15	60
Divinely D'lish Veritas Granola	200	11	4	0	0	22	4	4	0
Gracious Granola	220	13	5	0	0	22	4	4	20
Ener-G Granola & Trail Mix, 1/3 cup	260	16	3	0	0	20	4	12	5
Familia Swiss Museli	250	3	1	0	0	45	5	16	0
Swiss Museli, No Sugar Added	200	3	2	0	0	41	5	8	0
Michaelene's Gourmet Granola, all (avg)	103	2	0	0	0	18	3	5	11

Food	Cal	Fat	Sat	TFat	Chol	Carb	Fib	Sug	Sod
GRANOLA AND MUSELI (CONT'D)									
Natural Ovens Great Granola, 1/4 cup	110	4	1	0	0	18	5	3	10
Nature's Path Granola									
Ginger Zing or FlaxPlus (avg)	140	5	1	0	0	21	2	5	17
HempPlus	140	5	0	0	0	20	3	5	25
Acai Apple or PomegranPlus	130	5	1	0	0	21	2	7	35
SoyPlus or Peanut Butter (avg)	135	5	1	0	0	21	2	6	40
Heritage, Raspberry	130	3	0	0	0	22	3	5	45
Northern Gold Honey Almond Granola	250	9	2	0	0	36	5	8	0
Cashews & Raisins Granola	240	8	1	0	0	38	5	11	5
Blueberry & Raspberry Granola	230	5	1	0	0	41	4	12	60
Quaker 100% Natural Granola (avg)	230	9	4	0	0	34	3	16	20

CEREAL - HOT

NOTE: There is a difference between "instant" and "quick cooking" cereals. Generally, instant has upwards of 200mg sodium per serving; quick-cooking averages 2mg.

Wheat cereal, regular, cooked, 1 cup	160	1	0	0	0	33	4	0	0
Instant, 1 serv	130	0	0	0	0	30	1	14	210
Oat cereal, regular or quick cooked, 1 cup ..	147	2	0	0	0	25	4	1	2
Instant, flavored, 1 cup	257	3	0	0	0	24	4	23	36
Rice cereal, cooked, 1 cup	127	0	0	0	0	28	0	0	3
Farina, cooked, 1 cup	112	0	0	0	0	24	0	0	5
Grits, regular or quick, cooked, 1 cup	143	0	0	0	0	31	1	0	5
Instant, 1 cup	167	0	0	0	0	37	2	0	515

BRANDS . . .

INSTANT (*1 PACKAGE/SERVING UNLESS NOTED*)

Arrowhead Mills Organic, 1 oz	140	2	0	0	0	26	3	5	45
Erewhon Organic w/Added Bran	130	3	1	0	0	25	4	1	0
Raisin, Dates & Walnuts	130	3	1	0	0	24	3	1	40
Mother's Instant	150	3	1	0	0	27	4	2	0
Nu-World Foods Berry Delicious, 1 cup ..	91	1	0	0	0	21	3	2	9

REGULAR/QUICK

Most brands are within the generic range.

CEREAL, GRANOLA AND BREAKFAST BARS

(Also see Diet, Energy and Nutritional Bars, pg 144)

Cereal bar, mixed fruit, 1 oz	104	2	0	0	0	20	1	9	83
Granola bar, oats, fruits & nuts, 1 oz	111	2	0	0	0	22	2	12	70
Granola bar, choc chip, 1 oz	118	5	3	0	0	19	1	9	76

33

BREAKFAST PRODUCTS
Cereal, Granola and Breakfast Bars

Food	Cal	Fat	Sat	TFat	Chol	Carb	Fib	Sug	Sod
CEREAL, GRANOLA AND BREAKFAST BARS (CONT'D)									
Breakfast bar, oat, raisin, coconut, 1 oz	130	5	4	0	0	19	1	8	78
Granola bar, peanut butter, 1 oz	119	4	1	0	0	18	1	9	115

BRANDS . . . *(1.3 OZ BAR UNLESS NOTED)*

There are many low-sodium cereal and granola bars, the following have 90mg or less per serving.

Food	Cal	Fat	Sat	TFat	Chol	Carb	Fib	Sug	Sod
Aunt Candice Breakfast, Strawberry, 2 oz .	230	8	1	0	0	32	2	10	65
Barbara's Bakery Granola, all, 0.8 oz (avg)	80	2	0	0	0	14	1	7	0
Cereal Bars, Multigrain, all	120	2	0	0	0	25	2	13	65
Puffins, Blueberry or Strawberry Yogurt	140	2	1	0	0	24	3	8	85
Divinely D'lish Granola Bars, 1.9 oz (avg)	220	10	4	0	0	34	4	12	3
EnviroKidz Crispy Rice, Peanut Butter, 1 oz	110	3	1	0	0	20	1	7	80
Crispy Rice, Berry or Choc	110	3	0	0	0	20	1	7	90
Fibar Chewy & Nutty Granola Bars, 1.2 oz									
Milk Choc Almond Crunch	140	5	3	0	0	23	1	11	20
Health Valley									
Moist & Chewy, Wild Berry, 1 oz	100	1	0	0	0	22	2	10	5
FF Raspberry, Strawberry, Raisin, Date									
Almond, Blueberry, or Choc Chip	140	0	0	0	0	35	3	14	10
Fruit Bars, Apricot or Apple, 1.5 oz	140	0	0	0	0	35	3	14	10
Breakfast Bakes, Raisin, Date, or Apple, 1 oz	70	0	0	0	0	19	3	11	30
Cereal Bars, LF Strawberry, Blueberry,									
Fig, or Apple Cobbler	130	2	0	0	0	27	1	13	50
Cafe Creations, Choc Raspberry, 1.4 oz ..	130	3	0	0	0	27	2	16	50
Choc Espresso, 1.4 oz	130	3	0	0	0	27	2	17	60
Cinnamon Danish, 1.4 oz	130	3	0	0	0	27	2	17	80
Moist & Chewy, Dutch Apple or									
Peanut Crunch, 1 oz	110	3	0	0	0	19	2	10	80
Tarts, LF Strawberry, Raspberry, Red									
Cherry, Blueberry, or Baked Apple	130	2	0	0	0	28	1	14	80
Creme Sandwich Bar, Vanilla or Bavarian .	130	2	0	0	0	28	1	14	80
Hershey's Snack Barz	130	6	3	0	0	17	0	11	80
Cookies 'n' Creme or S'mores (avg)	115	5	3	0	0	17	0	11	90
Kashi TLC Granola Bars									
Peanut Peanut Butter, 1 oz	130	5	1	0	0	20	4	5	65
Trail Mix, 1 oz	130	5	1	0	0	30	4	6	90
Kellogg's Nutri-Grain Cereal & Milk Bars									
Fruit Loops, 0.8 oz	95	3	2	0	0	16	1	10	75
Rice Krispie Treats, Double Chocolatey									
Chunk, 0.8 oz	100	4	3	0	0	15	1	9	75

Food	Cal	Fat	Sat	TFat	Chol	Carb	Fib	Sug	Sod
CEREAL, GRANOLA AND BREAKFAST BARS (KELLOGG'S CONT'D)									
Split Stix, Original, 1 oz	120	5	3	0	0	20	1	12	80
Cocoa Krispies, 0.8 oz	100	3	2	0	0	17	0	11	80
Kudos Choc Chip or Snickers (avg)	100	4	2	0	0	18	1	10	70
Peanut Butter	130	6	3	0	0	18	1	10	75
M&Ms	100	3	2	0	0	17	1	9	80
Nature's Choice, all, 0.7 oz (avg)	120	2	0	0	0	25	2	13	65
Nature's Path									
Cranberry Granola Bar, 1.4 oz	160	4	2	0	0	27	3	13	75
Apricot & Nut Granola Bar, 1.4 oz	160	5	2	0	0	26	2	12	85
Flax Plus Granola Bar, 1.4 oz	150	4	1	0	0	27	2	12	90
Nature's Promise, all, 1 oz	140	0	0	0	0	35	3	14	10
Quaker									
Trail Mix Bars, Mixed Nuts	160	6	1	0	0	23	1	11	45
Choc, Raisin & Peanut	150	5	2	0	0	25	1	14	45
Cranberry, Raisin & Almond	150	5	1	0	0	24	1	10	50
Chewy, Choc Chip, 25% less sugar, 1 oz	100	4	1	0	0	17	3	6	50
Choc Chip, 1 oz	120	4	2	0	0	20	1	9	60
Honey Nut, 1 oz	110	2	1	0	0	22	1	9	65
Oatmeal Raisin or 'Smores, 1 oz	110	2	1	0	0	22	1	10	70
Maple Brown Sugar	110	2	1	0	0	22	1	9	70
Peanut Butter Choc Chunk, less sugar	100	3	1	0	0	17	3	5	75
Fruit 'n Crunch, all, 1.4 oz	160	4	1	0	0	31	2	13	75
Chewy, Choc Chip Cookies & Milk	120	4	2	0	0	20	1	10	80
Cookies & Cream or Choc Chunk (avg)	115	3	1	0	0	21	1	8	80
Dipps, Choc Chip, 1.1 oz	150	6	5	0	0	21	1	13	85
Breakfast Bars, Apple Crisp, 1.3 oz	130	3	1	0	0	27	1	9	90
Skippy									
Snack Bars, Triple Nut	170	9	2	0	0	19	2	8	80
Peanut Butter & Marshmallow	140	7	2	0	0	18	1	11	80
Sunbelt, most, 1.5 oz (avg)	120	5	2	0	0	19	1	9	65

(DOUGHNUTS)

(see Doughnuts, pg 77)

(FRENCH TOAST)

(also see Breakfast Meals, pg 90)

French toast, ready-to-heat, 2 slices, 4.2 oz	352	8	3	0	96	38	2	10	584

BRANDS . . . *(2 SLICES UNLESS NOTED)*
Most brands are within the generic range.

35

Food	Cal	Fat	Sat	TFat	Chol	Carb	Fib	Sug	Sod

PANCAKES AND WAFFLES

(also see Breakfast Meals, pg 90)

Food	Cal	Fat	Sat	TFat	Chol	Carb	Fib	Sug	Sod
Pancake, plain, frozen, 2.9 oz (2)	185	4	1	0	15	32	2	8	414
Waffle, plain, frozen, 2.5 oz (2)	200	7	1	0	10	30	3	7	447
Pancake or waffle, plain, 2.7 oz mix (2)	147	2	0	0	9	28	2	8	477
Potato pancake, med, 2.6 oz (2)	199	11	2	0	70	21	5	2	565

BRANDS . . .

FROZEN/REFRIGERATED *(2 PANCAKES OR WAFFLES UNLESS NOTED)*

Food	Cal	Fat	Sat	TFat	Chol	Carb	Fib	Sug	Sod
Eggo Waffles, Banana Bread	200	7	1	0	0	32	2	5	280
Special K, FF	120	0	0	0	0	26	1	4	280
Kineret Potato Latkes, 3 oz	140	6	2	0	0	18	2	18	200
Tio Pepe's Churro Waffle Sticks, 1 oz	110	5	2	0	15	14	2	5	100
Van's Mini, Original, Blueberry, or									
Choc Chip, 2 sets of 4	116	4	0	0	0	18	2	4	114
Gourmet Original or Blueberry (avg)	150	4	0	0	0	24	2	4	152
Belgian, Original or Blueberry (avg)	178	4	0	0	0	31	2	4	196
Organic, Original	190	5	0	0	0	30	6	4	230
Hearty Oats, all (avg)	200	8	1	0	0	31	4	6	280
Organic, Soy-Flax	230	11	2	0	0	26	6	4	290

MIX *(1/3 CUP MIX UNLESS NOTED)*

Food	Cal	Fat	Sat	TFat	Chol	Carb	Fib	Sug	Sod
Arrowhead Mills Pancake Mixes									
Kamut, 1/4 cup	140	2	0	0	0	24	4	0	200
Authentic Foods Pancake & Baking	130	2	0	0	0	24	0	1	170
Baker Mills Flapjack & Waffle	130	1	0	0	0	27	4	2	216
'Cause You're Special Hearty									
Pancake-Waffle, 1 pancake	52	0	0	0	0	12	0	1	153
Classique Fare Belgian, 1/3 cup mix	70	1	0	0	40	13	0	5	160
The Cravings Place, 1 oz	97	0	0	0	0	22	1	0	43
Dixie Diner Pancake & Waffle	17	0	0	0	0	3	2	0	158
Flax Z Snax Pancake/Waffle, Blueberry	110	4	3	0	0	17	9	1	170
Buttermilk	110	4	3	0	5	17	9	1	180
Martha's FF Cinn Apple Pancakes,									
sugar free, 4	130	2	0	0	0	25	2	2	200
Streits NSA Potato Pancake Mix, 3	60	0	0	0	0	14	1	1	15
Sweet N'Low Pancake	150	0	0	0	0	36	1	0	20

SHELF-STABLE

Food	Cal	Fat	Sat	TFat	Chol	Carb	Fib	Sug	Sod
LaNouba Low Carb Belgian Waffles									
Choc or Coffe (avg)	133	8	3	-	0	17	1	0	1
Vanilla	264	23	6	-	0	56	4	0	2

Food	Cal	Fat	Sat	TFat	Chol	Carb	Fib	Sug	Sod

PANCAKE AND WAFFLE SYRUP

Food	Cal	Fat	Sat	TFat	Chol	Carb	Fib	Sug	Sod
Maple syrup, 1/4 cup	210	0	0	0	0	54	0	48	7
Fruit syrup, 1/4 cup	210	0	0	0	0	52	0	50	50
Pancake syrup, 1/4 cup	184	0	0	0	0	48	0	26	64
Sugar free, 1/4 cup	30	0	0	0	0	12	0	0	115
Lite, 1/4 cup	98	0	0	0	0	27	0	9	120

BRANDS . . . *(1/4 CUP UNLESS NOTED)*
Most syrups are within the generic range, the following have less than the generic:

Food	Cal	Fat	Sat	TFat	Chol	Carb	Fib	Sug	Sod
DaVinci Sugar Free Pancake	0	0	0	0	0	0	0	0	35
Knott's Berry Farm Fruit, all (avg)	100	0	0	0	0	25	0	25	20
Maple Grove Fruit Syrup, all (avg)	210	0	0	0	0	53	0	52	0
Smucker's Fruit Syrup (avg)	210	0	0	0	0	52	0	50	0
Sorrell Ridge	120	0	0	0	0	29	0	20	25
Spring Tree Sugar Free	30	0	0	0	0	11	0	0	35
Steel's Fruit, No Sugar Added (avg)	60	0	0	0	0	20	0	0	20

PASTRIES AND COFFEECAKES

(also see Snack Cakes, Pies and Sweet Snacks, pg 87)

Food	Cal	Fat	Sat	TFat	Chol	Carb	Fib	Sug	Sod
Strudel, apple, 1 oz	78	3	1	-	2	12	1	7	76
Coffeecake, creme-filled w/choc frosting, 1 oz	94	3	1	-	20	15	1	-	92
Coffeecake, cheese, 1 oz	96	4	2	-	24	13	0	-	96
Eclair, custard-filled w/choc glaze, 1 oz	74	5	1	-	36	7	0	2	96
Cream puff, custard-filled, 1 oz	73	4	1	-	38	6	0	3	97
Coffeecake, cinnamon w/crumb topping, 1 oz	119	7	2	-	9	13	1	-	100
Danish pastry, fruit, 1 oz	105	5	1	-	32	16	1	8	100
Sweet roll, cheese, 1 oz	102	5	2	-	22	12	0	-	101
Danish pastry, nut, 1 oz	122	7	2	-	13	13	1	7	103
Danish pastry, cinnamon, 1 oz	114	6	2	-	6	13	0	-	105
Coffeecake, fruit, 1 oz	88	3	1	-	2	15	1	-	109
Sweet roll, cinnamon w/raisins, 1 oz	106	5	1	-	19	14	1	9	109
Danish pastry, cheese, 1 oz	106	6	2	-	5	11	0	2	128
Cinnamon roll w/frosting, 1 oz	94	3	1	-	0	15	0	-	217
Popovers, mix, 1 oz	105	1	0	-	0	20	0	-	257

BRANDS . . . *(2 OZ UNLESS NOTED)*

FROZEN/REFRIGERATED

Food	Cal	Fat	Sat	TFat	Chol	Carb	Fib	Sug	Sod
Athens or *Apollo* Maple Walnut Baklava	210	10	1	-	0	28	0	17	50
Oatmeal Raisin Baklava	180	5	1	-	0	34	1	19	50
Soy Nut Baklava	190	6	1	-	0	29	2	17	60
Apple Fillo Pocket Pastry, 6 oz	340	7	1	-	0	65	3	27	140

BREAKFAST PRODUCTS
Toaster Foods and Pastries

Food	Cal	Fat	Sat	TFat	Chol	Carb	Fib	Sug	Sod
PASTRIES AND COFFEECAKES (CONT'D)									
Aunt Trudy's Baklava, all, 2 oz (avg)	210	10	1	-	0	28	0	17	50
The Fillo Factory Raspberry Baklava	270	11	2	-	0	35	0	22	85
Choc Baklava	260	10	2	-	0	35	1	23	85
Walnut Baklava	270	12	3	-	5	33	0	20	105
Sara Lee Coffee Cake, 1.9 oz	190	8	2	-	20	30	1	18	150
Pecan Coffee Cake, 1.9 oz	140	13	3	-	20	23	1	9	150
MIX									
Chébé Cinnamon Roll-ups	73	0	0	0	0	18	0	0	100
The Cravings Place									
Cinnamon Crumble Coffee Cake, 1/9	204	1	0	-	0	49	1	27	17
Gluten Free Pantry Coffee Cake	210	2	0	0	5	46	1	21	160
SHELF-STABLE									
Ener-G Choc Cinnamon Rolls, 2.9 oz	190	6	0	-	0	32	7	9	105
Pepperidge Farm Peach Dumplings	320	11	3	-	0	50	4	15	150
Otis Spunkmeyer Cinnamon Rolls, 1	140	-	-	-	-	17	0	10	95
Wolferman's English Walnut Povitica	190	10	3	0	35	22	1	11	65
Cream Cheese or Strawberry Povitica (avg)	160	9	4	0	40	20	0	10	95
Rugelach, 1.2 oz	160	0	2	0	25	17	1	14	110

TOASTER FOODS AND PASTRIES

Food	Cal	Fat	Sat	TFat	Chol	Carb	Fib	Sug	Sod
Toaster pastry, fruit, frosted, 1.8 oz	204	5	1	0	0	37	1	11	218
Toaster pastry, cinnamon, 1.8 oz	206	7	2	0	0	34	1	11	212
BRANDS . . .									
FROZEN/REFRIGERATED *(1 SERVING UNLESS NOTED)*									
Amy's Toaster Pops, 2 oz									
Apple or Strawberry	140	3	0	0	0	26	1	8	130
SHELF-STABLE *(1 SERVING UNLESS NOTED)*									
Kellogg's									
Go Tarts									
Brown Sugar Cinn or Strawberry	140	4	2	0	0	25	1	14	140
Frosted Choc Fudge	140	4	2	0	0	24	1	13	160
Pop Tarts									
Cinn Roll	210	7	2	0	0	35	1	15	160
Apple Strudel	200	6	3	0	0	35	1	16	160
Nabisco *Kool Stuf*									
Screamin' Strawberry	180	5	1	0	0	33	1	13	160
Nature's Path Blueberry Frosted	200	4	2	0	0	38	1	20	125
Apple Frosted	210	5	2	0	0	39	1	21	130
Strawberry Frosted	210	4	2	0	0	40	1	19	140

Food	Cal	Fat	Sat	TFat	Chol	Carb	Fib	Sug	Sod

CONDIMENTS AND SAUCES

CAPERS

Food	Cal	Fat	Sat	TFat	Chol	Carb	Fib	Sug	Sod
Capers, 1 tbsp	2	0	0	0	0	0	0	0	255

BRANDS . . .

Food	Cal	Fat	Sat	TFat	Chol	Carb	Fib	Sug	Sod
Giant Nonpareilles	5	0	0	0	0	1	0	0	35

CHUTNEY AND FRUIT RELISHES

Food	Cal	Fat	Sat	TFat	Chol	Carb	Fib	Sug	Sod
Cranberry sauce, whole or jellied, 1/4 cup	105	0	0	0	0	27	1	26	20
Cranberry/orange relish, 1/4 cup	122	0	0	0	0	32	0	27	22
Mango chutney, 1 tbsp	60	0	0	0	0	14	0	9	170

NOTE: While most chutneys average 170mg per tablespoon, some chutneys have as much as 900mg.

BRANDS . . .

CRANBERRY SAUCE AND RELISH *(1 TBSP UNLESS NOTED)*
Most brands are within the generic range.

OTHER CHUTNEYS AND FRUIT RELISHES

Food	Cal	Fat	Sat	TFat	Chol	Carb	Fib	Sug	Sod
American Spoon Cherry Gooseberry	35	0	0	0	0	10	0	9	35
Roast Apple and Onion Relish	45	0	0	0	0	11	0	10	55
Busha Browne's Banana Chutney	40	0	0	0	0	10	0	9	0
Crosse & Blackwell Apple Curry	25	0	0	0	0	7	0	5	25
Cranberry	40	0	0	0	0	10	0	9	0
Floribbean Papaya Chutney w/Rum	38	0	0	0	0	10	0	9	0
Fox's Fine Foods Cranberry Apple	33	0	0	0	0	9	0	8	0
Gloria's Depoe Bay Cranberry Chutney	50	0	0	0	0	14	0	12	0
Shady Grove Apple Chutney	30	0	0	0	0	7	0	5	15
Kozlowski Farms Peach Chutney	30	0	0	0	0	7	0	3	0
Neera's, all (avg)	20	0	0	0	0	5	0	2	26
Prairie Thyme Raspberry Jalapeño Ambrosia or Peach Habanero	35	0	0	0	0	9	0	8	5
Roland Major Grey's Extra Spicy Mango	40	0	0	0	0	11	0	9	40
Steel's Mango Ginger	5	0	0	0	0	1	0	1	2
Wild Thymes Chutneys (avg)	14	0	0	0	0	6	0	5	0

COOKING WINE

Food	Cal	Fat	Sat	TFat	Chol	Carb	Fib	Sug	Sod
Cooking wine, 1 fl oz	14	0	0	0	0	2	0	0	182

BRANDS . . .
Most brands are within the generic range.

Food	Cal	Fat	Sat	TFat	Chol	Carb	Fib	Sug	Sod

COOKING WINE (CONT'D)
NOTE: Instead of cooking wines, use madeira, sherry, etc. from the wine department, which have little or no sodium (see Wine and Champagne, pg 13).

(HOLLANDAISE SAUCE)

(see Hollandaise and Bernaise Sauce, pg 52)

(HORSERADISH)

Food	Cal	Fat	Sat	TFat	Chol	Carb	Fib	Sug	Sod
Horseradish, 1 tsp	2	0	0	0	0	1	0	0	16

BRANDS . . . *(1 TSP UNLESS NOTED)*
Most brands are within the generic range.

(JAMS, JELLIES AND FRUIT SPREADS)

Food	Cal	Fat	Sat	TFat	Chol	Carb	Fib	Sug	Sod
Fruit butter, 1 tbsp	29	0	0	0	0	7	0	6	3
Jam or jelly, 1 tbsp	56	0	0	0	0	14	0	10	6

BRANDS . . .
Most brands are within the generic range.

(KETCHUP)

Food	Cal	Fat	Sat	TFat	Chol	Carb	Fib	Sug	Sod
Ketchup, 1 tbsp	15	0	0	0	0	4	0	3	167

BRANDS . . . *(1 TBSP UNLESS NOTED)*

Food	Cal	Fat	Sat	TFat	Chol	Carb	Fib	Sug	Sod
Chef Allen Mango	20	0	0	0	0	5	0	4	25
Estee Imitation, SF	15	0	0	0	0	3	0	2	0
Heinz NSA	20	0	0	0	0	5	0	4	0
Hunt's NSA	20	0	0	0	0	4	0	4	0
Steel's Rocky Mountain	16	0	0	0	0	2	0	0	40
Tree of Life Organic	10	0	0	0	0	3	0	3	25
Westbrae Natural Fruit Sweetened, NSA	10	0	0	0	0	3	0	2	5
Unsweetened Un-Ketchup	5	0	0	0	0	1	0	0	60

(MARASCHINO CHERRIES)

Food	Cal	Fat	Sat	TFat	Chol	Carb	Fib	Sug	Sod
Cherries, 1	8	0	0	0	0	2	0	2	0

BRANDS . . .
Most brands are within the generic range.

(MAYONNAISE AND SANDWICH SPREADS)

Food	Cal	Fat	Sat	TFat	Chol	Carb	Fib	Sug	Sod
Mayonnaise, 1 tbsp	103	12	2	0	0	0	0	0	73
Light, 1 tbsp	49	5	1	0	0	1	0	1	107
Mayonnaise-type salad dressing, 1 tbsp	57	5	1	0	4	4	0	1	105
FF, 1 tbsp	13	0	0	0	0	2	0	2	118

Food	Cal	Fat	Sat	TFat	Chol	Carb	Fib	Sug	Sod
MAYONNAISE AND SANDWICH SPREADS (CONT'D)									
Sandwich Spread, 1 tbsp	58	5	1	0	11	3	0	2	150
BRANDS . . . *(1 TBSP UNLESS NOTED)*									
Gefen Lite	50	5	1	0	5	1	0	0	15
Hain Eggless, NSA	100	11	2	0	0	1	0	1	0
Kraft Light Mayo	45	4	0	0	5	0	0	0	90
La Costena	100	12	2	0	15	0	0	0	65
Saffola	100	11	1	0	10	0	0	0	70
Spectrum Roasted Garlic	100	11	2	0	19	0	0	0	30
Organic or Wasabi	100	11	2	0	10	0	0	0	65
Lite Canola or Lite Canola Eggless	35	4	0	0	0	0	0	0	65
Vegenaise, all (avg)	90	9	1	0	0	1	0	0	80
SANDWICH SPREAD *(1 TBSP UNLESS NOTED)*									
Beano's All American	50	4	1	0	5	3	0	2	105

MUSTARD

Food	Cal	Fat	Sat	TFat	Chol	Carb	Fib	Sug	Sod
Honey mustard, 1 tsp	10	0	0	0	0	2	0	1	25
Yellow mustard, 1 tsp	3	0	0	0	0	0	0	0	56
Dijon-type mustard, 1 tsp	5	0	0	0	0	0	0	0	120
BRANDS . . . *(1 TSP UNLESS NOTED)*									
DIJON-TYPE MUSTARD									
Annie's Naturals	0	0	0	0	0	0	0	0	65
Gold's	0	0	0	0	0	0	0	0	40
Grey Poupon Honey	10	0	0	0	0	2	0	1	5
Plochman's Honey	3	0	0	0	0	1	0	1	0
Temeraine NSA	7	1	0	0	0	0	0	0	7
HONEY MUSTARD									
Most brands are within the generic range.									
YELLOW MUSTARD									
Brad's Gourmet Spicy or Pretzel Dip (avg)	15	1	0	0	0	2	0	0	0
Cherchies Champagne	10	0	0	0	0	2	0	2	0
East Shore, all	15	0	0	0	0	2	0	0	0
Haus Barhyte Sweet & Sour	15	0	0	0	0	3	0	3	20
HoneyCup Uniquely Sharp or Stone Ground	15	1	0	0	0	3	0	1	0
Inglehoffer Sweet Hot Mustard	15	1	0	0	0	2	0	0	30
Raye's Hot & Spicy	5	0	0	0	0	0	0	0	10
Westbrae Natural Stone Ground NSA	0	0	0	0	0	0	0	0	0

NUT BUTTERS

Food	Cal	Fat	Sat	TFat	Chol	Carb	Fib	Sug	Sod
Tahini, 2 tbsp	179	16	2	0	0	6	3	0	35

41

Food	Cal	Fat	Sat	TFat	Chol	Carb	Fib	Sug	Sod
NUT BUTTERS (CONT'D)									
Almond butter, 2 tbsp	203	19	2	0	0	7	1	2	144
Peanut butter, 2 tbsp	188	16	3	0	0	6	2	3	147
Cashew butter, 2 tbsp	188	16	3	0	0	9	1	2	196
BRANDS . . . *(2 TBSP UNLESS NOTED)*									
Adams Natural, Unsalted	210	16	3	0	0	6	2	1	5
Arrowhead Mills									
Creamy or Crunchy	190	17	3	0	0	6	2	1	0
Crazy Richard's Natural Creamy	200	17	2	0	0	6	0	2	0
Eastwind, all (avg)	210	16	3	0	0	10	2	3	10
Estee SF	180	16	3	0	0	6	2	2	0
Fifty50, No Sugar Added	190	16	2	0	0	7	3	1	0
Kettle									
Organic Peanut Butter	170	14	3	0	0	5	2	2	0
Cashew, NSA or Hazelnut, NSA (avg)	185	16	2	0	0	8	2	2	0
Sunflower Butter, Roasted, NSA	160	14	2	0	0	5	0	2	1
Almond Butter	180	17	2	0	0	6	2	0	55
MaraNatha									
Cashew Macadamia, NSA	200	18	3	0	0	8	1	2	0
Macadamia, NSA	230	24	4	0	0	5	3	1	0
Almond, NSA or Peanut Butter, NSA (avg)	195	17	1	0	0	6	3	2	0
Tahini, NSA or Cashew, NSA (avg)	200	16	2	0	0	10	2	0	5
Peanut Butter w/Salt	190	16	3	0	0	7	2	2	80
Natural Value Nut Butters, NSA	200	15	3	0	0	6	1	1	0
Nutella	200	11	2	0	0	23	2	20	15
Peanut Wonder LS	100	3	0	0	0	13	0	2	95
Peter Pan LS	190	17	3	0	0	5	2	2	10
Simply Jif	190	16	3	0	0	6	2	2	65
Smucker's Natural NSA	210	16	3	0	0	6	2	7	0
Woodstock Farms Cashew	180	15	3	0	0	9	0	2	0

OLIVES

Food	Cal	Fat	Sat	TFat	Chol	Carb	Fib	Sug	Sod
Black, 0.5 oz	16	2	0	0	0	1	0	0	122
Green, 0.5 oz	15	2	0	0	0	1	1	0	225
Kalamata, 0.5 oz	40	4	0	0	0	1	0	0	240
BRANDS . . . *(0.5 OZ UNLESS NOTED)*									
Black Pearls Sliced Ripe	25	2	0	0	0	1	0	0	95
Kalamata Gold									
Organic Kalamata	45	4	1	0	0	2	0	0	100
Lindsay LS, med	25	3	2	0	0	1	0	0	40

Food	Cal	Fat	Sat	TFat	Chol	Carb	Fib	Sug	Sod

PATÉS AND SPREADS

(also see Cream Cheese and Spreads, pg 62; Sandwich Spreads, pg 134, Dips and Spreads, pg 142)

Food	Cal	Fat	Sat	TFat	Chol	Carb	Fib	Sug	Sod
Chicken liver paté, 1 oz	57	4	1	0	111	2	0	0	109
Goose liver paté, smoked, 1 oz	131	12	4	0	43	1	0	0	198

BRANDS . . .

MIX *(1 TSP MIX UNLESS NOTED)*

Food	Cal	Fat	Sat	TFat	Chol	Carb	Fib	Sug	Sod
The Original Bagel Spreads (avg)	10	0	0	0	0	3	0	1	10

READY-TO-EAT *(1 OZ UNLESS NOTED)*

Food	Cal	Fat	Sat	TFat	Chol	Carb	Fib	Sug	Sod
Bonavita Vegetarian Paté	60	4	0	0	0	4	0	0	140
Meditalia									
Roasted Eggplant Tapenade	20	2	1	0	2	0	0	0	12
Sun-Dried Tomato Tapenade	40	3	1	0	0	1	0	0	80
Roasted Red Pepper Tapenade	20	3	1	0	0	1	0	0	120
Green or Black Olive Tapenade	50	6	2	0	0	0	0	0	140
Sabra Vegetarian Liver Paté	70	7	1	0	14	1	1	1	87
Tartex Shiitake Paté	52	4	3	0	0	2	1	0	130
Walden Farms Bruschetta Pesto, 1 tsp	10	1	0	0	0	0	0	0	20

PICKLED AND SPECIALTY VEGETABLES

(also see Chili Peppers, pg 114)

Food	Cal	Fat	Sat	TFat	Chol	Carb	Fib	Sug	Sod
Corn relish, 1 tbsp	20	0	0	0	0	5	0	2	40
Sun-dried tomatoes in oil, 1/4 cup	59	4	1	0	0	6	2	0	73
Giardiniera, 1/4 cup	5	0	0	0	0	0	0	1	170
Cocktail onions, 0.5 oz	5	0	0	0	0	0	0	0	220
Hot banana peppers, 1 oz	5	0	0	0	0	1	1	0	378
Jalapeños, 1 oz	18	0	0	0	0	4	0	0	441
Pepperoncini, 1 oz	8	0	0	0	0	2	1	0	453
Red peppers, 1 oz	10	0	0	0	0	2	1	0	480

BRANDS . . . *(1 OZ UNLESS NOTED)*

Food	Cal	Fat	Sat	TFat	Chol	Carb	Fib	Sug	Sod
Aunt Nellie's Pickled Beets, Sliced	20	0	0	0	0	5	0	3	100
B&G									
Sweet Peppers, Unsalted Slices	20	0	0	0	0	5	0	3	7
Sandwich Toppers	20	0	0	0	0	5	0	3	75
Hot Chopped Sandwich, 1 tbsp	5	0	0	0	0	1	0	1	120
Cento Roasted Peppers	5	0	0	0	0	1	0	1	65
Delallo Sun-Dried Tomatoes in Oil	90	5	0	0	0	9	3	3	30
Gaea Roasted Red Peppers, 1/2 cup	10	0	0	0	0	2	0	1	120

CONDIMENTS AND SAUCES
Pickles and Pickle Relish

Food	Cal	Fat	Sat	TFat	Chol	Carb	Fib	Sug	Sod
PICKLED AND SPECIALTY VEGETABLES (CONT'D)									
Haddon House									
Roasted Red Peppers, 5 oz	0	0	0	0	0	5	0	1	20
Jok 'n' Al Tomato Relish	17	0	0	0	0	4	0	2	105
La Squisita Roasted Peppers, 1/2 cup	25	0	0	0	0	4	1	2	140
Mother Teresa's Mediterranean, Giardiniera	15	1	0	0	0	2	0	0	45
Mushrooms	15	1	0	0	0	2	0	0	130
VEGETABLE RELISH AND SPREADS									
Alberto's Sweet Zucchini Relish	30	0	0	0	0	7	0	0	0
American Spoon									
Red Spoon Pepper	30	0	0	0	0	7	0	6	50
Sweet Tomato Relish	15	0	0	0	0	3	0	3	65
Roasted Veg Relish	20	2	0	0	0	2	1	1	65
Mediterranean Relish	30	3	0	0	0	1	0	0	70
Portabello Mushroom Relish	20	1	0	0	0	2	1	1	105
B&G Piccalilli	20	0	0	0	0	4	0	4	120
Cains Sweet Pepper Relish	20	0	0	0	0	5	0	4	45
Howard's Hot Pepper Relish	20	0	0	0	0	5	0	5	55
Green Tomato Piccalilli	15	0	0	0	0	3	1	2	100
Mezzetta Sweet Bell Pepper Relish, 1 tbsp	25	0	0	0	0	6	0	5	55
Deli-Style Hot Bell Pepper Relish	25	0	0	0	0	6	0	5	60
Peloponnese Sweet Pepper Spread, 1 tbsp	15	2	0	0	0	0	0	0	90
Prairie Thyme Roasted Tomato	20	0	0	0	0	5	0	5	38
Private Harvest Bread Toppers									
Tomato Basil	25	2	0	0	0	2	0	2	65
Spicy Red Bell Pepper	25	2	0	0	0	2	0	1	70
Susan's Gourmet Foods Tuscan Tepenade									
w/Sun-Dried Tomatoes	17	1	0	0	0	3	1	1	46

PICKLES AND PICKLE RELISH

PICKLES

Food	Cal	Fat	Sat	TFat	Chol	Carb	Fib	Sug	Sod
Bread & butter pickles, 1 oz	23	0	0	0	0	5	0	3	188
Sweet pickles, 1 oz	33	0	0	0	0	9	0	4	263
Sweet gherkin, 1 oz	35	0	0	0	0	10	0	4	282
Dill pickles, 1 oz	5	0	0	0	0	1	0	1	359
Slice, 1	1	0	0	0	0	0	0	0	90
BRANDS . . . *(1 OZ UNLESS NOTED)*									
BREAD AND BUTTER									
B&G Unsalted	25	0	0	0	0	6	0	6	0
Cains	25	0	0	0	0	7	0	6	110

Food	Cal	Fat	Sat	TFat	Chol	Carb	Fib	Sug	Sod
PICKLES AND PICKLE RELISH (CONT'D)									
Frog Ranch Zesty	30	0	0	0	0	8	–	–	100
Heinz Sandwich Slices	25	0	0	0	0	6	0	4	135
Mt Olive Sandwich Stuffers	20	0	0	0	0	6	0	4	105
Sandwich Stuffers, No Sugar Added	20	0	0	0	0	1	0	0	105
Zesty Strips	20	0	0	0	0	6	0	4	105
DILL PICKLES									
B&G Unsalted Crunchy Dills	10	0	0	0	0	2	0	1	0
Ba-Tampte Half Sour	0	0	0	0	0	1	0	0	135
Cascadian Farm Kosher Dill, LS	5	0	0	0	0	1	0	0	135
Mt Olive									
Kosher Dill Strips, Reduced Sodium	0	0	0	0	0	1	0	0	135
SWEET PICKLES									
Cains Sweet Crickles or									
Sweet Cucumbers	30	0	0	0	0	7	0	6	110
Farman's Sweet	25	0	0	0	0	7	0	7	70
Sweet Gherkins	30	0	0	0	0	7	0	7	90
Heinz Kosher Sweet Gherkins	23	0	0	0	0	5	0	5	129
Haddon House Sweet Midgets, 5	40	0	0	0	0	11	0	10	25
Mt Olive Sweet	35	0	0	0	0	8	0	7	100
Sweet Gerkins or Midgets	35	0	0	0	0	8	0	7	100
PICKLE RELISH *(1 TBSP UNLESS NOTED)*									
Sweet pickle relish, 1 tbsp	20	0	0	0	0	5	0	2	122
Hamburger or hot dog relish, 1 tbsp	17	0	0	0	0	4	0	3	164
Dill pickle relish, 1 tbsp	5	0	0	0	0	1	0	1	240
BRANDS . . .									
B&G SF Sweet Relish	20	0	0	0	0	5	0	4	0
Hot Dog Relish	20	0	0	0	0	3	0	3	75
Cascadian Farm Sweet Pickle Relish	20	0	0	0	0	5	0	4	75
Claussen Sweet Pickle Relish	10	0	0	0	0	3	0	2	85
Farman's Sweet Pickle Relish	15	0	0	0	0	3	0	2	90
Gedney Hot Dog Relish	18	0	0	0	0	4	0	3	100
Gold's Sweet Hot Dog Relish	15	0	0	0	0	3	0	3	90
Heinz Hot Dog or Sweet Relish	20	0	0	0	0	5	0	3	95
Majestic Sweet Relish	20	0	0	0	0	4	0	2	80
Mt Olive Sweet Pickle Relish	20	0	0	0	0	4	0	2	80

(PIMENTO)

Pimento, 1 oz	6	0	0	0	0	1	0	1	3

Food	Cal	Fat	Sat	TFat	Chol	Carb	Fib	Sug	Sod

PIMENTO (CONT'D)

BRANDS . . .

Most brands are within the generic range.

(SALAD DRESSINGS)

Food	Cal	Fat	Sat	TFat	Chol	Carb	Fib	Sug	Sod
Vinegar & oil, 2 tbsp	144	16	3	0	0	1	0	0	0
Ranch dressing, 2 tbsp	145	15	2	0	10	2	0	1	245
Mix, to make 2 tbsp	120	0	0	0	0	1	0	0	135
FF, 2 tbsp	33	0	0	0	0	7	0	2	211
LF, 2 tbsp	66	5	0	0	6	5	0	1	280
French dressing, 2 tbsp	146	14	2	0	0	5	0	5	268
LF, 2 tbsp	74	4	0	0	0	9	0	5	257
Thousand island dressing, 2 tbsp	118	11	2	0	8	5	0	5	276
LF, 2 tbsp	61	4	0	0	0	7	0	5	249
Russian dressing, 2 tbsp	107	8	1	0	8	9	1	0	282
Caesar dressing, 2 tbsp	155	17	3	0	1	1	0	0	317
LF, 2 tbsp	33	1	0	0	0	6	0	5	323
Blue cheese or roquefort, 2 tbsp	151	16	3	0	5	2	0	1	328
LF, 2 tbsp	28	1	0	0	3	4	0	1	515
Italian dressing, 2 tbsp	86	8	1	0	0	3	0	2	486
FF, 2 tbsp	13	0	0	0	0	2	0	2	316
Mix, to make 2 tbsp	5	0	0	0	0	1	0	1	320
LF, 2 tbsp	23	2	0	0	2	1	0	1	410
Zesty Italian, 2 tbsp	109	11	1	0	0	2	0	1	505

BRANDS . . .

MIX

Most brands are within the generic range.

READY-TO-USE *(2 TBSP UNLESS NOTED)*

There are many low-sodium salad dressings, the following have less than 90mg per serving.

Food	Cal	Fat	Sat	TFat	Chol	Carb	Fib	Sug	Sod
American Spoon Raspberry Vinaigrette	70	4	0	0	0	10	0	9	45
Cherry Vinaigrette	90	3	0	0	0	16	0	15	80
Annie's Naturals Balsamic Vinaigrette	100	10	1	0	0	3	0	3	75
LF Raspberry Vinaigrette	35	2	0	0	0	5	0	4	75
Cannon's Cranberry Vinaigrette	80	0	0	0	0	20	0	18	25
Chelten House Raspberry Vinaigrette	60	6	1	0	0	3	0	2	70
Consorzio Raspberry & Marinade, Mango, or Raspberry & Balsamic (avg)	24	0	0	0	0	6	0	4	0
Edible Scents, all	170	17	2	0	0	5	0	4	0

Food	Cal	Fat	Sat	TFat	Chol	Carb	Fib	Sug	Sod
SALAD DRESSINGS (CONT'D)									
Emeril's House Herb Vinaigrette	100	10	2	0	0	1	0	1	70
Girard's Raspberry Vinaigrette	90	10	2	0	0	9	0	9	65
Gloria's Caribbean Sunshine	45	1	0	0	0	9	0	0	0
Raspberry Poppyseed	140	9	0	0	0	16	0	0	0
Raspberry Poppyseed, Oil Free	60	0	0	0	0	15	0	0	0
Roasted Red Pepper Vinaigrette, LS	65	7	0	0	0	2	0	0	70
Gunther's Lemon & Oregano	140	16	2	0	0	2	0	0	50
Roasted Garlic, Sun-Dried Tomato	180	20	2	0	0	0	0	0	50
Hail Caesar Balsamic Vinaigrette, FF	10	0	0	0	0	2	0	2	0
Raspberry Vinaigrette, FF	6	0	0	0	0	1	0	1	2
Italian Herb, FF	8	0	0	0	0	2	0	0	5
Pepper Vinaigrette, LF	50	6	2	0	0	0	0	0	6
Honey Dijon, FF	28	0	0	0	0	7	0	1	10
Basil Dijon Vinaigrette	76	8	1	0	0	0	0	0	44
Original Caesar	140	14	2	0	12	0	0	0	70
Island Grove									
Caribbean Garlic Dressing & Marinade	70	7	1	0	0	3	0	3	5
LF Raspberry Poppy	40	3	0	0	0	5	0	5	40
LF Vadalia Onion	35	2	0	0	0	5	0	5	55
Key Lime Vinaigrette	30	3	0	0	0	3	0	3	73
Tangy Honey Mustard Lite	100	10	1	0	0	0	0	0	85
Maple Grove Farms Poppyseed, FF	50	0	0	0	0	11	0	8	80
Marie's Raspberry Vinaigrette	35	0	0	0	0	8	0	5	35
Miko Dressing & Marinade, Ginger, all	70	6	0	0	0	3	0	2	50
Roasted Garlic Peanut	70	6	0	0	0	3	0	2	50
Naturally Fresh Cranberry Walnut	110	10	3	0	10	6	0	5	30
Poppyseed	140	13	2	0	0	6	0	6	60
Olde Cape Cod Poppyseed	80	4	0	0	0	11	0	10	6
Raspberry Vinaigrette	70	3	0	0	0	12	0	11	30
Balsamic Vinaigrette	25	0	0	0	0	6	0	6	60
Paula's Lemon & Dill or Lime & Cilantro	15	0	0	0	0	4	0	4	40
Tangerine & Mint	15	0	0	0	0	4	0	4	57
Orange & Basil	15	0	0	0	0	4	0	4	64
Honey Mustard	80	6	0	0	0	7	0	7	70
Roasted Garlic or Toasted Onion	10	0	0	0	0	3	0	3	80
Private Harvest Chinese Chicken Salad	140	13	1	0	0	5	0	5	70
Riverhouse Blue Cheese	130	13	8	0	0	3	1	3	85
Steel's Sweet Ginger Lime	136	14	0	0	0	2	2	0	22
Valley Grille Honey Mustard	130	12	1	0	0	6	0	5	85

CONDIMENTS AND SAUCES
Salad Toppings

Food	Cal	Fat	Sat	TFat	Chol	Carb	Fib	Sug	Sod

(SALAD TOPPINGS)

Food	Cal	Fat	Sat	TFat	Chol	Carb	Fib	Sug	Sod
Croutons, plain, 2 tbsp (7 grams)	28	0	0	0	0	5	0	0	49
Seasoned, 2 tbsp (7 grams)	33	1	0	0	0	4	0	0	87
Bacon bits, imitation, 1 tbsp	33	2	0	0	0	2	1	0	124

BRANDS . . .

BACON BITS
Most brands are within the generic brand.

CROUTONS (7 GRAMS OR 2 TBSP UNLESS NOTED)

PLAIN
Most plain croutons are within the generic range.

SEASONED

Food	Cal	Fat	Sat	TFat	Chol	Carb	Fib	Sug	Sod
Cardini's Caesar	35	2	0	0	0	4	0	0	50
Chatham Village Caesar	35	2	0	0	0	4	0	0	50
Edwards & Sons Lightly Salted. 0.5 oz	30	1	0	0	0	5	0	0	25
Ener-G, 0.5 oz	25	1	0	0	0	3	0	0	25
Fresh Gourmet Seasoned, most (avg)	25	2	0	0	0	3	0	0	55
FF Parmesan Ranch	15	0	0	0	0	3	0	0	55
Marzetti Caesar	35	2	0	0	0	4	0	1	50
Butter & Garlic	35	2	0	0	0	4	0	1	55
Cheese & Garlic	40	3	0	0	0	3	0	1	60
Old London Toastettes Toasted Onion	25	1	0	0	0	3	0	0	50
Cheese-Garlic, Caesar, Buttermilk-Ranch	25	1	0	0	0	3	0	0	55
Olivia's Croutons									
Butter & Garlic or Parmesan Pepper	40	1	1	0	5	4	0	0	50
Osem Onion Garlic, Garlic Paprika,									
Mediterranean Herb, or Toasted, 0.5 oz	50	2	0	0	0	8	0	0	45
Pepperidge Farm Whole Grain Caesar	35	1	0	0	0	5	0	1	50
Seasoned	30	1	0	0	0	5	1	1	55

OTHER TOPPINGS

Food	Cal	Fat	Sat	TFat	Chol	Carb	Fib	Sug	Sod
Durkee Salad Sensations Garden									
Style, 1 tbsp	35	2	0	0	0	3	1	1	70
French's French Fried Onions, 2 tbsp	45	4	1	-	0	3	0	0	60

(SAUCES)

BBQ/GRILLING SAUCES AND MARINADES *(also see Asian Sauces, pg 111)*

Food	Cal	Fat	Sat	TFat	Chol	Carb	Fib	Sug	Sod
Barbecue sauce, 2 tbsp	23	1	0	0	0	4	0	1	255
Marinade, 1 tbsp	10	1	0	0	0	1	0	1	380

Food	Cal	Fat	Sat	TFat	Chol	Carb	Fib	Sug	Sod

BBQ/GRILLING SAUCES AND MARINADES (CONT'D)

BRANDS . . .

There are many low-sodium barbecue/grilling sauces and marinades, the following have 100mg or less per serving.

MIX (2 TBSP PREP UNLESS NOTED)

Food	Cal	Fat	Sat	TFat	Chol	Carb	Fib	Sug	Sod
Adolph's Marinade in Minutes	5	0	0	0	0	2	0	0	0
Bernard BBQ, LS	40	0	0	0	0	10	0	6	5
Med-Diet Bar-B-Q	35	0	0	0	0	8	0	-	35

READY-TO-USE (2 TBSP UNLESS NOTED)

Food	Cal	Fat	Sat	TFat	Chol	Carb	Fib	Sug	Sod
A-1 Italian Herb Marinade, 1 tbsp	15	0	0	0	0	4	0	2	48
American Spoon Ginger Plum Grilling	70	0	0	0	0	18	0	15	5
Billy Bee Honey Garlic	80	0	0	0	0	20	0	20	30
Blue Crab Bay Co. Seafood Marinade & Grilling	120	12	2	0	0	6	0	6	40
Bronco Bob's Chipotle Sauce									
Wild Cherry	50	0	0	0	0	12	0	11	85
Tangy Apricot	45	0	0	0	0	11	1	10	100
Chef Allen Papaya Pineapple BBQ	30	0	0	0	0	8	0	2	50
Key Lime Mojo, 1 tbsp	5	0	0	0	0	2	0	1	55
Consorzio Tropical Grill, 1 tbsp	40	3	0	0	0	3	0	3	10
Diana's Grilling & Moisturizing Sauce									
Raspberry Chipotle	25	0	0	0	0	2	0	-	0
Lime Wasabi Grill Crazy	25	0	0	0	0	7	0	-	5
Earth & Vine Provisions									
Papaya Chipotle Pineapple	45	0	0	0	0	11	0	9	5
Raspberry Ancho Orange	45	0	0	0	0	11	1	8	15
Emeril's Marinades Ginger Maple Chipotle									
or Hickory Maple Chipotle, 1 tbsp	35	3	0	0	0	2	0	1	75
Orange Herb w/Poppy Seeds, 1 tbsp	80	8	1	1	0	2	0	1	85
Roasted Veg, 1 tbsp	70	7	1	0	0	1	0	0	90
Enrico's, all	36	2	0	0	0	6	0	-	8
Fischer & Wieser Papaya Lime Serrano	80	0	0	0	0	22	0	20	0
Charred Pineapple Bourbon	70	0	0	0	0	16	0	16	0
Seville Orange Cranberry Horseradish	50	0	0	0	0	14	0	12	0
Mango Ginger Habanero	80	0	0	0	0	22	0	20	0
Texas 1015 Onion Glaze	90	0	0	0	0	22	0	22	10
Hot Plum Chipotle	80	0	0	0	0	22	0	20	30
Floribbean Mango Garlic	40	0	0	0	0	10	0	8	5
Key Lime w/Ginger	40	0	0	0	0	10	0	7	5
Frotera Hot Sauces, all	5	0	0	0	0	1	0	0	35

CONDIMENTS AND SAUCES
Sauces (BBQ/Grilling Sauces and Marinades)

Food	Cal	Fat	Sat	TFat	Chol	Carb	Fib	Sug	Sod
BBQ/GRILLING SAUCES AND MARINADES (CONT'D)									
Garlic Survival Roasted Garlic Marinade .	5	0	0	0	0	1	0	0	0
Garlic Lemon Marinade	5	0	0	0	0	1	0	0	5
The Ginger People Dipping & Cooking									
Sweet Ginger Chili	60	0	0	0	0	15	0	15	0
Ginger Wasabi	40	4	0	0	0	1	0	1	35
Island Grove Hurricane Bay Florida Spice	25	0	0	0	0	6	0	6	45
Southwestern Marinade	47	0	0	0	0	12	0	12	47
Oriental Sweet Heet	25	0	0	0	0	5	0	5	95
Kona Coast Grilling & Dipping Sauces									
Sunset Sweet N/Sour	60	0	0	0	0	15	0	12	65
Aloha Sweet Onion	60	0	0	0	0	14	1	11	90
Lollipop Tree Mango Garlic	60	0	0	0	0	14	0	13	10
Lucas Marinating & Barbecue	10	0	0	0	0	2	0	0	0
Lum Taylor's Barbeque	110	0	0	0	0	27	0	27	15
Miko Dressing & Marinade	70	6	0	0	0	3	0	2	50
Ginger, all varieties	70	6	0	0	0	3	0	2	50
Roasted Garlic Peanut	70	6	0	0	0	3	0	2	50
Mr. Spice Honey	60	0	0	0	0	14	0	7	0
Honey Mustard	30	0	0	0	0	7	0	7	0
Hot Wing	24	0	0	0	0	6	0	3	0
Mrs. Dash 10-Min Marinades, 1 tbsp (avg)	25	2	0	0	0	2	0	1	0
Nellie & Joe's Key West Style									
Traditional Marinade, 1 tbsp	80	8	1	0	0	2	0	0	40
Oasis Foods Grilling Sauce & Marinade									
Sweet Papaya Lime Serrano, 1 tbsp	40	0	0	0	0	10	0	9	0
Honey Mango Ginger Habanero, 1 tbsp ..	40	0	0	0	0	11	0	10	0
Smokin' Mesquite Mustard, 1 tbsp	10	0	0	0	0	2	0	2	15
Plum Hot Chipotle BBQ, 1 tbsp	50	0	0	0	0	13	0	13	35
Roasted Raspberry Chipotle, 1 tbsp	40	0	0	0	0	10	1	9	65
Olde Cape Cod BBQ & Grilling Sauce									
Lemon Ginger	25	0	0	0	0	5	0	4	10
Cranberry or Honey Orange	70	0	0	0	0	18	0	17	75
Private Harvest									
Tequilla Lime Grilling, 1 tbsp	100	0	0	0	0	2	0	2	0
Robbies Hot or Mild	25	0	0	0	0	5	0	5	30
Steel's Rocky Mt BBQ	40	0	0	0	0	10	0	0	25
Superior Choice All-Purpose	25	0	0	0	0	6	0	0	10
Thai Kitchen Lemongrass Splash, 1 tbsp	10	0	0	0	0	1	0	1	77
Valley Grille Maple Grilling, 1 tbsp	40	3	0	0	0	4	0	3	45

Food	Cal	Fat	Sat	TFat	Chol	Carb	Fib	Sug	Sod
BBQ/GRILLING SAUCES AND MARINADES (CONT'D)									
Wing-Time Buffalo Wing Sauce									
Hot or Super Hot (avg)	45	5	1	0	0	2	0	1	40
Bar-B-Q	50	3	0	0	0	7	0	6	45
Mild or Med (avg)	50	5	1	0	0	2	0	1	50
Garlic	50	5	1	0	0	2	0	1	55

BEARNAISE SAUCE *(see Hollandaise and Bernaise Sauce, pg 52)*

BROWNING AND SEASONING SAUCE

Food	Cal	Fat	Sat	TFat	Chol	Carb	Fib	Sug	Sod
Browning & seasoning sauce, 1 tsp	15	0	0	0	0	3	0	0	10

BRANDS . . .
Most brands are within the generic range.

CHEESE SAUCE *(also see Alfredo Sauce, pg 100)*

Food	Cal	Fat	Sat	TFat	Chol	Carb	Fib	Sug	Sod
Cheese sauce, ready-to-serve, 1/4 cup	110	8	4	0	18	4	0	0	522
Mix, prep, 1/4 cup	60	3	2	0	4	8	0	1	685

BRANDS . . .
MIX *(1/4 CUP PREP UNLESS NOTED)*

Food	Cal	Fat	Sat	TFat	Chol	Carb	Fib	Sug	Sod
Bernard Diet	25	1	0	0	0	5	0	2	70
Med-Diet Cheddar Cheese	20	0	0	0	0	3	0	-	115

READY-TO-USE
Most brands are within the generic range.

CLAM SAUCE *(see Clam Sauce, pg 100)*

COCKTAIL/SEAFOOD SAUCE

Food	Cal	Fat	Sat	TFat	Chol	Carb	Fib	Sug	Sod
Cocktail sauce, 1/4 cup	80	2	0	0	0	16	1	14	680

BRANDS . . .
MIX *(1/4 TSP UNLESS NOTED)*
Blue Crab Bay

Food	Cal	Fat	Sat	TFat	Chol	Carb	Fib	Sug	Sod
Cocktail Sauce Blend (seasoning mix)	0	0	0	0	0	0	0	0	0

READY-TO-USE *(1/4 CUP UNLESS NOTED)*

Food	Cal	Fat	Sat	TFat	Chol	Carb	Fib	Sug	Sod
American Spoon Great Lakes Seafood	40	0	0	0	0	8	4	4	40
Great Impressions LS	84	0	0	0	0	20	0	-	24
Steel's	32	0	0	0	0	0	0	0	160
Uncle Dave's Kickin'	20	0	0	0	0	8	0	4	240

CURRY SAUCE

Food	Cal	Fat	Sat	TFat	Chol	Carb	Fib	Sug	Sod
Curry paste, ready-to-use, 1 tbsp	10	0	0	0	0	2	0	1	270
Curry mix, 1 tbsp	45	3	0	0	0	3	2	1	460

Food	Cal	Fat	Sat	TFat	Chol	Carb	Fib	Sug	Sod
CURRY SAUCE (CONT'D)									
BRANDS . . .									
Mr. Spice Indian, 2 tbsp	30	0	0	0	0	6	0	6	0
GRAVY									
Au jus, canned, 1/4 cup	10	0	0	0	0	1	0	0	30
Mix, 1 tsp	9	0	0	0	0	1	0	0	348
Turkey gravy, mix, prep, 1/4 cup	27	1	0	0	2	4	0	1	274
Canned, 1/4 cup	30	1	0	0	1	3	0	0	343
Beef gravy, canned, 1/4 cup	31	1	1	0	2	3	0	0	326
Brown gravy, mix, prep, 1/4 cup	25	1	0	0	1	4	0	1	339
Mushroom, canned, 1/4 cup	30	2	0	0	0	3	0	0	339
Chicken gravy, canned, 1/4 cup	47	3	1	0	1	3	0	0	343
BRANDS . . .									
MIX									
Med-Diet Premium Mushroom, Chicken, or Brown (avg)	15	0	0	0	0	3	0	-	40
Tony Chachere's Instant Roux	10	0	0	0	0	2	0	0	80
Instant White Gravy	20	0	0	0	0	4	0	0	150
Instant Brown Gravy	10	0	0	0	0	2	0	0	160
READY-TO-USE									
Hain Brown, 1/4 cup	15	0	0	0	0	3	0	1	125
HARD SAUCE									
Plum pudding hard sauce, 1 tbsp	180	8	5	0	15	26	0	25	65
BRANDS . . .									
Most brands are within the generic range.									
HOLLANDAISE AND BERNAISE SAUCE									
Bearnaise sauce, mix, 1 tsp	10	0	0	0	0	2	0	0	110
Hollandaise sauce, mix, 2 tsp	15	0	0	0	15	1	0	0	110
BRANDS . . . *(1 TSP UNLESS NOTED)*									
Spice Islands Hollandaise, 1 tbsp mix	10	0	0	0	5	1	0	0	35
Wagner's Hollaindaise, mix	15	1	0	0	10	2	0	0	75
HOT PEPPER SAUCE *(also see Hispanic Sauces, pg 117)*									
Hot sauce, 1 tsp	1	0	0	0	0	0	0	0	124
BRANDS . . . *(1 TSP UNLESS NOTED)*									
Dave's Gourmet Insanity	10	0	0	0	0	0	0	0	10
Island Grove Jamaican	10	0	0	0	0	1	0	1	25
West Indies Pepper	3	0	0	0	0	8	0	8	30
Marie Sharp's all (avg)	24	0	0	0	0	5	0	2	10

Food	Cal	Fat	Sat	TFat	Chol	Carb	Fib	Sug	Sod
HOT PEPPER SAUCE (CONT'D)									
McIlhenny Tabasco (red)	1	0	0	0	0	0	0	0	30
Mr. Spice Tangy Bang	2	0	0	0	0	0	0	0	0
Phamous Phloyd's	15	0	0	0	0	4	1	0	2
Pickapeppa	5	0	0	0	0	1	0	1	40
Santa Barbara Original Blend	1	0	0	0	0	0	0	0	55
Walkerswood Zesty Caribbean or Savory	5	0	0	0	0	1	0	0	40
Hot Jamaican Pepper	5	0	0	0	0	1	0	0	45
Watkins Calypso Hot or Caribbean Red	10	0	0	0	0	0	0	2	25
The Wizard's Hot Stuff	0	0	0	0	0	0	0	0	65

LIQUID SMOKE

Liquid smoke, 1 tsp	0	0	0	0	0	0	0	0	10

BRANDS . . .

Most brands are within the generic range.

MINT SAUCE

Mint sauce, 1 tsp	5	0	0	0	0	1	0	1	0

BRANDS . . .

Most brands are within the generic range.

PASTA AND PIZZA SAUCE *(see Pasta Sauce, pg 100; Pizza Sauce, pg 105)*

SLOPPY JOE SAUCE

Sloppy joe sauce, canned, 1/4 cup	30	0	0	0	0	6	1	5	370
Mix, 1/8 pkg	15	0	0	0	0	3	0	1	360

BRANDS . . .

Dixie Diner Sloppy Joe Complete, 7 oz	83	1	0	0	0	9	5	2	117

STEAK SAUCE

Steak sauce, 1 tbsp	14	0	0	0	0	4	0	2	262

BRANDS . . . *(1 TBSP UNLESS NOTED)*

Busha Browne's Planters	5	0	0	0	0	2	0	1	10
Chef Allen Orange Chipotle Blasting	5	0	0	0	0	10	0	0	20
Earp's Western Steak & Dinner	30	0	0	0	0	7	0	10	55
Mr. Spice	15	0	0	0	0	4	0	2	0
Newman's Own	20	1	0	0	0	4	0	1	85
Southern Comfort	15	0	0	0	0	3	0	3	60

TARTAR SAUCE

Tartar sauce, 1 tbsp	70	8	2	0	5	0	0	0	130

BRANDS . . .

Most brands are within the generic range.

CONDIMENTS AND SAUCES
Vinegar

Food	Cal	Fat	Sat	TFat	Chol	Carb	Fib	Sug	Sod
WORCESTERSHIRE SAUCE									
Worcestershire sauce, 1 tsp	4	0	0	0	0	1	0	1	55
BRANDS . . . *(1 TSP UNLESS NOTED)*									
Robbie's	0	0	0	0	0	1	0	1	15
World Harbors Angostura	5	0	0	0	0	1	0	1	20
(VINEGAR)									
Vinegar, 1 tbsp	2	0	0	0	0	1	0	0	0
Balsamic vinegar, 1 tbsp	5	0	0	0	0	2	0	2	0
Rice vinegar, unseasoned, 1 tbsp	0	0	0	0	0	0	0	0	0
Seasoned, 1 tbsp	20	0	0	0	0	5	0	5	240

BRANDS . . .
Most brands are within the generic range.

Food	Cal	Fat	Sat	TFat	Chol	Carb	Fib	Sug	Sod

DAIRY PRODUCTS AND ALTERNATIVES

BUTTER, MARGARINE AND SPREADS

Food	Cal	Fat	Sat	TFat	Chol	Carb	Fib	Sug	Sod
Butter spray, 2 sprays	0	0	0	0	0	0	0	0	5
Butter, stick, salted, 1 tbsp	102	12	7	0	31	0	0	0	82
Stick, unsalted, 1 tbsp	102	12	7	0	31	0	0	0	0
Whipped, salted, 1 tbsp	67	8	5	0	21	0	0	0	78
Margarine, stick, salted, 1 tbsp	99	11	2	3	0	0	0	0	115
Stick, unsalted, 1 tbsp	102	11	2	3	0	0	0	0	0
Trans-fat free, salted, 1 tbsp	80	9	2	0	0	0	0	0	100
Tub, salted, 1 tbsp	102	11	2	1	0	0	0	0	153

BRANDS . . .

BUTTER (*1 TBSP UNLESS NOTED*)

Most unsalted brands are within the generic range, the following are less than the generic.

Food	Cal	Fat	Sat	TFat	Chol	Carb	Fib	Sug	Sod
Land O Lakes Whipped, Unsalted	50	6	4	0	15	0	0	0	0
Honey	90	8	4	0	15	4	0	3	35
Whipped	50	6	4	0	15	0	0	0	50
Whipped, Light	35	4	3	0	10	0	0	0	55
Vermont Butter & Cheese Cultured	110	12	7	0	30	0	0	0	30

MARGARINE

Most unsalted brands are within the generic range. (NOTE: Fleischman's and Organic Valley are the most widely available.) The following are less than the generic.

Food	Cal	Fat	Sat	TFat	Chol	Carb	Fib	Sug	Sod
Land O Lakes Country Morning Blend, soft	100	11	3	2	0	0	0	0	80
Fresh Butter Taste Blend, soft	80	8	2	0	0	0	0	0	80
Promise Buttery Light	50	6	1	-	0	0	0	0	5

CHEESE – BLOCK, CHUNK AND WEDGES

(also see Cheese – Grated and Shredded, pg 59)

Although some of the following cheeses exceed sodium guidelines, they are less than the generic.

BLUE, GORGONZOLA, ROQUEFORT AND STILTON

Food	Cal	Fat	Sat	TFat	Chol	Carb	Fib	Sug	Sod
Stilton, 1 oz	110	9	5	0	30	0	0	0	220
Gorgonzola, 1 oz	100	8	5	0	20	1	0	0	350
Blue, 1 oz	100	8	5	0	21	1	0	0	395
Roquefort, 1 oz	105	9	6	0	26	1	0	0	513

DAIRY PRODUCTS AND ALTERNATIVES
Cheese – Block, Chunk and Wedges

Food	Cal	Fat	Sat	TFat	Chol	Carb	Fib	Sug	Sod
CHEESE – BLUE, GORGONZOLA, ROQUEFORT AND STILTON (CONT'D)									
BRANDS . . . *(1 OZ UNLESS NOTED)*									
Black River Blue or Gorgonzola	100	8	5	0	25	0	0	0	260
Denmark's Finest Blue	100	8	6	0	15	0	0	0	310
Rosenborg Bellablu	120	11	7	0	35	0	0	0	270
Noble Blue	130	12	8	0	35	0	0	0	300
Saga Classic Blue	130	12	8	0	15	0	0	0	210
Treasure Cave Gorgonzola, Crumbled	100	8	5	0	20	1	0	0	310
BRIE, CAMEMBERT AND LIMBURGER									
Brie, 1 oz	95	8	5	0	28	0	0	0	178
Limburger, 1 oz	93	8	5	0	26	0	0	0	227
Camembert, 1 oz	85	7	4	0	20	0	0	0	239
BRANDS . . . *(1 OZ UNLESS NOTED)*									
Merry Goat Round Brie	80	6	4	0	15	1	0	0	50
Rosenborg Danish Camembert	90	7	5	0	25	0	0	0	180
CHEDDAR AND COLBY									
Colby, 1 oz	112	9	6	0	27	1	0	0	171
Cheddar, 1 oz	114	9	6	0	30	0	0	0	176
Smoked cheddar, 1 oz	110	9	6	0	25	0	0	0	400
BRANDS . . . *(1 OZ UNLESS NOTED)*									
Black Diamond LS Cheddar	118	10	-	-	-	0	0	0	15
Heluva Good LS Cheddar	110	9	6	0	30	1	0	0	5
Horizon Reduced Fat Cheddar	80	6	4	0	20	1	0	0	140
Organic Valley Less Fat/Sodium Cheddar	90	6	4	0	15	1	0	0	125
Papa Cheese Cheddar, LF	100	7	4	0	20	0	0	0	100
Pearl Valley Reduced Fat, LS Colby	100	7	5	0	15	0	0	0	95
Tillamook Medium Cheddar	110	10	6	0	15	1	0	0	130
Tree of Life Cheddar, Natural, LS	110	9	6	0	24	0	0	0	110
EDAM, FONTINA AND GOUDA									
Fontina, 1 oz	110	9	5	0	33	0	0	0	227
Gouda, 1 oz	101	8	5	0	32	1	0	0	232
Edam, 1 oz	101	8	5	0	25	0	0	0	274
BRANDS . . . *(1 OZ UNLESS NOTED)*									
Bel Gioioso Fontina	100	8	4	0	25	0	0	0	170
Miller's Gouda, NSA	104	8	5	0	29	0	0	0	24
FARMER AND HOOP									
Hoop, FF, 4 oz (1/2 cup)	96	0	0	0	8	2	0	2	15
Farmer, 1 oz (2 tbsp)	50	3	2	0	10	0	0	0	120

Food	Cal	Fat	Sat	TFat	Chol	Carb	Fib	Sug	Sod
CHEESE – FARMER AND HOOP (CONT'D)									
BRANDS . . . *(4 OZ UNLESS NOTED)*									
FARMER									
Friendship Farmer, NSA, 2 tbsp	50	3	2	0	10	0	0	0	10
HOOP									
Most brands are within the generic range.									
FETA AND GOAT									
Goat cheese, hard, 1 oz	128	10	7	0	30	1	0	1	98
Soft, 1 oz	76	6	4	0	13	0	0	0	104
Semisoft, 1 oz	103	8	6	0	22	1	0	1	146
Feta, 1 oz	75	6	4	0	25	1	0	0	316
BRANDS . . . *(1 OZ UNLESS NOTED)*									
FETA									
Organic Creamery Crumbled	60	4	3	0	10	1	0	0	250
GOAT									
Le Chevrot Goat	70	6	0	0	13	1	0	0	50
Mountain Top Goat Bleu	90	7	5	0	15	1	0	0	30
Mozzarella Co. Goat	63	5	-	-	-	1	0	0	50
Vermont Butter & Chevre Chevre	80	6	4	0	20	1	0	1	45
HAVARTI AND BRICK									
Brick, 1 oz	105	8	5	0	27	1	0	0	159
Havarti/tilsit, 1 oz	96	7	5	0	29	1	0	0	213
BRANDS . . . *(1 OZ UNLESS NOTED)*									
The Deli Counter (Safeway)	120	10	6	0	30	1	0	0	135
Denmark's Finest									
Havarti w/Caraway	120	10	7	0	25	0	0	0	140
Havarti	120	10	7	0	25	0	0	0	150
Tilsit	90	7	5	0	20	1	0	0	160
MISCELLANEOUS CHEESES									
BRANDS . . . *(1 OZ UNLESS NOTED)*									
Ski Queen Gjetost	130	9	6	0	30	7	0	7	90
MONTEREY JACK AND MUENSTER									
Monterey jack, 1 oz	106	9	5	0	25	0	0	0	152
Muenster, 1 oz	104	9	5	0	27	0	0	0	178
BRANDS . . . *(1 OZ UNLESS NOTED)*									
Alpine Lace Reduced Sodium Muenster	100	9	5	0	25	1	0	0	85
Boar's Head Muenster, LS	100	8	5	0	20	0	0	0	75
Organic Valley Reduced Fat Jack	80	5	4	0	15	1	0	0	80

DAIRY PRODUCTS AND ALTERNATIVES
Cheese – Block, Chunk and Wedges

Food	Cal	Fat	Sat	TFat	Chol	Carb	Fib	Sug	Sod
MOZZARELLA AND PROVOLONE									
Mozzarella, part-skim, low moisture, 1 oz	86	6	4	0	15	1	0	0	150
Whole milk, 1 oz	85	6	4	0	22	1	0	0	178
Provolone, 1 oz	100	8	5	0	20	1	0	0	248
BRANDS . . . *(1 OZ UNLESS NOTED)*									
Alpine Lace Reduced Fat/Sodium Provolone	90	6	4	0	15	1	0	1	180
Bel Gioioso Fresh Mozzarella Balls	40	3	2	0	10	0	0	0	40
Fresh Mozzarella, Ciliegine	80	6	4	0	22	1	0	0	40
Fresh Mozzarella	80	6	4	0	20	0	0	0	85
Mild Provolone	100	8	5	0	25	0	0	0	120
Calabro, FF Mozzarella	40	0	0	0	0	1	0	1	110
Formaggio Fresh, Unsalted	80	6	4	0	20	1	0	0	60
Mozzarella Co. – has several unsalted and lightly salted mozzarellas									
Organic Valley Mozzarella	80	6	4	0	20	1	0	0	105
Polly-O Fresh Mozzarella	80	7	4	0	20	0	0	0	15
PARMESAN, ROMANO AND ASIAGO									
(also see Cheese – Grated and Shredded, pg 59)									
Romano, 1 oz	110	8	5	0	30	1	0	0	340
Asiago, 1 oz	110	9	5	0	0	1	0	1	400
Parmesan, 1 oz	111	7	5	0	19	1	0	0	454
BRANDS . . . *(1 OZ UNLESS NOTED)*									
Bella Rosa Parmigiano Reggiano	20	2	1	0	4	0	0	0	30
Organic Valley Romano	40	3	2	0	10	0	0	0	120
Orsinia Parmigiano Reggiano	10	6	5	0	20	0	0	0	220
QUESO (MEXICAN CHEESES)									
Chihuahua, 1 oz	106	8	5	0	30	2	0	0	175
Asadero, 1 oz	101	8	5	0	30	1	0	0	186
Anejo, 1 oz	106	8	5	0	30	1	0	0	321
BRANDS . . . *(1 OZ UNLESS NOTED)*									
Mozzarella Co. – has a lightly salted queso blanco and queso fresco.									
SWISS, GRUYERE AND JARLSBERG									
Swiss, 1 oz	108	8	5	0	26	2	0	0	54
Gruyere, 1 oz	117	9	5	0	31	0	0	0	95
BRANDS . . . *(1 OZ UNLESS NOTED)*									
Boar's Head Swiss, NSA	110	8	5	0	25	1	0	0	10
Lacey Swiss, Reduced Fat/Sodium	90	6	4	0	15	0	0	0	35
Gold Label Premium Imported Swiss	110	8	5	0	20	1	0	0	65
Dietz & Watson Swiss	110	8	5	0	28	0	0	0	30

Food	Cal	Fat	Sat	TFat	Chol	Carb	Fib	Sug	Sod
CHEESE – SWISS, GRUYERE AND JARLSBERG (CONT'D)									
Emmentaler Swiss	120	9	6	0	25	0	0	0	50
Hillandale Farms Swiss, NSA	100	8	5	0	25	1	0	0	10
Lucerne (Safeway) Swiss, NSA	100	8	5	0	25	1	0	0	10
Pearl Valley Smoked Swiss	110	8	5	0	30	1	0	0	60

CHEESE – GRATED AND SHREDDED

Food	Cal	Fat	Sat	TFat	Chol	Carb	Fib	Sug	Sod
Asiago, shredded, 1 tbsp	20	2	1	0	5	0	0	0	55
Swiss, shredded, 1/4 cup (1 oz)	100	8	5	0	25	0	0	0	60
Romano, grated, 1 tbsp	19	2	1	0	5	0	0	0	70
Parmesan, grated, 1 tbsp	23	2	1	0	4	0	0	0	75
Cheddar, shredded, 1/4 cup	100	9	6	0	30	0	0	0	180
Mozzarella, part skim, shredded, 1/4 cup	90	6	4	0	20	0	0	0	220

BRANDS . . . *(1/4 CUP OR 1 OZ UNLESS NOTED)*

CHEDDAR
Most brands are within the generic range.

MOZZARELLA

Food	Cal	Fat	Sat	TFat	Chol	Carb	Fib	Sug	Sod
Sorrento Whole Milk Mozzarella	90	7	5	0	25	1	0	0	120
Part Skim Mozzarella	80	6	4	0	15	1	0	0	150

PARMESAN, ROMANO AND ASIAGO *(1 TBSP UNLESS NOTED)*

Food	Cal	Fat	Sat	TFat	Chol	Carb	Fib	Sug	Sod
4C Imported Parmesan	20	2	1	0	5	0	0	0	70
Buitoni Fresh Shredded Romano	20	2	1	0	5	0	0	0	50
Fresh Shredded Parmesan	20	2	1	0	5	0	0	0	60
Horizon Shredded Parmesan	20	2	1	0	5	0	0	0	70
Kraft Romano/Parmesan, Reduced Fat........	20	1	0	0	1	2	0	0	75
Maggio Shredded Parmesan	20	1	1	0	0	0	0	0	35
Wisantigo Asiago, Shredded	20	2	1	0	5	1	0	0	55
Romano, Shredded	20	2	1	0	5	0	0	0	60
Parmesan, Shredded	25	2	1	0	5	0	0	0	70

SWISS
Most brands are within the generic range.

CHEESE SUBSTITUTES

Food	Cal	Fat	Sat	TFat	Chol	Carb	Fib	Sug	Sod
Parma! Parmesan seasoning	25	2	0	0	0	2	0	0	25

CHEESE – PACKAGED/SLICED

Food	Cal	Fat	Sat	TFat	Chol	Carb	Fib	Sug	Sod
Swiss, 0.8 oz	80	6	4	0	19	1	0	0	40
Monterey jack, 0.8 oz	78	6	4	0	19	0	0	0	113
Cheddar, 0.8 oz	85	7	4	0	22	0	0	0	130
Muenster, 0.8 oz	77	6	4	0	20	0	0	0	132

DAIRY PRODUCTS AND ALTERNATIVES
Cheese – Shelf-Stable

Food	Cal	Fat	Sat	TFat	Chol	Carb	Fib	Sug	Sod
CHEESE – PACKAGED AND SLICED (CONT'D)									
Provolone, 0.8 oz	74	6	4	0	14	1	0	0	184
American/Processed, 0.8 oz	69	5	3	0	20	2	0	2	280

BRANDS . . . *(0.8 OZ SLICE UNLESS NOTED)*

SWISS CHEESE

Most "natural," "aged," or "deli style" brands are within the generic range; "processed" varieties may have as much as 290mg per slice.

OTHER CHEESE VARIETIES

Alpine Lace									
Muenster, Reduced Sodium	110	9	5	0	25	1	0	0	85
The Deli Counter (Safeway)									
Havarti	120	10	6	0	30	1	0	0	135
Smoked Fontina, 0.75 oz	110	9	6	0	25	1	0	0	150
Horizon Provolone, 0.8 oz	70	6	4	0	15	0	0	0	140
Sara Lee									
Hot Pepper Monterey Jack & Jalapeño	80	6	4	0	20	0	0	0	125
Sargento									
Provolone, Deli Style, Thin Slice, 0.7 oz	70	5	4	0	15	0	0	0	135
Provolone, Reduced Fat	50	4	2	0	10	0	0	0	140

CHEESE – SHELF-STABLE

Processed, boxed, 1 oz	60	6	4	0	25	3	0	2	410
Processed spread, jar, 2 tbsp	90	7	3	0	10	4	0	2	480

BRANDS . . .
Most brands are within the generic range.

CHEESE – STRING

String cheese, 1 oz	90	6	4	0	20	1	0	0	190

BRANDS . . . *(1 OZ UNLESS NOTED)*

Organic Valley Stringles									
Organic String	60	4	3	0	10	1	0	1	110
Colby Jack	80	7	4	0	20	1	0	0	125
Cheddar	80	7	5	0	20	0	0	0	135

CHEESE SUBSTITUTE/NON-DAIRY

Soy-based, parmesan, grated, 2 tsp	15	1	0	0	0	1	0	0	85
Soy-based, mozzarella or american, 1 slice (avg)	20	0	0	0	0	3	0	1	220

BRANDS . . .
Most brands are within the generic range.

Food	Cal	Fat	Sat	TFat	Chol	Carb	Fib	Sug	Sod

COTTAGE CHEESE AND RICOTTA

COTTAGE CHEESE

Food	Cal	Fat	Sat	TFat	Chol	Carb	Fib	Sug	Sod
Cottage cheese w/fruit, 4 oz (1/2 cup)	110	4	3	0	15	5	0	3	389
Cottage cheese, 4 oz (1/2 cup)	116	5	3	0	17	3	0	3	458
LF, 4 oz (1/2 cup)	81	1	0	0	5	3	0	3	459

BRANDS . . . *(4 OZ UNLESS NOTED)*

Food	Cal	Fat	Sat	TFat	Chol	Carb	Fib	Sug	Sod
Friendship LF, NSA	90	1	1	0	5	4	0	3	50
Hood LF, NSA	90	1	1	0	15	6	0	5	55
Lucerne NSA	80	1	1	0	5	4	0	3	40

RICOTTA

Food	Cal	Fat	Sat	TFat	Chol	Carb	Fib	Sug	Sod
Ricotta cheese, 2 oz (1/4 cup)	107	8	5	0	31	2	0	2	52
Part skim, 2 oz (1/4 cup)	86	5	3	0	19	3	0	3	77

BRANDS . . . *(1/4 CUP UNLESS NOTED)*

Food	Cal	Fat	Sat	TFat	Chol	Carb	Fib	Sug	Sod
Calabro FF	25	0	0	0	0	1	0	1	30
Miceli's Lite	60	3	2	0	15	3	0	3	55
Mozzarella Co.	74	5	2	0	15	2	0	0	36
Polly-O Part Skim	90	6	2	0	20	0	0	0	65
Precious LF	70	3	2	0	15	3	0	3	45
Sargento Light	60	3	2	0	15	3	0	3	55
FF	50	0	0	0	10	5	0	2	65
Sorrento FF	60	0	0	0	5	5	0	4	60

CHEESE SAUCE

(see Cheese Sauce, pg 51)

CHEESE TOPPERS

BRANDS . . . *(2 TBSP UNLESS NOTED)*

Food	Cal	Fat	Sat	TFat	Chol	Carb	Fib	Sug	Sod
Private Harvest Cranberries & Wine	45	0	0	0	0	10	0	8	0
Pear	45	0	0	0	0	11	0	10	20
Caramel Nut	130	7	1	0	0	14	1	13	30
Tomato, Apple & Raisin	40	0	0	0	0	10	0	9	40
Sun-Dried Tomato	70	5	2	0	5	2	0	1	95

COFFEE CREAMERS AND FLAVORINGS

(see Coffee Creamers and Flavorings, pg 15)

CREAM

Food	Cal	Fat	Sat	TFat	Chol	Carb	Fib	Sug	Sod
Light whipping cream, 1 tbsp	44	5	3	0	17	0	0	0	5

Food	Cal	Fat	Sat	TFat	Chol	Carb	Fib	Sug	Sod
CREAM (CONT'D)									
Half & half, 1 tbsp	20	2	1	0	6	1	0	1	6
FF, 1 tbsp	9	0	0	0	0	1	0	1	22
Light cream, 1 tbsp	29	3	2	0	10	1	0	0	6
Heavy whipping cream, 1 tbsp	52	6	4	0	21	0	0	0	6

BRANDS . . .
Most brands are within the generic range.

(CREAM – SOUR)

Food	Cal	Fat	Sat	TFat	Chol	Carb	Fib	Sug	Sod
Sour cream, regular, 2 tbsp	64	6	4	0	13	1	0	0	16
Reduced fat, 2 tbsp	54	4	1	0	11	2	0	0	21
FF, 2 tbsp	22	0	0	0	3	5	0	0	42

BRANDS . . . *(2 TBSP UNLESS NOTED)*

REGULAR AND REDUCED FAT
Most brands are within the generic range.

FAT FREE

Food	Cal	Fat	Sat	TFat	Chol	Carb	Fib	Sug	Sod
Breakstone's FF	30	0	0	0	5	5	0	2	25
Daisy FF	20	0	0	0	0	1	0	1	15
Friendship FF	25	0	0	0	0	4	0	2	20
Hood FF	25	0	0	0	0	4	0	2	25

SOUR CREAM ALTERNATIVES

Food	Cal	Fat	Sat	TFat	Chol	Carb	Fib	Sug	Sod
Imitation sour cream, 2 tbsp	59	6	5	0	0	2	0	2	29

BRANDS . . .
Most brands are within the generic range.

(CREAM CHEESE AND SPREADS)

Food	Cal	Fat	Sat	TFat	Chol	Carb	Fib	Sug	Sod
Mascarpone, 1 oz	124	13	7	0	36	1	0	0	16
Cream cheese, 1 oz	100	9	6	0	40	1	0	1	100
Whipped, 2 tbsp	60	6	4	0	20	1	0	1	90
Favored, 1 oz	90	8	5	0	30	5	0	4	120
Light, 1 oz	70	5	4	0	20	2	0	2	160
FF, 1 oz	30	0	0	0	5	2	0	1	200
Neufchatel, 1 oz	70	6	4	0	20	1	0	1	120

BRANDS . . . *(1 OZ UNLESS NOTED)*

CREAM CHEESE (FLAVORED)

Food	Cal	Fat	Sat	TFat	Chol	Carb	Fib	Sug	Sod
Bruegger's Strawberry	100	9	5	0	20	3	0	2	70
Light, Garden Veggie	60	4	3	0	15	2	0	1	75
Onion & Chive	100	9	6	0	25	2	0	1	75
Light, Herb & Garlic	70	5	3	0	15	3	0	2	85

Food	Cal	Fat	Sat	TFat	Chol	Carb	Fib	Sug	Sod
CREAM CHEESE AND SPREADS (BRUEGGER'S CONT'D)									
Honey Walnut	110	8	5	0	25	5	0	2	85
Wildberry	100	9	5	0	25	4	0	2	85
Olive Pimento	100	9	4	0	30	2	0	1	90
Garden Veggie	90	8	5	0	25	3	1	2	95
Jalapeno	100	9	5	0	30	3	0	2	100
Bacon Scallion	100	8	5	0	30	4	0	1	105
Smoked Salmon	100	9	5	0	25	2	0	1	105
Certified Kosher Gourmet									
Scallion	90	9	6	0	30	0	0	0	100
Lox Spread	80	8	5	0	25	0	0	0	105
Crystal Farms									
Blueberry or Raspberry	100	9	6	0	30	5	0	4	100
Marzetti Fruit Dip	70	3	2	0	10	10	0	9	85
Philadelphia									
Whipped									
Cinnamon 'n Brown Sugar	70	6	4	0	20	3	0	2	55
Mixed Berry	70	5	3	0	15	3	0	3	55
Garlic 'n Herb	60	6	4	0	20	1	0	1	100
Blueberry	90	7	5	0	30	5	0	5	110
Swirls Peaches 'n Cream	90	7	4	0	30	5	0	4	110
CREAM CHEESE (PLAIN)									
Bruegger's Plain	90	8	5	0	25	4	0	1	85
Light, Plain	70	5	2	0	15	3	1	2	90
Lucerne (Safeway) Whipped, 2 tbsp	70	7	5	0	20	1	0	1	65
Morning Select Whipped, 2 tbsp	67	7	4	0	20	1	0	1	60
Mozzarella Co. – has an unsalted and lightly salted cream cheese									
Nancy's Plain	95	9	6	0	35	2	0	2	35
Richfood Whipped, 2 tbsp	70	7	5	0	20	1	0	1	65
TempTee, Soft, 2 tbsp	80	8	5	0	25	1	0	1	70
MASCARPONE									
Most brands are within the generic range.									
NEUFCHATEL									
Most brands are within the generic range.									

CREAM CHEESE ALTERNATIVES
BRANDS . . . *(2 TBSP UNLESS NOTED)*

Food	Cal	Fat	Sat	TFat	Chol	Carb	Fib	Sug	Sod
Cascade Fresh									
Mediterranean Style Yogurt	60	6	4	0	15	2	0	2	20
Soya Kaas	100	9	2	0	0	0	0	0	115
Tofutti Better Than Cream Cheese	80	8	2	0	0	1	0	0	135

DAIRY PRODUCTS AND ALTERNATIVES
Eggs and Egg Substitutes

Food	Cal	Fat	Sat	TFat	Chol	Carb	Fib	Sug	Sod
CREAM CHEESE AND SPREADS (CONT'D)									
SPREADS									
BRANDS . . . *(2 TBSP UNLESS NOTED)*									
Alouette Garlic & Herbs, Light	50	4	3	0	15	2	0	2	60
Spinach Artichoke	70	6	4	0	15	1	0	1	70
Savory Vegetable	70	6	5	0	15	1	0	1	80
Sun-Dried Tomato & Basil	80	7	5	0	15	1	0	1	95
Triple Onion or Garlic & Herbs (avg)	80	7	5	0	20	1	0	1	100
Elegante Roasted Sweet Peppers	90	9	6	0	30	2	0	1	140
Elegante Sun-Dried Tomato & Garlic	90	9	6	0	30	2	0	1	140
Cibo Naturals									
Fresh Herb & Garlic	130	13	8	0	35	1	0	1	135
Basil & Roasted Walnut	130	13	8	0	35	1	0	1	140
Smoked Jalapeño	130	13	8	0	40	1	0	1	140
Rising Sun Farms Cheese Tortas									
Marionberry	120	11	5	0	20	5	0	3	45
Mild Curry w/Apricots & Cranberries	110	9	5	0	20	7	0	3	45
Key Lime w/Cranberries	110	10	5	0	20	5	0	3	50
Roasted Garlic	100	8	5	0	20	6	1	2	70
Mediterranean	90	7	5	0	20	5	0	3	85
Pesto Dried Tomato	100	9	5	0	25	3	0	2	90
Gorgonzola	110	9	5	0	20	4	0	3	100
Rondele									
Bagel Temptations, Strawberry	90	8	5	0	30	4	0	3	75
Bagel Temptations, Plain	110	10	7	0	35	1	0	1	115
Salsa	60	6	4	0	20	1	0	1	110
Toasted Onion	70	7	4	0	25	2	0	1	125
Peppercorn Parmesan	70	7	4	0	25	1	0	1	130
Bagel Temptations, Mixed Berry	110	9	6	0	35	4	0	3	130
Roasted Garlic & Artichoke	70	7	5	0	25	1	0	1	135
Pub Cheese, Zesty Salsa	60	6	4	0	20	1	0	1	140
EGGS AND EGG SUBSTITUTES									
Egg yolk, large, 1	55	5	2	0	212	0	0	0	8
Egg, whole, small, 1	54	4	1	0	157	0	0	0	52
Medium, 1	65	4	1	0	186	1	0	0	62
Large, 1	74	5	2	0	212	0	0	0	70
Egg white, large, 1	17	0	0	0	0	0	0	0	55
Egg substitute, 1/4 cup (1 egg)	53	2	0	0	1	0	0	0	111

Food	Cal	Fat	Sat	TFat	Chol	Carb	Fib	Sug	Sod

EGGS AND EGG SUBSTITUTES (CONT'D)

BRANDS . . .

EGGS
Most brands are within the generic range.

EGG SUBSTITUTES *(also see Eggs – Dried/Powdered, pg. 5)*

Kineret Light 'n Tasty, 1/4 cup	30	0	0	0	0	1	0	1	80

(MILK PRODUCTS AND NON-DAIRY ALTERNATIVES)

(also see Milk and Milk Substitutes – Canned and Powdered, pg 8)

BUTTERMILK

Buttermilk, LF, 1 cup	98	2	1	0	10	12	0	12	257

BRANDS . . . *(1 CUP UNLESS NOTED)*

Friendship Buttermilk, LF	120	4	3	0	15	12	0	12	125

MILK

Milk, whole, 1 cup	146	8	5	0	24	11	0	11	98
2%, 1 cup	122	5	3	0	20	11	0	11	100
1%, 1 cup	102	2	2	0	12	12	0	12	107
NF, 1 cup	101	1	0	5	0	12	0	12	145
Goat milk, 1 cup	168	10	7	0	27	11	0	11	122

BRANDS . . . *(1 CUP UNLESS NOTED)*
Most brands are within the generic range.

MILK – FLAVORED

Eggnog, ready-to-drink, 1 cup	343	19	11	0	150	34	0	21	137
Mix, prep w/whole milk, 1 cup	258	8	5	0	30	39	0	34	150
Choc milk, ready-to-drink, 1 cup	208	8	5	0	30	26	2	24	150
LF, 1 cup	158	3	2	0	8	26	1	25	153

BRANDS . . .

Hood Golden or Vanilla (avg)	180	9	5	0	65	22	0	20	100
Light	140	4	3	0	45	22	0	21	100

NON-DAIRY ALTERNATIVES

Soy Milk, 8 fl oz	80	5	1	0	0	15	0	13	85
Rice Milk, 8 fl oz	120	2	0	0	0	25	0	11	90

BRANDS . . . *(8 FL OZ UNLESS NOTED)*

MIX

Ener-G Soy Quik powder, 2 tbsp	50	2	0	0	0	4	2	2	0

READY-TO-DRINK

Bolthouse Farms Perfectly Protein	160	3	1	0	0	25	0	21	60

DAIRY PRODUCTS AND ALTERNATIVES
Whipped Toppings

Food	Cal	Fat	Sat	TFat	Chol	Carb	Fib	Sug	Sod
NON-DAIRY ALTERNATIVES (CONT'D)									
Power Dream, Java Jolt, 11 fl oz	240	5	1	0	0	26	2	24	70
Rice Dream Horchata	170	3	0	0	0	37	0	22	5
Westsoy Soy Drink, Plain, Unsweetened ..	90	5	0	0	0	5	4	0	30
Vanilla, Unsweetened	100	5	1	0	0	5	4	0	30

WHIPPED TOPPINGS

(also see Sauces and Toppings, pg 86)

Food	Cal	Fat	Sat	TFat	Chol	Carb	Fib	Sug	Sod
Whipped topping, ready-to-eat, 1 tbsp	13	1	1	0	0	1	0	1	1
Powder, prep, 1 tbsp	8	0	0	0	0	1	0	1	3
Pressurized, 1 tbsp	8	0	0	0	2	0	0	0	4

BRANDS ...
Most brands are within the generic range.

YOGURT

Food	Cal	Fat	Sat	TFat	Chol	Carb	Fib	Sug	Sod
Yogurt, plain, 8 oz	138	7	5	0	30	11	0	11	104
LF, 8 oz	143	4	2	0	15	16	0	16	159
FF, 8 oz	127	0	0	0	5	17	0	17	175
Yogurt, fruit, LF, 8 oz	238	3	2	0	14	42	0	7	132
NF, 8 oz	213	0	0	0	0	43	0	43	132
Vanilla, NF, 8 oz..	98	0	0	0	5	17	0	17	134
LF, 8 oz	193	3	2	0	11	31	0	31	150

BRANDS ... *(8 OZ UNLESS NOTED)*

PLAIN

Food	Cal	Fat	Sat	TFat	Chol	Carb	Fib	Sug	Sod
Cascade Fresh FF, Plain	110	0	0	0	5	16	0	10	120
Colombo FF, Plain	100	0	0	0	10	16	0	10	100
Light, Plain	130	3	2	0	15	16	0	19	125
Horizon Organic FF Plain, 6 oz	80	0	0	0	0	12	1	11	120
Mountain High FF Plain	120	0	0	0	0	19	0	15	150
Plain, LF	150	2	1	0	15	22	0	15	150
Stonyfield Farm Organic, LF Plain	120	2	2	0	10	18	3	15	150
All Natural, FF Plain	100	0	0	0	0	18	3	16	150
Total Plain, Whole Milk	250	12	6	0	25	29	0	29	80
Plain, FF	80	0	0	0	0	6	0	6	110

FRUIT/FLAVORED YOGURT
Blue Bunny

Food	Cal	Fat	Sat	TFat	Chol	Carb	Fib	Sug	Sod
Carb Freedom, all, 6 oz (avg)	903	2	0	0	15	5	0	5	70
Lite 85, 6 oz (avg)	80	0	0	0	5	14	0	8	90
Breyers Light FF, Strawberry	120	0	0	0	0	22	0	17	100
Light FF, Apple Cinnamon	120	0	0	0	0	22	0	16	105

Food	Cal	Fat	Sat	TFat	Chol	Carb	Fib	Sug	Sod
FRUIT/FLAVORED YOGURT (BREYERS CONT'D)									
Light FF, Berry Banana	120	0	0	0	0	22	0	16	105
Black Cherry, LF	240	3	2	0	15	46	0	44	115
Brown Cow Cream at the Top									
Cherry Vanilla	240	8	5	0	30	38	0	35	95
Peach or Raspberry	220	8	5	0	30	31	0	29	100
Cascade Fresh									
FF, Flavored, all, 6 oz	110	0	0	0	0	20	0	16	90
LF, all, 6 oz	140	2	1	0	10	23	0	19	90
Colombo									
Classic, Fruit on the Bottom, all	220	2	2	0	15	47	0	36	115
Light, all	120	0	0	0	5	21	0	15	110
Dannon Carb Control, all, 4 oz	60	3	2	0	10	3	0	3	30
LaCreme Mousse, all, 2.5 oz (avg)	90	3	2	0	10	15	0	14	45
Light 'n Fit w/Fiber, all, 4 oz	70	0	0	0	5	13	3	8	55
Activa, Vanilla, 4 oz	110	2	2	0	10	19	0	17	70
Creamy Fruit Blends, 4 oz	110	1	1	0	5	20	0	18	70
Activa, fruit flavored, 4 oz	110	2	1	0	5	19	0	17	75
LaCreme, Strawberry, 4 oz	140	5	3	0	20	20	0	18	75
LaCreme, Vanilla, 4 oz	140	5	3	0	20	20	0	18	75
Light 'n Fit, Vanilla, 6 oz	90	0	0	0	5	16	0	12	95
All Natural, all, 6 oz	150	3	2	0	10	25	0	25	100
Horizon Organic FF, all, 6 oz (avg)	140	0	0	0	5	27	1	26	105
Stonyfield Farm									
Organic, 6 oz									
Wild Berry	170	6	4	0	20	24	2	22	85
Strawberries & Cream	170	6	4	0	20	24	2	22	90
Vanilla Truffle	210	5	3	0	20	37	2	33	90
French Vanilla	190	6	4	0	25	27	3	24	95
Blueberry, LF or Strawberry, LF	130	2	1	0	5	25	2	22	95
Peachy, LF	130	2	1	0	5	25	2	23	95
LF Maple Vanilla or Vanilla (avg)	135	2	1	0	5	23	2	22	100
Mocha Latte, LF	140	2	1	0	5	25	2	22	105
Raspberry, LF	130	2	1	0	5	25	3	22	105
All Natural, 6 oz									
Apricot Mango, FF or Blueberry, FF	130	0	0	0	0	26	2	23	100
Raspberry, FF	130	0	0	0	0	25	2	23	100
Choc Underground, FF	170	0	0	0	0	37	3	34	100
Black Cherry, LF	130	0	0	0	0	26	2	23	105
Light, all (avg)	100	0	0	0	0	28	3	17	105

Food	Cal	Fat	Sat	TFat	Chol	Carb	Fib	Sug	Sod
FRUIT/FLAVORED YOGURT (CONT'D)									
Wallaby Organic, all, 6 oz	140	3	2	0	15	24	0	21	105
Yoplait Whips, fruit flavors, 4 oz	140	3	2	0	10	25	0	21	75
Light, fruit flavors, 6 oz	100	0	0	0	5	19	0	14	85
Light, other flavors, 6 oz	110	0	0	0	5	20	0	15	90

NON-DAIRY YOGURT ALTERNATIVES

Bᴿᴬɴᴅꜱ . . . *(6 OZ UNLESS NOTED)*

Nancy's Cultured Soy

Food	Cal	Fat	Sat	TFat	Chol	Carb	Fib	Sug	Sod
Plain	150	3	0	0	0	25	2	15	20
Vanilla	120	3	0	0	0	19	3	10	20
Blackberry, Blueberry, or Raspberry	140	4	0	0	0	24	4	13	20
Strawberry,	140	4	0	0	0	22	3	12	20
Key Lime	160	3	0	0	0	31	4	21	20
Mango	170	3	0	0	0	33	3	23	20
O'Soy Choc	160	3	0	0	30	28	4	22	30
Blueberry	170	2	0	0	0	33	4	27	35
Peach or Strawberry	170	2	0	0	0	32	4	27	35
Vanilla	150	2	0	0	0	26	4	21	40
Raspberry	170	2	0	0	0	32	4	27	45
Silk Soy Yogurt, all (avg)	150	2	0	0	0	29	1	21	25

(YOGURT – FROZEN)

(see Frozen Yogurt, pg 78)

(YOGURT DRINKS)

Food	Cal	Fat	Sat	TFat	Chol	Carb	Fib	Sug	Sod
Fruit flavored, 10 oz	240	0	0	0	0	48	0	44	150
Bᴿᴬɴᴅꜱ . . . *(10 OZ UNLESS NOTED)*									
Brown Cow LF Smoothie, Strawberry	170	2	1	0	5	31	0	27	125
Dannon									
Light 'n Fit Smoothie, 6.9 oz									
Strawberry	80	0	0	0	0	14	0	13	85
Raspberry	80	0	0	0	0	15	1	13	95
Frusion, Banana Berry	270	4	2	0	15	52	0	49	130
Kemps Yo-J, all, 8 oz	150	0	0	0	0	34	0	32	55
Lifeway Kefir, LF, all, 8 oz	174	2	2	0	10	25	3	21	125
Old Home Light Smoothie, all, 8 oz (avg)	85	0	0	0	5	15	4	9	110
Yogurt Smoothie, all, 10 oz (avg)	280	4	2	0	15	55	1	51	135
Weight Watchers Smoothie, all, 7 oz	80	0	0	0	5	13	2	10	100
Yoplait Light Smoothie, all, 8 oz	90	0	0	0	5	16	3	9	120

Food	Cal	Fat	Sat	TFat	Chol	Carb	Fib	Sug	Sod

DESSERTS AND SWEETS

BROWNIES AND DESSERT BARS

Food	Cal	Fat	Sat	TFat	Chol	Carb	Fib	Sug	Sod
Brownie, ready-to-eat, 1 oz	115	5	1	-	5	18	1	10	88
Mix, 1 oz	123	4	1	-	0	22	0	17	120
Lemon bar, mix, 1 oz	150	4	1	-	0	29	0	24	90

BRANDS . . .

Although there are many low sodium brownies and dessert bars, the following have less than 100mg.

FROZEN/REFRIGERATED

Food	Cal	Fat	Sat	TFat	Chol	Carb	Fib	Sug	Sod
Sara Lee Cheesecake Bites, 3.9 oz	100	7	5	0	15	8	0	6	55
Brownie Bites, 1.4 oz	180	8	4	0	10	24	1	16	60

MIX *(1 PIECE UNLESS NOTED)*

Food	Cal	Fat	Sat	TFat	Chol	Carb	Fib	Sug	Sod
Arrowhead Mills Wheat Free	90	2	1	0	0	21	1	13	40
Brownie	90	2	1	0	0	21	1	14	45
Aunt Candice	47	1	1	0	0	9	0	1	66
Bernard Butterscotch or Choc	70	0	0	0	0	20	0	7	10
Betty Crocker Sunkist Lemon Bars	130	3	1	1	0	24	0	17	80
Walnut Choc Chunk	130	4	1	1	0	24	1	17	85
Triple Chunk or Choc Chunk (avg)	130	3	2	1	0	24	1	18	90
Pecan	120	4	1	1	0	22	0	15	90
Canturbury Naturals Choc	130	3	1	0	0	27	1	19	80
'Cause You're Special Choc Fudge	125	1	0	0	0	29	1	19	82
The Cravings Place Ooey Gooey Choc	113	3	2	0	0	23	1	15	22
Firenza Triple Choc	160	2	1	0	0	23	1	17	70
Gluten-Free Pantry Brownie Mix	150	3	2	0	0	30	0	22	65
Hodgson Mill	120	1	1	0	0	28	2	19	80
Hol-grain Choc	90	0	0	0	0	22	1	17	70
Krusteaz Pecan or Raspberry Bars	130	4	0	0	0	22	1	11	70
Lemon or Lime Bars, 0.8 oz	150	3	0	0	0	29	0	24	80
Manischewitz Choc w/Fudge Frosing	150	4	2	0	0	27	1	20	75
Namaste Brownies	160	7	1	0	20	22	0	15	95
Nature's Path Hemp Plus	140	2	0	0	0	31	3	20	55
Double Fudge	150	3	2	0	0	31	3	21	65
Oetker Choc, 1.5 oz	160	1	0	0	0	36	0	26	90
Pillsbury Choc Extreme	120	3	2	-	0	22	1	16	60
Choc Chunk	120	4	2	-	0	22	1	15	60
White Fudge Chunk	120	4	2	-	0	21	1	15	65
Milk Choc	110	2	0	-	0	23	1	16	70

DESSERTS AND SWEETS
Cakes

Food	Cal	Fat	Sat	TFat	Chol	Carb	Fib	Sug	Sod
BROWNIES (PILLSBURY CONT'D)									
Traditional Fudge or Fudge Toffee	120	3	1	-	0	23	1	16	75
Double Choc	110	2	1	-	0	23	1	16	75
Walnut	140	5	1	-	0	24	1	16	85
Cheesecake Swirl	130	5	2	-	6	21	1	14	85
Choc or Vanilla Frosted	140	4	1	-	0	27	1	19	90
Hot Fudge Swirl or Caramel Swirl (avg) ..	125	3	2	-	0	23	1	16	90
Southern Gourmet Fudge	110	0	0	0	0	28	1	26	10
SHELF-STABLE									
Golden Star Frosted, 2.5 oz	107	0	0	0	0	24	0	16	30
Hostess Brownie Bites, 1.3 oz	170	9	2	-	30	25	1	17	80

(CAKES)

(also see Cheesecakes, pg 71; Snack Cakes, Pies and Sweet Snacks, pg 87)

Food	Cal	Fat	Sat	TFat	Chol	Carb	Fib	Sug	Sod
Sponge cake, 1 oz	82	1	0	0	29	17	0	10	69
Fruitcake, 1 oz	92	3	0	0	1	17	1	8	77
Pound cake w/butter, 1 oz	116	6	4	0	66	15	0	13	119
Marble cake, pudding-type, mix, 1 oz	118	3	1	0	0	22	1	16	147
Carrot cake, pudding-type, mix, 1 oz	118	3	0	0	0	22	1	16	161
German choc, pudding-type, mix, 1 oz	114	3	1	0	0	23	1	14	182
Gingerbread, mix, 1 oz	124	4	1	0	0	21	1	13	186
Yellow cake, mix, 1 oz	122	3	1	0	1	22	0	12	186
Mix, pudding-type, 1 oz	120	3	1	0	0	23	0	13	195
White cake, mix, 1 oz	121	3	1	0	0	22	0	15	188
Angel food cake, 1 oz	72	0	0	0	0	16	0	15	210
Choc cake, mix, 1 oz	121	4	1	0	0	21	1	13	234
Pudding-type, mix, 1 oz	112	3	1	0	0	22	1	14	253
BRANDS . . .									
FROZEN/REFRIGERATED									
Awrey Bakeries Raspberry Nut, 2.8 oz....	310	17	4	2	30	38	1	27	115
Pepperidge Farm Strawberry Stripe, 1/8 .	250	12	4	-	15	32	1	21	110
Mango, 1/8 (2.5 oz)	190	5	2	-	15	35	0	22	110
Coconut, 1/8 (2.5 oz)	250	11	3	-	25	35	1	24	115
Golden or Vanilla, 1/8 (2.5 oz)	250	12	3	-	25	33	1	21	120
Sara Lee Strawberry Swirl Pound, 3 oz	290	11	3	0	60	44	1	25	140
Weight Watchers Carrot Cake, 1 oz	80	3	0	0	10	16	2	11	90
Choc Cake, 1 oz	80	3	1	0	5	15	2	10	110
MIX *(1 OZ UNLESS NOTED)*									
Authentic Foods Lemon	110	1	0	0	0	24	1	14	45
Choc	100	1	0	0	0	23	1	14	105

Food	Cal	Fat	Sat	TFat	Chol	Carb	Fib	Sug	Sod
CAKES (CONT'D)									
Bob's Red Mill Gluten Free, Choc	110	1	0	0	0	24	2	12	85
Canterbury Naturals Choc Orange Pound	150	6	4	0	15	24	1	22	50
'Cause You're Special Choc Pound, 2 oz	217	1	1	0	0	58	3	30	120
Golden Pound, 2 oz	207	0	0	0	0	50	1	27	120
Fran Gare's Choc Bake Mix	93	3	0	0	0	10	4	0	106
Manischewitz Sponge	130	0	0	0	0	33	0	23	5
Sweet 'N Low, all, 1/5 pkg	160	3	1	0	0	36	1	1	30
Sylvan Border Farm Lemon, 2.9 oz	280	11	1	0	55	42	1	19	95
SHELF-STABLE *(1 OZ UNLESS NOTED)*									
Kuchen Meister Marzipan Stollen, 1.8 oz	203	9	3	0	3	29	1	16	60
Cakes, all, 1.8 oz (avg)	220	10	5	0	35	29	14	12	100
CHEESECAKES									
Cheesecake, ready-to-eat, 2 oz	182	13	5	0	31	14	0	12	117
No-bake, mix, prep, 2 oz	155	7	4	0	16	20	1	19	215
BRANDS . . .									
FROZEN/REFRIGERATED									
David Glass Ultimate, 2.2 oz									
Milk Choc Mousse	270	20	10	-	27	20	1	11	76
Choc Covered	217	14	8	-	65	19	0	15	86
New York	203	13	8	-	60	18	0	14	91
Key Lime Mousse	200	13	6	-	21	18	1	13	140
Sara Lee Choc-Dipped Bites, 3.9 oz (2)	100	7	5	0	15	8	0	6	55
Choc-Dipped Pecan Bites, 3.9 oz (2)	90	6	4	0	15	8	1	6	55
Weight Watchers Smart Ones									
New York Style w/Black Cherry									
Swirl, 1 cheesecake	150	5	3	0	15	21	1	17	140
MIX									
Sans Sucre Cheesecake, all	60	2	1	0	5	8	0	4	80

COFFEECAKES *(see Pastries and Coffeecakes, pg 37)*

CAKE FROSTING, ICING AND DECORATIONS

(see Frosting, Icing and Decorations, pg 6)

CANDY AND CHEWING GUM

Food	Cal	Fat	Sat	TFat	Chol	Carb	Fib	Sug	Sod
Breath savers, 1 pc	10	0	0	0	0	2	0	0	0
Sweet choc candy, 1 oz	143	10	6	0	0	15	2	12	0
Gumdrops, 1 oz	34	0	0	0	0	9	0	21	4
Jelly beans, 1 oz	104	0	0	0	0	26	0	18	7

Food	Cal	Fat	Sat	TFat	Chol	Carb	Fib	Sug	Sod
CANDY AND CHEWING GUM (CONT'D)									
Choc coated fondant, 1 oz	102	3	2	0	0	22	0	21	7
Choc coated raisins, 1 oz	109	4	2	0	1	19	1	17	10
Lollipop, 0.6 oz (1)	60	0	0	0	0	16	0	12	10
Hard candy, 1 oz	106	0	0	0	0	28	0	20	11
Butterscotch, 1 oz	112	1	0	0	3	2	0	24	12
Choc coated peanuts, 1 oz	145	9	4	0	3	14	1	11	12
Caramels, choc-flavored roll, 1 oz	103	2	0	0	0	22	0	19	24
Caramel, 1 oz	108	2	2	0	2	22	0	24	70

BRANDS ...

Most brands are within the generic range.

CANDY BARS

Food	Cal	Fat	Sat	TFat	Chol	Carb	Fib	Sug	Sod
Sweet choc bar, 1.5 oz	207	14	8	0	0	24	2	21	7
Milk choc bar w/almonds, 1.5 oz	216	14	7	0	8	22	3	18	30
Milk choc bar, 1.6 oz	235	13	6	0	10	26	2	23	35
Milk choc w/rice cereal, 1.5 oz	223	12	7	0	9	29	2	25	65

BRANDS ...

Most brands are within the generic range.

CHEWING GUM

Food	Cal	Fat	Sat	TFat	Chol	Carb	Fib	Sug	Sod
Chewing gum, 1 stick	5	0	0	0	0	1	0	1	0

BRANDS ...

Most brands are within the generic range.

PEANUT BARS *(see Peanut Bars, pg 146)*

(COFFEECAKES)

(see Pastries and Coffeecakes, pg 37)

(COOKIES)

Food	Cal	Fat	Sat	TFat	Chol	Carb	Fib	Sug	Sod
Sugar wafers w/creme filling, 1 oz	145	7	1	-	0	20	0	10	42
Ladyfingers, 1 oz	103	3	1	-	103	17	0	11	42
Marshmallow, choc coated, 1 oz	119	5	1	0	0	19	1	13	48
Coconut macaroons, 1 oz	115	4	3	-	0	21	1	20	70
Graham crackers, choc covered, 1 oz	137	7	4	-	0	19	1	12	82
Wafers, vanilla, 1 oz	125	4	1	2	0	21	1	11	88
Choc, 1 oz	123	4	1	-	1	21	1	8	164
Choc chip cookies, soft, 1 oz	130	7	2	-	0	17	1	8	92
Mix, 1 oz	141	7	2	-	0	19	0	14	82
Refrg dough, 1 oz	126	6	2	-	7	17	1	10	59

Food	Cal	Fat	Sat	TFat	Chol	Carb	Fib	Sug	Sod
COOKIES (CONT'D)									
Fig Bar, 1 oz	99	2	0	0	0	20	1	13	99
Sandwich:									
Vanilla w/creme filling, 1 oz	137	6	1	-	0	20	0	11	99
Peanut butter, 1 oz	136	6	1	0	0	19	1	10	104
Choc w/creme filling, 1 oz	132	5	1	2	0	20	1	12	137
Butter cookies, 1 oz	132	5	3	0	33	20	0	6	100
Sugar cookies, 1 oz	136	6	2	-	15	19	0	13	101
Refrg dough, 1 oz	124	6	1	-	8	17	0	7	120
Oatmeal cookies, 1 oz	128	5	1	0	0	19	1	7	109
Refrg dough, 1 oz	120	5	1	7	-	17	1	-	83
Mix, 1 oz	131	5	1	0	0	19	-	-	134
Animal cookies, 1 oz	125	4	1	2	0	21	0	8	114
Peanut butter, 1 oz	135	7	1	0	0	17	1	9	118
Refrg dough, 1 oz	130	7	2	-	8	15	0	9	113
Prep from recipe, 1 oz	135	7	1	0	9	17	0	9	147
Shortbread, 1 oz	142	7	2	-	6	18	1	4	129
Molasses, 1 oz	122	4	1	-	0	21	0	12	130
Gingersnaps, 1 oz	118	3	1	2	0	22	1	10	185
BRANDS . . .									
FROZEN/REFRIGERATED (1 OZ UNLESS NOTED)									
Nestle Toll House Choc Chip	140	6	2	-	10	20	0	13	100
Pillsbury Cookie Dough									
Sugar Cookie Sheets, 2 cookies	160	8	2	3	5	22	0	12	60
Easy Open, Peel Apart, Gingerbread	140	5	1	2	10	12	0	6	70
Choc Chip	120	7	2	2	5	15	1	9	85
Sugar	140	6	2	2	10	19	0	10	85
Ready-to-Bake, Choc Candy	120	5	2	1	5	16	0	11	70
Sugar	120	6	2	2	5	15	0	8	70
S'Mores	120	5	2	1	5	16	0	10	75
Choc Chip, Choc Chip w/Walnuts,									
or Mint Choc Chip (avg)	120	7	2	1	5	14	1	9	80
Choc Chunk or Doublc Choc Chip									
& Chunk (avg)	120	7	2	2	5	17	1	10	85
Choc Chip, Sugar Free	90	4	1	1	5	16	3	0	85
The Upper Crust Peanut Butter, 1 oz (2)	130	7	3	0	16	18	2	13	38
Choc Fudge, 1.8 oz (3)	230	4	2	0	15	31	8	12	49
Ginger, 1 oz (2)	130	5	4	0	20	16	1	10	60
Choc Chip, 1 oz (2)	130	6	4	0	20	16	1	11	60
Sugar, 1 oz (2)	130	5	4	0	20	16	0	10	60

DESSERTS AND SWEETS
Cookies

Food	Cal	Fat	Sat	TFat	Chol	Carb	Fib	Sug	Sod

COOKIES (CONT'D)

MIX *(1 OZ UNLESS NOTED)*

Food	Cal	Fat	Sat	TFat	Chol	Carb	Fib	Sug	Sod
Betty Crocker Choc Chip	120	3	2	-	0	21	0	13	60
Sugar	120	3	1	-	0	22	0	12	65
Pouch Mix Sugar	120	3	1	1	0	22	0	13	65
'Cause You're Special									
Classic Sugar, 1	51	0	0	0	0	12	0	4	27
Choc Chip, 0.5	66	1	0	0	0	14	0	7	56
The Cravings Place									
Create-Your-Own Cookie Mix	34	0	0	0	0	7	0	0	4
Peanut Butter	68	0	0	0	0	16	0	8	5
Choc Chunk	78	1	1	-	0	17	1	9	8
Double Choc Chunk	76	1	1	-	0	16	1	9	8
Raisin Spice	82	0	0	0	0	20	0	12	9

SHELF-STABLE *(1 OZ UNLESS NOTED)*

There are many low-sodium cookies, the following have 50mg or less per serving.

Food	Cal	Fat	Sat	TFat	Chol	Carb	Fib	Sug	Sod
Afrika Dark Choc Wafers, 1.1 oz (8)	170	10	6	0	5	12	1	9	20
Almondina Biscuits, 1.1 oz	140	5	1	-	0	21	1	13	10
Andre's Carbo-Save, all	130	9	5	-	15	3	1	1	5
Archway Coconut Macaroon, 0.7 oz	100	6	5	0	0	12	1	10	40
Aunt Gussie's Choc Chip Square, 0.6 oz	70	4	0	0	0	10	0	6	40
Pecan Meltaways, all, 1.4 oz	200	11	6	0	20	20	1	12	45
Choc Chip	120	8	5	0	15	16	1	8	45
Choc Chip Dipped, 1.3 oz	180	10	6	0	20	20	1	12	50
Bahlsen Waffleletten	160	9	6	-	5	18	1	10	40
Choco Leibniz Dark Choc	140	7	4	0	5	18	1	10	50
Barbara's Bakery Fig Bars, all, 0.7 oz (avg)	65	0	0	0	0	14	1	9	20
Choc Chip, 0.6 (1)	80	4	2	0	10	9	1	5	40
Double Dutch, 0.6 (1)	80	4	3	0	10	9	1	4	45
Tradtional Shortbread, 0.6 (1)	80	4	3	0	10	9	1	3	45
Barry's Bakery Merangos, 12 (avg)	105	1	1	0	0	24	0	23	20
French Twists, 1 (avg)	40	2	0	0	0	7	0	4	25
Mini Peaks, 100 pcs	100	0	0	0	0	24	0	24	45
Bonne Mamam Pecan Shortbread, 0.7 oz	100	6	3	-	15	10	0	5	45
BP Gourmet Meringues (avg)	90	0	0	0	0	27	0	0	0
Dreams (avg)	100	0	0	0	0	25	0	25	35
Carr's Chococcines	150	9	6	-	0	16	1	12	20
Dark Choc Imperials	150	7	5	-	5	18	2	10	40
Petits Bijoux	140	5	2	-	0	21	1	9	40
Milk Choc Imperials	150	7	5	-	5	18	1	12	50

Food	Cal	Fat	Sat	TFat	Chol	Carb	Fib	Sug	Sod
COOKIES (CONT'D)									
DeBenkelaer Pirouline	130	4	3	0	15	23	1	13	50
Delacre Matadi Creme-Filled Wafers	190	11	7	-	5	20	1	15	15
Marquisettes	140	7	4	-	5	17	1	7	45
Duchy Originals Lemon Biscuits	160	8	5	-	25	20	1	8	11
Ener-G Cinnamon	160	9	5	0	0	21	0	9	10
Coconut Macaroon, 0.6 oz	80	5	3	0	0	8	1	7	10
Lemon Sandwich	160	9	4	1	0	21	0	13	10
White Choc Chip Macadamia, 0.6 oz	80	4	1	0	15	10	0	6	15
Ginger, 0.5 oz	50	2	1	0	0	9	0	5	15
Choc, 0.6 oz	60	3	2	0	5	9	0	4	20
Almond Butter, 0.5 oz	50	3	0	0	0	6	0	3	25
Choc Hazelnut, 0.6 oz	80	4	1	0	15	11	0	6	25
Vanilla or Vanilla Lemon Cream, 0.6 oz (avg)	105	4	2	0	5	15	0	9	25
Choc Vanilla Cream Sandwich	110	4	2	0	5	16	0	10	25
French Almond, 0.8 oz	70	4	0	0	0	18	1	15	30
Choc Chip Potato, 0.6 oz	80	4	1	0	0	11	0	6	30
Vanilla Choc Cream Sandwich	110	5	2	0	5	16	0	8	35
Vanilla, 0.6 oz	90	4	0	0	10	11	0	5	45
Estee Creme Wafers, Vanilla	175	9	2	0	0	22	0	0	20
Creme Wafers, Choc	170	9	2	0	0	22	0	0	30
Choc Sandwich	140	7	3	0	0	18	0	11	50
Fifty/50 Strawberry Wafers	150	9	2	0	0	20	1	0	15
Vanilla Sandwich, 1.3 oz	170	7	2	0	0	27	0	10	20
Duplex Sandwich, 1.3 oz	160	7	2	0	0	26	1	10	25
Peanut Butter	160	7	2	0	0	19	1	8	25
Vanilla Wafers	150	9	2	0	0	20	1	0	35
Choc Sandwich, 1.3 oz	160	7	2	0	0	26	1	10	35
Coconut	160	10	3	0	0	18	1	6	45
Choc Wafers	160	9	2	0	0	20	1	0	45
Choc Chip	170	10	3	0	0	17	1	7	50
Glutano Luxury Ginger, 0.6 oz	100	5	0	0	0	12	1	7	25
Choc Creme Wafer	150	9	6	0	0	16	1	8	25
Tarteletts, 0.9 oz	122	6	3	0	0	17	1	4	29
Caramel Crunch or Choc Chip Biscuit (avg)	130	7	3	0	5	16	1	8	30
G-Man, 0.6 oz	80	3	2	0	0	12	0	3	35
Half-covered Choc	134	7	4	0	0	17	1	3	44
Hazelnut, 0.6 oz	111	7	2	0	0	12	1	5	45
Health Valley Choc Chip Oatmeal, 0.8 oz	100	4	1	0	0	14	1	7	50
Oatmeal Raisin, 0.8 oz	90	4	0	0	0	14	1	8	50
Heavenly Desserts Meringues, 1 (avg)	0	0	0	0	0	1	0	0	0

DESSERTS AND SWEETS
Cookies (Biscotti)

Food	Cal	Fat	Sat	TFat	Chol	Carb	Fib	Sug	Sod
COOKIES (CONT'D)									
Josef's Fancy Vanilla, 2 oz	230	7	1	1	20	40	2	13	15
Sugar, 1.3 oz	190	6	0	0	20	33	0	18	20
Graham Crackers	100	5	2	0	0	12	1	4	50
Keebler Sugar Wafers (4)	160	8	2	4	0	21	0	14	25
Fudge Shoppe, Caramel Filled (2)	160	8	5	1	0	20	0	13	30
Fudge Sticks (3)	150	8	5	2	0	19	0	15	30
Chips Deluxe, Coconut, 0.6 oz (1)	80	5	2	2	0	9	1	4	40
Sandies, Choc Chip & Pecan or									
Pecan Shortbread, 0.6 (avg)	80	5	1	2	0	9	0	4	50
Chips Deluxe, Peanut Butter Cups, 0.6 oz	90	5	2	2	0	10	1	5	50
Lu Le Chocolatier	150	8	7	-	0	17	1	11	10
Le Truffe, Praline/Choc, 1.2 oz	170	9	7	-	0	20	2	15	15
Le Petit Ecolier, Dark Choc	120	6	4	-	5	17	1	9	50
Manischewitz Meringue, 30 (avg)	120	2	1	0	0	28	0	25	20
Miss Meringue, Meringues (avg)	120	2	1	0	0	26	1	25	20
Madeleines (avg)	160	9	6	0	55	18	1	11	25
Murray Sugar Free Wafers	130	10	2	0	0	19	0	0	15
Nabisco Mallomars	120	5	3	0	0	18	1	2	40
Choc Covered Nutter Butter, 0.6 oz	90	5	2	0	0	12	0	7	45
Chips Ahoy! Chunky, 0.6 oz (1)	80	4	2	0	0	10	1	6	50
Natural Ovens Carob Chip, 1.3 oz	90	4	0	0	0	16	3	6	15
Oatmeal Raisin, 1.3 oz	90	3	0	0	0	15	3	6	15
Pamela's Lemon Shortbread, 0.8 oz	120	6	4	0	15	15	1	5	50
Papadopoulos Caprice Creme-Filled									
Wafers, 1.1 oz (avg)	150	7	3	0	0	20	1	15	40
Pepperidge Farm Lido	90	5	2	-	5	10	0	5	40
Raspberry Milano	130	7	3	-	5	16	1	8	40
Choc or Vanilla Filled Pironette (avg)	135	6	3	-	5	19	1	14	45
Mint Choc Filled Pironette	130	5	3	-	5	20	1	13	50
Reko Pizzelle Anise, Lemon, Maple, or Vanilla	150	6	1	-	15	20	0	8	20
Snackwell's Devil's Food, 0.6 oz	50	0	0	0	0	12	0	7	30
Stella D'oro Anginetti, 1.1 oz	140	4	2	-	40	23	1	17	10
Tree of Life Toasted Almond Butter, 0.9 oz	70	0	0	0	0	16	1	7	35
BISCOTTI									
Biscotti, 1 oz	110	0	0	0	0	24	0	15	95
BRANDS . . . *(1 OZ UNLESS NOTED)*									
Alex & Dani's Totally Choc	130	5	3	-	28	20	1	12	55
Amazing Almond	130	6	3	-	25	17	1	8	55

Food	Cal	Fat	Sat	TFat	Chol	Carb	Fib	Sug	Sod
BISCOTTI (AUNT GUSSIE'S CONT'D)									
Aunt Gussie's most (avg)	140	7	1	0	20	17	1	8	10
Freida's Kitchen all	80	0	0	0	0	18	0	6	25
Health Valley Amaretto or Choc	120	3	0	0	0	23	3	7	50
Scotto's, all (avg)	90	0	0	0	0	19	0	5	20
Stella D'oro									
Choc Chunk, 0.7 oz	90	4	2	0	5	14	0	8	35
Choc Almond, 0.7 oz	90	4	1	0	5	13	1	7	40
Almond, 0.7 oz	100	5	1	0	5	13	1	6	45
French Vanilla, 0.7 oz	90	4	1	0	10	15	0	7	55
The Upper Crust all (avg)	110	4	0	-	19	15	1	7	41

DOUGHNUTS

Food	Cal	Fat	Sat	TFat	Chol	Carb	Fib	Sug	Sod
French cruller, glazed, 1.5 oz	169	8	2	-	5	24	1	14	141
Yeast, glazed, 1.5 oz	169	10	2	-	3	19	1	10	144
Cake, plain, sugar or glazed, 1.5 oz	175	9	2	-	13	21	1	10	165
Cake, choc-coated or frosted, 1.5 oz	204	13	3	-	26	21	1	10	184
Cake, plain, 1.5 oz	173	9	1	-	15	20	1	9	224
Yeast, jelly-filled, 3 oz	289	16	4	-	22	33	1	18	249
Yeast, creme-filled, 3 oz	307	21	5	-	20	26	1	12	263

BRANDS . . .
Most brands are within the generic range.

FROZEN DESSERTS AND PASTRIES

(also see Pastries and Coffeecakes, pg 37; Ice Cream, Ices and Frozen Yogurt, pg 78)

BRANDS . . .

Food	Cal	Fat	Sat	TFat	Chol	Carb	Fib	Sug	Sod
Delizza Choc Dipped Cream Puffs, 3.6 oz	375	25	16	0	130	34	1	26	68
Mini Cream Puffs, 2.7 oz	291	24	14	0	111	15	1	10	77
Mini Eclairs, 3.6 oz	333	21	13	0	63	32	1	20	128
The Fillo Factory Apple Strudel, 4.5 oz	290	10	1	-	0	47	2	15	110
Apple Turnover, 3.8 oz	220	6	0	0	0	39	1	11	120
Michael Angelo's Cannoli, 1.3 oz	140	7	3	0	10	14	1	7	30
Nancy's Petite Souffle									
Belgian Choc, 1.5 oz (3)	170	10	6	0	55	18	2	10	115
Choc Caramel, 1.5 oz (3)	170	15	6	0	60	18	1	12	125
Rich's Bavarian Creme Eclair, 2 oz	190	9	8	-	40	24	0	18	80
New York Hazelnut Eclair, 2 oz	220	12	10	-	36	26	0	20	85
Weight Watchers Smart Ones									
Double Fudge Brownie Parfait, 3.9 oz	220	3	2	0	10	44	1	20	95
Choc Chip Cookie Dough Sundae 2.7 oz	190	5	2	0	5	35	1	15	120

DESSERTS AND SWEETS
Ice Cream, Ices and Frozen Yogurt

Food	Cal	Fat	Sat	TFat	Chol	Carb	Fib	Sug	Sod

(GELATIN)

(see Puddings and Gelatins, pg 84)

(ICE CREAM, ICES AND FROZEN YOGURT)

FROZEN YOGURT

Food	Cal	Fat	Sat	TFat	Chol	Carb	Fib	Sug	Sod
Choc, 1/2 cup	110	3	2	0	11	19	1	19	55
All other flavors, 1/2 cup	127	4	2	0	13	22	0	21	63

BRANDS . . .
Most frozen yogurt is within the generic range.

ICE CREAM

Food	Cal	Fat	Sat	TFat	Chol	Carb	Fib	Sug	Sod
Strawberry, 1/2 cup	127	6	3	0	19	18	1	15	40
Choc, 1/2 cup	143	7	4	0	22	19	1	17	50
Vanilla, 1/2 cup	145	8	5	0	32	17	1	15	58
Sugar-free, 1/2 cup	105	5	3	0	18	15	1	4	65
Fat-free, 1/2 cup	99	0	0	0	0	22	1	5	70

BRANDS . . . *(1/2 CUP UNLESS NOTED)*
Most ice cream is low in sodium, the following have 40mg or less.

Ben & Jerry's

Food	Cal	Fat	Sat	TFat	Chol	Carb	Fib	Sug	Sod
Body & Soul, Cherry Garcia	170	9	6	0	35	22	2	16	40
Organic, Strawberry	210	12	8	0	55	21	0	19	40

Blue Bunny *Premium*

Food	Cal	Fat	Sat	TFat	Chol	Carb	Fib	Sug	Sod
Double Strawberry	140	6	4	0	25	20	0	18	40
Bordeaux Cherry Choc	160	8	5	0	25	20	0	17	40

Breyer's

Food	Cal	Fat	Sat	TFat	Chol	Carb	Fib	Sug	Sod
CarbSmart, Neapolitan	120	9	6	0	40	9	3	0	10
Strawberry or Vanilla (avg)	120	9	6	0	25	10	3	4	30
All Natural									
Choc	140	8	5	0	20	17	1	16	30
Peach or Strawberry (avg)	120	5	3	0	15	17	0	16	30
Black Raspberry Choc	160	7	5	0	15	20	0	20	35
Extra Creamy Choc	140	7	5	0	20	17	1	15	35
Lactose Free Vanilla	130	7	5	0	20	14	0	14	35
Vanilla & Choc	140	7	5	0	20	16	0	15	35
Vanila Ice Cream & Orange Sherbet	130	5	3	0	15	21	0	17	35
Vanilla, Choc, Strawberry	130	7	5	0	20	16	0	15	35
Cherry Vanilla	140	6	4	0	20	17	0	16	40
Coffee	130	7	5	0	20	15	0	14	40
Choc Chip or Mint Choc Chip (avg)	160	8	6	0	20	17	1	16	40

Food	Cal	Fat	Sat	TFat	Chol	Carb	Fib	Sug	Sod
ICE CREAM (BREYER'S CONT'D)									
Natural Vanilla	140	7	5	0	20	15	0	15	40
Vanilla Swiss Almond	150	9	5	0	20	16	0	15	40
Double Churned									
Creamy Choc	140	7	5	0	20	17	1	15	35
Strawberries & Cream	130	6	4	0	15	16	0	14	35
Mint Choc Chip	160	9	6	0	20	18	1	15	40
Vanilla, Choc, Strawberry	140	7	5	0	20	17	0	14	40
A&W Root Beer Float	130	5	3	0	15	20	0	16	35
Choc Overload	170	9	6	0	15	21	1	18	40
Very Choc Cherry	150	7	5	0	15	19	0	17	40
Light, Creamy Choc	110	4	2	0	10	17	1	13	40
Mint Choc Chip	130	5	4	0	10	18	1	16	40
Vanilla, Choc, Strawberry	100	4	2	0	10	16	0	13	40
Dreyer's / Edy's									
Grand, Real Strawberry	130	6	4	0	20	16	0	15	30
Toasted Almond	150	9	5	0	25	15	0	12	30
Vanilla Choc	150	8	5	0	25	16	0	14	30
Vanilla Bean	140	8	5	0	25	15	0	14	35
Vanilla	150	10	6	0	35	14	0	11	35
Rocky Road	170	10	5	0	30	19	0	14	35
Neapolitan	140	7	5	0	25	16	0	14	35
French Vanilla	150	9	5	0	50	16	0	11	35
Choc	150	8	5	0	25	17	0	15	35
Cherry Vanilla	140	7	4	0	25	17	0	14	35
Double Vanilla	140	7	5	0	35	16	0	15	40
Coffee	140	8	5	0	25	15	0	13	40
Andes Cool Mint	170	9	6	0	25	19	0	16	40
Cherry Choc Chip	160	8	5	0	20	19	0	16	40
Spumoni	150	8	5	0	25	16	0	13	40
Slow Churned									
Orange & Cream	100	3	2	0	15	19	0	14	35
Strawberry	110	4	2	0	15	18	0	13	40
Rocky Road	120	4	2	0	20	17	0	12	40
Neapolitan	100	3	2	0	20	15	0	11	40
Carb Benefit									
Choc Chip or Mint Choc Chip	160	11	8	0	30	14	6	2	30
Vanilla Bean	140	9	6	0	30	13	6	2	30
Choc	150	10	6	0	30	13	7	2	35
Good Humor Orange Cream	120	4	3	0	10	20	0	15	40
Choc	120	6	4	0	15	16	1	14	40

DESSERTS AND SWEETS
Ice Cream, Ices and Frozen Yogurt (Non-Dairy Alternatives)

Food	Cal	Fat	Sat	TFat	Chol	Carb	Fib	Sug	Sod
ICE CREAM (CONT'D)									
Häagen-Dazs *Light*, Cherry Fudge Truffle ...	230	7	4	0	50	37	0	33	40
Hood Strawberry	130	7	4	0	25	17	0	13	40
New England Creamery									
Maine Blueberry & Sweet Cream	140	6	4	0	25	19	0	16	40
Stonyfield Farm Choc Raspberry Swirl	230	13	8	0	50	25	0	24	30
After Dark Choc	250	17	10	0	60	21	0	20	35
Cookies 'N Dream	270	18	11	0	55	27	1	25	40
Turkey Hill *Premium*									
Orange Cream Swirl	140	6	-	0	20	19	0	-	25
Black Cherry	140	7	-	0	25	18	0	-	30
Choc Marshmallow	160	7	-	0	30	24	0	-	30
Dutch Choc	150	8	-	0	30	19	0	-	30
Neapolitan	150	8	-	0	30	18	0	-	30
Strawberries & Cream	140	6	-	0	25	19	0	-	30
Black Raspberry or Columbian Coffee (avg)	140	7	-	0	30	18	0	-	35
Original Vanilla or Vanilla Bean	140	8	-	0	30	16	0	-	35
Vanilla & Choc	150	8	-	0	30	17	0	-	35
Light, Choc Chip	110	4	-	0	10	17	0	-	30
CarbIQ Vanilla Bean or Choco Mint									
Chip (avg)	120	9	-	0	30	16	0	-	30
NON-DAIRY ALTERNATIVES									
(also see Specialties – Bars, Pops and Sandwiches [Non-Dairy Alternatives], pg 82)									
BRANDS . . . *(1/2 CUP UNLESS NOTED)*									
Soy Delicious Twisted Vanilla Orange	120	2	0	0	0	24	3	18	40
Choc Velvet	130	4	1	0	0	23	1	14	50
Creamy Vanilla	130	3	0	0	0	24	3	13	55
Mint Marble Fudge	140	3	1	0	0	27	2	17	55
Neapolitan	120	4	1	0	0	23	2	13	55
Strawberry	120	3	0	0	0	23	3	13	55
Choc Peanut Butter	140	5	1	0	0	23	2	13	60
Purely Decadent									
Cherry Nirvana	190	9	2	0	0	32	5	17	15
Choc Obsession	210	9	2	0	0	36	5	20	15
Swinging Anna Banana	230	13	4	0	0	31	5	22	15
Purely Vanilla	170	8	1	0	0	29	6	18	20
Chunky Mint Madness	200	8	2	0	0	35	6	16	30
Mint Choc Chip	190	8	2	0	0	27	5	21	45
Mocha Almond Fudge	200	9	1	0	0	32	6	22	45
Peanut Butter Zig Zag	230	13	3	0	0	32	5	16	50
Praline Pecan	210	10	1	0	0	33	5	15	50

Food	Cal	Fat	Sat	TFat	Chol	Carb	Fib	Sug	Sod
SHERBET AND SORBET									
Sherbet, orange, 1/2 cup	107	1	1	0	0	23	2	18	34
BRANDS . . .									
Most brands are within the generic range.									
SPECIALTIES – BARS, POPS AND SANDWICHES									
Bar, fruit & juice, 1 bar	80	0	0	0	0	19	1	16	4
Yogurt bar, choc, 1 bar	120	0	0	0	0	22	0	15	45
Bar, choc covered, 2.2 oz bar	220	15	11	-	15	18	0	15	55
Bar, drumstick, 3.4 oz	340	20	11	-	20	34	1	23	85
Sandwich, 2.3 oz	180	7	4	-	20	26	0	12	160
BRANDS . . .									
FRUIT AND JUICE BARS *(1 BAR UNLESS NOTED)*									
Most brands are within the generic range.									
ICE CREAM AND YOGURT BARS *(1 BAR UNLESS NOTED)*									
Blue Bunny Root Beer Float	80	2	2	0	10	14	0	11	25
Star Bar	110	7	6	0	5	11	0	9	30
Big Star Bar	130	8	7	0	5	13	0	11	40
English Toffee	130	9	7	0	15	12	0	9	40
Heath	190	13	10	0	20	16	0	13	40
Breyers Light, Creamy Fudge	90	3	2	0	10	14	1	11	40
CarbSmart, Almond	180	15	10	0	15	9	2	5	40
Fruitful Cream-Based Bars (avg)	130	5	3	0	15	24	0	15	25
Choc Yogurt-Based Bar	160	0	0	0	0	33	0	15	65
Good Humor Toasted Almond	180	10	3	2	10	22	1	17	30
Milk Choc	180	13	9	0	15	15	1	13	30
Häagen-Dazs Raspberry Sorbet &									
Vanilla Yogurt	90	0	0	0	0	21	1	15	15
Mint & Dark Choc Ice Cream	290	20	12	0	65	23	1	20	30
Choc & Dark Choc Ice Cream	300	21	13	0	70	24	1	22	40
Healthy Choice Raspberry Orange Sorbet	90	1	1	0	5	18	1	14	35
Hood Ice Cream Bar	150	11	9	0	15	12	1	9	30
Orange Cream or Java Smoothie (avg)	95	2	1	0	8	18	0	12	40
Choc Fudge, No Sugar Added	50	2	1	0	5	12	2	3	40
Klondike Choc	250	17	13	0	20	21	1	18	45
Dark Choc, York, or Neapolitan (avg)	250	17	13	0	20	22	1	17	50
The Original or Original Vanilla	250	17	13	0	20	22	0	19	55
Whitehouse Cherry	250	17	13	0	20	24	0	21	55
Popsicle CarbSmart Creamsicle	25	1	0	0	0	5	2	0	0
Creamsicle	70	2	1	0	5	13	0	9	20
Creamsicle, No Sugar Added	45	1	0	0	5	10	2	2	25

DESSERTS AND SWEETS
Ice Cream Cones

Food	Cal	Fat	Sat	TFat	Chol	Carb	Fib	Sug	Sod
SPECIALTIES — ICE CREAM AND YOGURT BARS (POPSICLE CONT'D)									
Pudding Pops	90	3	3	0	0	15	0	10	40
Fudgsicle	60	2	2	0	0	12	0	9	45
DRUMSTICKS AND SANDWICHES *(1 SANDWICH OR DRUMSTICK UNLESS NOTED)*									
Breyers CarbSmart, Cone	210	16	10	0	20	14	3	3	40
CarbSmart, Sandwich	80	4	2	0	10	10	1	2	55
Hood LF Vanilla Sandwich	80	2	1	0	5	15	2	2	70
NON-DAIRY ALTERNATIVES									
Soy Delicious Purely Decadent Bars (avg)	210	10	3	0	0	26	4	22	10
Fudge Bar	140	4	0	0	0	25	2	16	25
Vanilla Bar	260	13	6	0	0	31	1	15	25
Vanilla & Almonds Bar	300	17	7	0	0	32	2	15	30
Sweet Nothings All (avg)	100	0	0	0	0	23	0	12	8
Tofutti Totally Fudge Pops	95	2	0	0	0	19	0	14	53
Delights Bar	120	7	2	0	0	7	0	0	80
Choc Fudge or Coffee Break Treats Bar	30	0	0	0	0	6	0	1	86
Hooray Hooray Bar	150	9	2	0	0	10	0	0	90
Monkey Bar or Marry Me Bars	220	13	8	0	0	22	0	18	105
SANDWICHES									
Soy Delicious Choc Chip Sandwich	260	10	4	0	0	41	2	8	60
Mint Choc Chip Sandwich	260	10	4	0	0	41	2	8	70
Li'l Buddies, Choc or Vanilla Sandwich (avg)	160	3	1	-	0	27	2	12	105
Li'l Buddies, Peanut Butter Sandwich	160	5	1	-	0	27	2	12	115
Li'l Buddies, Mint Sandwich	150	3	1	-	0	28	2	13	125
Mocha Mania Sandwich	265	14	6	0	0	32	2	19	130
Vanilla Cookie or Mint Mania Sandwich	265	14	6	0	0	32	2	18	130
Tofutti Cuties									
Vanilla Sandwich, No Sugar Added	100	5	1	0	0	11	0	0	86
Mint Choc Chip or Coffee Break Sandwich	120	5	1	0	0	19	0	11	110
Choc or Totally Vanilla Sandwich	130	5	1	0	0	16	0	9	110
Wild Berry, Jazzy, or Vanilla Sandwich	120	5	1	0	0	17	0	9	121
Blueberry, Strawberry, or Choc Wave Sandwich	140	6	2	0	0	20	0	12	130
Cookies 'N Cream Sandwich	120	6	1	0	0	17	0	9	135
Peanut Butter Sandwich	165	8	2	0	0	20	0	10	135

(ICE CREAM CONES)

Food	Cal	Fat	Sat	TFat	Chol	Carb	Fib	Sug	Sod
Cone, cake or wafer-type, 1	17	0	0	0	0	3	0	3	6
Sugar cone, 1	40	0	0	0	0	8	0	3	32
Ice cream cone, waffle, 1 oz cone	121	2	0	0	0	23	1	2	41

Food	Cal	Fat	Sat	TFat	Chol	Carb	Fib	Sug	Sod

ICE CREAM CONES (CONT'D)

BRANDS . . .

Most brands are within the generic range.

TOPPINGS

(see Sauces and Toppings, pg 86)

(PASTRIES)

(see Pastries and Coffeecakes, pg 37)

(PIES AND COBBLERS)

(also see Snack Cakes, Pies and Sweet Snacks, pg 87)

Food	Cal	Fat	Sat	TFat	Chol	Carb	Fib	Sug	Sod
Choc creme pie, 1/6	344	22	6	-	6	38	2	-	154
Coconut creme pie, 1/6	191	11	4	-	0	24	1	23	163
Lemon meringue pie, 1/6	303	10	2	-	51	53	1	27	165
Cherry pie, 1/6	304	13	3	-	0	47	1	17	288
Pumpkin pie, 1/6	229	10	2	-	22	30	3	15	307
Apple pie, 1/6	277	13	4	-	0	40	2	18	311
Peach pie, 1/6	261	12	2	-	0	39	1	7	316
Banana creme pie, no-bake mix, prep, 1/6	309	16	9	-	36	39	1	-	357
Blueberry pie, 1/6	271	12	2	-	0	41	1	12	380
Pecan pie, 1/6	452	21	4	-	36	65	4	32	479

BRANDS . . .

FROZEN/REFRIGERATED

Food	Cal	Fat	Sat	TFat	Chol	Carb	Fib	Sug	Sod
Amy's Apple Pie, 4 oz	230	8	5	0	25	37	2	15	135
Door Country Apple Crisp, 4 oz	180	8	3	0	7	43	2	23	76
Edwards Sundae Singles, 2.7 oz	300	19	9	-	13	29	0	20	120
Jeff Nathan Creations									
Apple Cobbler, 1/2	310	13	3	-	0	47	2	30	25
Mrs. Smith's									
Blueberry Crisp, 1/6	280	6	2	-	0	-	2	-	150
Boston Cream, 1/10	210	9	2	-	25	31	0	23	160
Strawberry Crisp, 1/6	290	7	2	-	0	-	2	-	160
Pet-Ritz Choc Drizzle Cream, 1/4	330	-	-	-	-	39	1	25	150
Racine Danish Kringles Raspberry, 1/8	170	8	2	-	5	24	0	15	105
Sara Lee									
Signature Strawberries & Cream, 1/8	400	27	15	-	5	33	2	20	60
Signature Key West Lime, 1/8	400	25	12	-	5	41	2	30	95
Dulce de Leche Caramel Swirl, 1/8	400	26	15	-	5	37	2	20	100
Tangy Lemon Meringue, 1/6	220	5	3	-	0	41	1	37	160

DESSERTS AND SWEETS
Puddings and Gelatins

Food	Cal	Fat	Sat	TFat	Chol	Carb	Fib	Sug	Sod
PIES AND COBBLERS (CONT'D)									
Weight Watchers Smart Ones									
Mississippi Mud, 2.8 oz	160	4	2	0	5	27	1	15	85
Key Lime Pie, 2.8 oz	190	5	2	0	10	33	1	25	85
MIX									
Chef Hans Apple Crisp, 1/2 cup	280	1	0	0	0	64	0	45	85
Concord Foods Apple Crisp, 1/8	110	0	0	0	0	28	0	20	0

(PUDDINGS AND GELATINS)

GELATIN

Food	Cal	Fat	Sat	TFat	Chol	Carb	Fib	Sug	Sod
Unflavored gelatin, 1 envl	23	0	0	0	0	0	0	0	14
Regular gelatin, 1/2 cup	80	0	0	0	0	19	0	18	98
Sugar free, 1/2 cup	13	0	0	0	0	5	0	0	55

BRANDS ...

MIX

Food	Cal	Fat	Sat	TFat	Chol	Carb	Fib	Sug	Sod
Calorie Control, all, 1/2 cup	10	0	0	0	0	1	0	0	0

PUDDING

Food	Cal	Fat	Sat	TFat	Chol	Carb	Fib	Sug	Sod
Custard, mix for 1/2 cup serv	86	1	0	0	54	17	0	12	59
Chocolate pudding:									
Regular (cooked), mix for 1/2 cup serv	97	1	0	0	0	22	1	17	88
Ready-to-eat, 1/2 cup	157	5	1	0	3	26	1	20	146
FF, 1/2 cup	110	0	0	0	0	23	1	17	192
Instant, mix for 1/2 cup serv	94	0	0	0	0	22	1	13	357
Lemon pudding:									
Regular (cooked), mix for 1/2 cup serv	76	0	0	0	0	19	0	12	106
Ready-to-eat, 1/2 cup	142	3	0	0	0	28	0	19	159
Instant, mix for 1/2 cup serv	95	0	0	0	0	24	0	14	333
Vanilla pudding:									
Regular (cooked), mix for 1/2 cup serv	83	0	0	0	0	21	0	17	166
Ready-to-eat, 1/2 cup	147	4	2	0	8	25	0	23	153
Ready-to-eat, FF, 1/2 cup	105	0	0	0	0	26	0	18	170
Instant, mix for 1/2 cup serv	94	0	0	0	0	23	0	23	360
Banana pudding:									
Regular (cooked), mix for 1/2 cup serv	83	0	0	0	0	20	0	16	173
Ready-to-eat, 1/2 cup	144	4	1	0	0	24	0	15	157
Instant, mix for 1/2 cup serv	92	0	0	0	0	23	0	19	375
Plum pudding, mix, 1/3 pkg	460	10	3	0	1	87	5	58	241
Coconut cream:									
Reg (cooked), mix for 1/2 cup serv	109	3	3	0	0	20	1	20	171
Instant, mix for 1/2 cup serv	109	3	3	0	0	21	1	16	260

Food	Cal	Fat	Sat	TFat	Chol	Carb	Fib	Sug	Sod
PUDDING (CONT'D)									
BRANDS ...									
FROZEN/REFRIGERATED									
Weight Watchers Smart Ones									
Choc Mousse, 2.8 oz	180	4	4	0	5	28	3	13	100
MIX *(FOR 1/2 CUP SERVING UNLESS NOTED)*									
Bird's Dessert Mix	25	0	0	0	0	6	0	0	30
Calorie Control Mousse, all	50	3	1	0	0	6	0	0	25
Key Lime Pie Filling & Mousse	60	3	2	0	0	7	0	0	40
Custard	20	0	0	0	0	4	0	3	40
Cheesecake, all	60	2	1	0	5	7	0	4	80
Pistachio, Lemon, or Strawberry	70	2	1	0	0	10	1	8	110
Butterscotch, Banana, or Coconut	70	2	1	0	0	10	1	8	110
Choc, Choc Mint, or Choc Almond	70	2	1	0	0	10	1	8	110
Vanilla or Pumpkin Pie Filling	70	2	1	0	0	10	1	8	110
Con-Gelli Caramel Custard Flan	60	0	0	0	0	19	0	15	45
Junket Custard, 0.4 oz mix (avg)	44	0	0	0	0	10	0	10	0
Mori Nu all, 1/4 pkg (avg)	110	3	2	0	0	22	1	18	5
Nestle Mousse European Style, 1/4 pkg									
Dark Choc	80	4	3	0	0	13	2	9	70
Milk Choc	80	3	2	0	0	14	1	11	75
Noh Hawaiian Coconut, 1/8 pkg	100	4	3	0	0	16	1	9	15
Oetker									
Pistachio Delight	100	2	2	0	0	19	0	18	25
Choc or Creme	40	0	0	0	0	9	0	1	30
Vanilla	40	0	0	0	0	10	0	4	45
Creme Caramel	100	0	0	0	15	23	0	21	45
Mousse, Choc	100	4	3	0	0	15	0	13	45
Mousse, Strawberry	75	3	2	0	0	13	0	11	55
French Vanilla Mousse Light	35	2	2	0	0	3	0	2	75
Tiramisu	150	5	3	1	5	24	0	14	80
Creme Brûlée	110	2	1	-	10	23	0	18	90
RC Bavarian or Mousse, all	90	4	4	0	0	13	0	12	35
Sans Sucre Mousse									
Mocha Cappuccino or Strawberry	50	2	1	0	0	7	0	0	25
French Vanilla, Lemon, or Choc (avg)	50	2	1	0	0	8	0	0	25
Key Lime	60	3	2	0	0	7	0	0	40

NOTE: Most of the above pudding mixes do not include milk or other added ingredients.

Food	Cal	Fat	Sat	TFat	Chol	Carb	Fib	Sug	Sod
PUDDING (CONT'D)									
READY-TO-EAT *(1/2 CUP UNLESS NOTED)*									
Ambrosia Custard	130	4	2	0	5	21	0	15	50
American Spoon Lemon, Lime, or									
Passion Fruit Curd, 1 tbsp	45	2	1	0	40	7	0	6	20
Hunt's Snack Pack Lemon Meringue	130	3	1	0	0	26	0	21	55
Imagine Natural Lemon, 1 cup	150	3	0	0	0	31	1	18	35
Banana, 1 cup	140	3	0	0	0	28	0	17	40
Butterscotch, 1 cup	140	3	0	0	0	28	1	16	55
Choc, 1 cup	160	3	0	0	0	34	1	21	85
Kozy Shack Creme Caramel Flan	150	4	3	0	35	27	0	16	85
RICE PUDDING AND TAPIOCA									
Rice pudding:									
Ready-to-eat, 1/2 cup	185	9	1	0	1	25	0	19	96
Mix for 1/2 cup serv	102	0	0	0	0	25	0	15	99
Tapioca pudding:									
Mix for 1/2 cup serv	85	0	0	0	0	22	0	15	110
Ready-to-eat, 1/2 cup	134	4	1	0	1	22	0	20	180
BRANDS . . .									
MIX *(1/2 CUP PREP UNLESS NOTED)*									
Minute Tapioca, 1 1/2 tsp	20	0	0	0	0	5	0	0	0
Uncle Ben's French Vanilla Rice	120	0	0	0	0	28	1	10	90
READY-TO-EAT *(3.5 OZ UNLESS NOTED)*									
Hunt's Snack Pack, Tapioca	130	5	1	0	0	21	0	13	130
Kraft Handi-Snacks, Tapioca	120	4	1	0	0	21	0	14	120

SAUCES AND TOPPINGS

(also see Whipped Toppings, pg 66)

Food	Cal	Fat	Sat	TFat	Chol	Carb	Fib	Sug	Sod
Strawberry, 2 tbsp	107	0	0	0	0	28	0	12	9
Pineapple, 2 tbsp	106	0	0	0	0	28	0	9	18
Marshmallow cream, 2 tbsp	91	0	0	0	0	22	0	13	23
Choc fudge sauce, 2 tbsp	133	3	2	0	1	24	1	13	131
Butterscotch or caramel sauce, 2 tbsp	103	0	0	0	0	27	0	9	143
BRANDS . . .									
FRUIT TOPPINGS									
Most brands are within the generic range.									
BUTTERSCOTCH AND CARAMEL TOPPINGS									
Wagner Butterscotch, 2 tbsp	150	2	2	5	0	33	1	21	65

DESSERTS AND SWEETS

Snack Cakes, Pies and Sweet Snacks

Food	Cal	Fat	Sat	TFat	Chol	Carb	Fib	Sug	Sod
SAUCES AND TOPPINGS (CONT'D)									
OTHER TOPPINGS									
MIX *(1 OZ UNLESS NOTED)*									
Whippet Original	100	5	3	0	0	20	0	8	45
Raspberry	150	5	3	0	0	25	0	9	50
SHELF-STABLE									
Steel's Classic Fudge Sauce, all (avg)	110	6	0	0	15	13	1	12	10
Nature Sweet, Butterscotch	60	0	0	0	0	21	0	0	10
Nature Sweet, Praline	80	3	0	0	0	18	0	0	10
Choc Fudge (Splenda)	45	3	2	0	10	5	2	0	15
Caramel (Splenda)	90	8	5	0	15	3	1	1	15
Wax Orchards Fudge Sauces, all	90	0	0	0	0	20	4	18	40

SNACK CAKES, PIES AND SWEET SNACKS

(also see Cakes, pg 70; Pastries and Cofeecakes, pg 37; Pies and Cobblers, pg 83)

Food	Cal	Fat	Sat	TFat	Chol	Carb	Fib	Sug	Sod
Cake, sponge, creme-filled, 1.5 oz	157	5	1	-	7	27	0	17	157
Cupcake, choc w/frosting, 1.5 oz	131	2	0	-	0	29	2	-	178
Cupcake, choc w/frosting, creme-filled, 1.8 oz	188	7	1	-	9	30	0	17	213
Pie, fruit filled, fried, 4.6 oz (avg)	404	21	3	-	0	55	3	27	479
BRANDS . . .									
FROZEN/REFRIGERATED									
Kraft									
Snack Bites									
Choc Covered Strawberry, 1 oz	130	7	3	0	10	15	0	10	55
Turtle, 1 oz	130	7	4	0	10	14	0	10	70
Snack Bars									
Strawberry Cheesecake, 1.5 oz	180	9	3	0	10	22	0	13	80
Classic Cheesecake, 1.5 oz	190	11	3	0	15	20	0	12	85
Marble Brownie, 1.5 oz	170	9	4	0	25	20	1	14	110
SHELF-STABLE									
Dolly Madison Raspberry Zinger, 1.5 oz	160	7	3	-	5	24	0	20	100
Devil's Food Zinger w/Icing	150	5	3	-	10	25	0	18	140
Drake's Coffee Cakes, 1.1 oz	130	6	2	0	5	18	1	12	80
LF Coffee Cakes, 1.1 oz	100	-	-	-	-	20	0	11	105
Pick-m-Ups, 1	250	-	-	-	-	30	1	12	125
Mini Coffee Cakes, 1.8 oz	210	-	-	-	-	32	1	17	130
Entenmann's									
Devil's Food Cookie Cake, 0.5 oz	60	1	0	0	0	13	0	8	40
Hostess									

87

DESDERTS AND SWEETS
Snack Cakes, Pies and Sweet Snacks

Food	Cal	Fat	Sat	TFat	Chol	Carb	Fib	Sug	Sod
Brownie Bites, 1.3 oz (3)	170	9	2	-	30	22	1	17	80
Mini-Muffins, Choc, 1.2 oz	160	9	3	-	20	17	0	9	100

Food	Cal	Fat	Sat	TFat	Chol	Carb	Fib	Sug	Sod
Cinnamon Crumb Cake, LF, 1 oz	80	1	0	-	0	19	0	9	105
Crumb Coffee Cake, 1 oz	130	5	2	-	10	19	0	10	110
Mini-Muffins, Blueberry, 1.2 oz	150	8	1	-	25	18	0	8	110
Mini-Muffins, Banana Walnut, 1.2 oz	230	14	2	-	30	24	1	15	125
Glazed Donettes, 1.5 oz (3)	210	12	6	-	0	22	0	19	140
Lance Fig Cake, LF, 1 oz	90	2	0	0	0	18	1	11	100
Dunking Stick, 1.4 oz	180	9	3	0	5	22	1	15	130
Little Debbie Sugar Wafers	120	6	2	2	0	17	0	13	50
German Choc Rings	140	7	5	0	0	18	1	11	65
Marshmallow Supremes, 1 pkg	140	5	1	0	0	22	1	15	65
Stars/Stripes Marshmallow Puffs, 1.3 oz	170	6	2	0	0	28	0	20	65
Star Crunch Cookies, 1.1 oz	150	6	4	0	0	22	1	13	75
Pecan Pinwheels, 1 oz	100	4	1	0	0	16	0	7	80
Caramel Cookie Bar, 1.2 oz	160	8	2	0	0	22	0	16	85
Fudge Rounds, 1.2 oz	150	4	1	0	0	23	1	14	85
Choc Chip Cream Pies, 1.2 oz	150	6	2	0	0	23	0	13	95
Jelly Creme Pies, 1.2 oz	160	7	2	0	0	23	0	15	100
Frosted Fudge Cake, 1.5 oz	200	10	3	0	5	25	1	18	105
Choc Marshmallow Pie, 1.5 oz	180	7	4	0	0	28	0	15	105
Creme Filled Lemon Cupcakes, 1	210	-	-	-	-	29	0	20	110
Creme Filled Orange Cupcakes, 1	210	-	-	-	-	29	0	22	110
Raisin Creme Pies, 1.2 oz	140	5	1	0	-	23	0	16	120
Smart Snack Angel Cakes, 2 oz	130	-	-	-	-	29	0	23	125
Nutty Bars, 2 oz (2)	310	18	7	0	0	33	1	22	115
Frosted Fudge Cakes, 1.5 oz	190	9	5	0	5	26	1	19	125
Fudge Brownies, 2.1 oz	270	12	3	0	10	39	1	22	140
Rice Dream Vanilla Pie, 1	290	-	-	-	-	37	2	12	70
Salerno Scooter Pie, 1.2 oz	140	5	3	0	-	23	0	14	80
Tastykake									
Kreamies, Banana, 1.5 oz	170	8	2	2	5	25	0	18	100
Kandy Kakes, Choc, 2 oz	270	15	9	2	0	35	2	25	115
Kandy Kakes, Peanut Butter, 2 oz	270	16	8	0	15	30	2	22	115
Kreamies, Choc, 1.5 oz	190	9	3	2	50	26	0	18	130

Food Food	Cal	Fat	Sat	TFat	Chol	Carb	Fib	Sug	Sod

DINNERS, ENTREES AND SIDE DISHES

APPETIZERS AND SNACKS

	Cal	Fat	Sat	TFat	Chol	Carb	Fib	Sug	Sod
Egg roll, 3 oz	160	4	1	0	0	23	2	0	390
Pizza snacks, cheese, 3 oz	210	8	3	0	10	25	1	4	420
Chicken wings, spicy, 3 oz	240	16	4	0	70	10	0	1	300
Cheese nuggets, 3 oz (6)	210	11	4	0	10	20	2	3	950

BRANDS . . .

FROZEN/REFRIGERATED

Athens Fillo Hors D'oeuvres

	Cal	Fat	Sat	TFat	Chol	Carb	Fib	Sug	Sod
Artichoke & Cheese, 1 oz (2)	50	4	2	0	10	2	0	0	140

Health is Wealth

	Cal	Fat	Sat	TFat	Chol	Carb	Fib	Sug	Sod
Spinach Munchies, 1 oz (2)	60	3	0	0	0	9	1	0	105
Mexican Munchies, 1 oz (2)	49	1	0	0	0	8	1	0	110
Spinach & Feta Munchies, 1 oz (2)	70	3	1	0	5	9	1	0	115
Nancy's Mini Cheese Souffle, 1 oz (2)	127	10	6	0	187	4	0	1	107

Twin Marquis

	Cal	Fat	Sat	TFat	Chol	Carb	Fib	Sug	Sod
Thai Curry Samosas, 1.3 oz (2)	50	6	1	0	10	8	2	2	70

BLINTZES AND CREPES

	Cal	Fat	Sat	TFat	Chol	Carb	Fib	Sug	Sod
Fruit, 2.2 oz	100	3	1	0	3	13	3	6	130
Cheese, 2.2 oz	100	3	1	0	10	15	2	4	155
Potato, 2.2 oz	95	3	1	0	5	16	2	2	265

BRANDS . . . *(2.2 OZ UNLESS NOTED)*

FROZEN/REFRIGERATED

CREPES

	Cal	Fat	Sat	TFat	Chol	Carb	Fib	Sug	Sod
Tuv Taam Apple Cinnamon Crepes	110	2	-	-	0	21	-	-	90

FRUIT BLINTZES

Most brands are within the generic range, the following have less than the generic.

	Cal	Fat	Sat	TFat	Chol	Carb	Fib	Sug	Sod
Flaum Cheese & Blueberry, 3 oz	135	4	-	0	0	22	-	-	105
Ratner's Cherry or Blueberry (avg)	90	1	0	25	0	19	0	6	95

OTHER BLINTZ VARIETIES

Flaum Potato, Potato Spinach, or

	Cal	Fat	Sat	TFat	Chol	Carb	Fib	Sug	Sod
Cheese, 3 oz (avg)	110	4	-	0	-	16	-	-	110
Golden Cheese	80	2	1	0	13	13	2	5	135
Potato	90	4	1	0	5	-	2	2	170
Kineret Potato	70	2	0	0	0	12	0	0	110
Cheese	65	1	0	0	0	12	0	1	120

89

DINNERS, ENTREES AND SIDE DISHES
Breakfast Meals

Food	Cal	Fat	Sat	TFat	Chol	Carb	Fib	Sug	Sod
BLINTZES AND CREPES - OTHER BLINTZ VARIETIES (CONT'D)									
King Kold Apple, 2.2 oz	80	1	0	-	25	13	0	4	100
Cheese, 2.5 oz	90	2	1	-	30	13	0	5	160
Ratner's Potato, 2.5 oz	80	3	0	0	25	13	0	0	170
Tuv Taam Apple Cinnamon Crepes	110	2	-	-	0	21	-	-	90
Diet Cheese/Cherry Blintzes	100	3	-	-	0	15	-	-	90
Cheese Blintzes, Sugar Free	70	3	-	-	0	12	-	-	105
Cheese Blintzes	95	3	-	-	0	13	-	-	110
Potato Blintzes	115	4	-	-	0	18	-	-	110

BREAKFAST MEALS

(also see French Toast, pg 35; Pancakes & Waffles, pg 36)

Food	Cal	Fat	Sat	TFat	Chol	Carb	Fib	Sug	Sod
Breakfast burrito, ham/cheese, 3.5 oz	212	7	2	0	192	28	1	-	405
French Toast & sausage, 5.6 oz	415	23	7	0	98	38	2	-	502
Scrambled eggs & sausage w/hash brown potatoes, 6.3 oz	361	27	7	0	283	17	1	-	772
Sausage biscuit, 3.4 oz	385	22	7	0	32	23	1	-	881

BRANDS . . .

FROZEN/REFRIGERATED

Food	Cal	Fat	Sat	TFat	Chol	Carb	Fib	Sug	Sod
Amy's									
Tofu Scramble Pocket Sandwich, 4 oz	180	6	0	0	0	23	1	2	520
Breakfast Burrito, 6 oz	250	7	1	0	0	38	5	4	540
Bob Evans Brunch Bowls Stuffed French Toast, Apples & Cream Cheese, 10 oz	460	17	9	0	125	70	2	42	480
Cedarlane Zone, Spinach & Mushroom Omelette, 10.1 oz	320	13	7	0	30	29	2	4	510
Chef's Omelet Western Style, 4.4 oz	150	9	3	0	130	6	0	0	440
Health is Wealth									
Breakfast Munchies, all, 1 oz (avg)	70	4	0	0	0	9	1	1	190
Hot Pockets Bacon, Egg & Cheese, 2.3 oz	170	9	4	0	45	17	1	6	260
Sausage, Egg, Cheese, 2.3 oz	180	10	4	0	35	16	1	6	260
LF Bacon, Egg & Cheese, 2.3 oz	150	5	2	0	40	21	2	2	280
Jimmy Dean French Toast & Sausage Sandwich, 3.7 oz	300	18	6	0	85	25	3	9	410
Lean Pockets Sausage/Egg/Cheese, 9 oz	140	5	2	0	45	19	2	4	310
Purnell's Sausage & Biscuits, 3 oz	280	16	5	0	30	30	1	2	250
South Beach Diet									
Veg Medley Wrap, 4.6 oz (1)	160	6	3	0	5	26	15	2	430
Southwestern Style Wrap, 4.6 oz (1)	160	5	2	0	10	26	15	2	520

Food Food	Cal	Fat	Sat	TFat	Chol	Carb	Fib	Sug	Sod
BREAKFAST MEALS (CONT'D)									
Swanson *Great Starts*									
Sausage Burrito, 3.5 oz	240	12	4	0	90	24	1	2	500
Bacon Burrito, 3.5 oz	250	11	4	0	90	27	1	3	540
Swift Premium *Morning Makers*									
Sausage, Egg & Cheese, 3.5 oz	250	10	5	0	55	31	3	5	370
Weight Watchers Smart Ones									
English Muffin Sandwich, 4 oz	200	5	2	0	15	27	2	2	480

⬡ ENTREES AND MEALS – CANNED

	Cal	Fat	Sat	TFat	Chol	Carb	Fib	Sug	Sod
Beef stew, 8.3 oz	220	12	5	0	37	16	4	2	947
Spaghetti & meatballs, 8.6 oz	247	10	4	0	19	30	7	10	1003
Macaroni & cheese, 8.7 oz	200	6	2	0	15	28	1	1	1027

BRANDS . . .
Most brands are within the generic range.

⬡ ENTREES AND MEALS – FROZEN/REFRIGERATED

ASIAN

DINNERS

	Cal	Fat	Sat	TFat	Chol	Carb	Fib	Sug	Sod
Chicken chow mein w/egg roll, 9 oz	210	7	4	0	30	28	3	3	850
Oriental beef, 9 oz	250	7	4	0	30	31	3	3	960
Chicken teriyaki rice bowl, 10.9 oz	430	6	1	0	25	77	1	-	1210
BRANDS . . . *(10 OZ UNLESS NOTED)*									
Amy's Organic *Lite in Sodium*, Brown Rice									
& Veg Bowl	250	8	1	0	0	36	5	7	250
Thai Stir Fry, 9.5 oz	310	11	7	0	0	45	5	2	420
Healthy Choice Mandarin Chicken	280	4	1	0	35	43	4	9	520
Lean Cuisine									
Asian Style Beef, 9.3 oz	200	3	2	0	25	29	3	8	550
Organic Classics Chicken Thai Curry	390	17	6	0	55	42	2	4	330

SKILLET MEALS AND DINNER HELPERS

BRANDS . . .	Cal	Fat	Sat	TFat	Chol	Carb	Fib	Sug	Sod
Annie Chun's *Noodle Express*, 3.7 oz									
Thai Peanut	200	7	1	0	0	39	1	5	300
Spicy Szechuan	170	3	0	0	0	29	1	4	470
Teriyaki or Chinese Chow Mein (avg)	160	3	0	0	0	29	1	4	510
Singapore Curry	160	3	0	0	0	28	2	3	550
Bird's Eye									
Voila! Garlic Shrimp, 6.4 oz	220	8	2	2	10	27	2	6	510

DINNERS, ENTREES AND SIDE DISHES
Dinners and Entrees – Frozen/Refrigerated (Fish and Seafood)

Food	Cal	Fat	Sat	TFat	Chol	Carb	Fib	Sug	Sod
FISH AND SEAFOOD									
DINNERS									
Baked lemon pepper fish dinner, 9.1 oz	220	6	2	0	40	55	7	10	630
Seafood scampi, 12 oz	410	12	5	0	75	56	5	5	1050
BRANDS . . .									
Michelino's Lean Gourmet									
Shrimp w/Pasta & Vegetables, 8 oz	260	6	4	0	55	38	2	5	530
Mrs Paul's Sweet/Sour Shrimp Bowl, 11 oz	310	1	1	0	95	65	1	16	500
PREPARED ENTREES									
Fish sticks, breaded, 3 oz	195	10	2	0	23	17	0	2	315
Fillets, battered or breaded, 3 oz	280	18	3	0	28	20	0	4	568
Popcorn shrimp, 3.2 oz	240	12	4	0	55	24	0	2	630
Crab cakes, 3 oz.......................................	233	14	3	0	115	7	0	-	688
BRANDS . . . *(4 OZ UNLESS NOTED)*									
Dr. Praeger's									
Minced Fish Sticks, 1.7 oz	110	6	1	0	15	10	1	0	170
Fishies, Breaded Fillets, or Sticks, 2.9 oz .	150	6	2	0	15	16	1	1	290
Gorton's Grilled Fillets									
Lemon Butter or Char Grilled, 3.9 oz	100	3	1	0	60	1	0	0	250
Caesar Parmesan, 3.9 oz	100	3	1	0	60	1	0	0	250
Garlic Butter or Italian Herb, 3.9 oz (avg) ..	100	3	1	0	60	1	0	0	275
Grilled Salmon, Classic Grilled, 3.2 oz	100	4	1	0	20	1	0	1	310
Cajun Blackened, 3.9 oz	100	3	1	0	60	1	0	0	330
Ian's Fish Sticks, 3.3 oz (5)	190	6	1	0	15	24	1	3	310
Kineret Crunchy Fish Portions, 2	260	10	2	-	35	29	1	1	270
Fish Cakes, 2	160	6	1	-	5	23	1	0	310
Mrs. Pauls Flounder Fillets, 2.8 oz (1)	150	7	4	0	25	12	0	1	190
Tenders, Beer Battered, 2.8 oz	130	2	0	0	20	19	0	3	320
PubHouse Battered Halibut, 4 oz	200	9	1	0	25	12	2	2	250
SeaPak									
Coconut Shrimp, Oven, 3.7 oz	310	14	4	0	65	36	1	19	140
Coconut Shrimp, Fry Only, 3.9 oz	220	4	3	0	85	30	2	9	150
Van de Kamp's									
Fish Sticks, Crunchy Breaded, 3.6 oz (6) .	240	12	2	0	25	20	0	2	330
Crunchy Fish Fillets, 3.5 oz (2)	250	15	3	0	25	19	0	2	350
SKILLET MEALS AND DINNER HELPERS									
Shrimp scampi, 12 oz	500	25	10	0	95	39	3	0	1230
BRANDS . . .									
Bird's Eye *Voila!* Garlic Shrimp, 6.4 oz	220	8	2	0	10	27	2	6	510
Chef's Choice Shrimp Linguini, 1 1/3 cup ..	170	1	0	-	40	30	4	2	450

Food	Cal	Fat	Sat	TFat	Chol	Carb	Fib	Sug	Sod
HISPANIC									
DINNERS									
Beef enchiladas w/beans & rice, 11 oz	360	11	5	0	20	55	9	7	1390
Tamales, beef enchiladas w/beans & rice, 13.4 oz	508	20	7	0	26	68	8	5	1812
BRANDS...									
Cedarlane									
LF Bean/Tofu Enchilada Meal, 9 oz	220	3	0	0	0	42	6	3	390
Zone, Cheese/Veg Enchiladas, 9.6 oz	300	12	4	0	15	32	7	6	540
Lean Cuisine Chicken Enchilada, 9 oz	270	5	2	0	20	47	3	7	510
PREPARED ENTREES									
Bean and cheese burrito, 5 oz	340	9	3	0	4	52	8	0	600
Beef and bean chimichanga, 5 oz	380	17	6	0	25	32	2	1	810
BRANDS...									
Amy's Organic *Lite in Sodium*									
Black Bean Enchilada, 4.75 oz	160	6	1	0	0	22	3	2	190
Cedarlane Garden Veg Enchilada, 4.5 oz	140	3	2	0	10	20	3	4	310
Chicken Taquitos, Corn, 5 oz (5)	300	10	2	0	25	37	1	1	340
Zone, Bean & Cheese Burrito, 6 oz	350	13	5	0	15	37	8	3	380
Cheese Enchilada, 4.8 oz	270	17	9	0	45	19	2	3	390
LF Veg Enchilada, 5 oz	180	3	2	0	10	26	2	2	390
Quesadilla w/Pico de Gallo, 3 oz (1)	250	11	6	-	25	27	0	4	420
Beef Taquitos, Corn, 5 oz (5)	260	10	2	0	30	31	2	1	420
Delimex Seasoned Beef & Cheddar Rolled Tacos, 5 oz (5)	360	16	5	0	15	44	8	1	370
El Monterey Bean/Cheese Burrito, 4.6 oz	220	6	2	0	5	34	4	1	360
Beef & Cheese Chimichanga, 5 oz	330	15	5	0	30	35	1	1	350
Steak & Cheese Burrito, 5 oz	290	10	4	0	30	37	1	1	370
Grilled Chicken Fajita, 5 oz	280	7	2	0	20	44	2	1	410
Grilled Chicken & 3 Cheese Quesadilla, 3.5 oz (1)	260	14	8	0	35	20	1	1	420
Charbroiled Steak Burrito, 5 oz	290	9	3	0	25	39	1	1	460
Health is Wealth Quesadilla Rolls, 3 oz	130	3	1	0	5	18	3	0	270
Jose Ole Beef & Cheese Mini Tacquitos, 3 oz (4)	180	8	2	0	5	21	2	1	390
Beef/Cheese Mini Tacos, 3 oz (4)	200	11	4	0	20	19	3	1	390
Beef/Cheese Taquitos, Flour 3 oz (2)	220	10	3	0	10	24	1	1	430
Chicken Taquitos, 3 oz (3)	180	8	1	0	10	23	2	0	430
Chicken/Cheese Taquitos, Flour 3 oz (2)	220	10	3	0	15	25	1	1	430
Shredded Beef Taquitos, Corn 3 oz (3)	180	7	2	0	5	24	2	0	440

DINNERS, ENTREES AND SIDE DISHES

Dinners and Entrees – Frozen/Refrigerated (International/Middle Eastern)

Food	Cal	Fat	Sat	TFat	Chol	Carb	Fib	Sug	Sod
HISPANIC - FROZEN ENTREES (CONT'D)									
Reser's Spicy Chicken Burrito, 4 oz	250	7	2	0	15	37	2	0	380
Senor Felix's Sonora Style Burrito, 1	280	8	2	0	10	45	3	4	240
SKILLET MEALS									
BRANDS ...									
Tyson Chicken Fajitas, 3.8 oz (1)	130	4	1	0	15	17	2	3	350
Chicken Quesadilla, 4 oz (1)	250	10	-	0	35	26	-	-	430
INTERNATIONAL/MIDDLE EASTERN									
DINNERS									
BRANDS ...									
Ethnic Gourmet Shahi Paneer, 12 oz	510	25	10	0	30	52	4	16	500
Lemongrass & Basil Chicken, 11 oz	400	11	7	0	40	53	4	11	540
PREPARED ENTREES									
Pierogi, potato & cheese, 4 oz	250	8	2	-	35	38	1	10	430
BRANDS ...									
Deep Indian Gourmet									
Dal Masala Curry, 5 oz	200	9	1	0	0	24	7	5	420
Golden Gourmet Pierogies									
Potato & Onion, 4 oz (3)	182	3	1	0	36	34	1	9	195
Potato & Cheese, 4 oz (3)	240	5	2	0	5	33	1	2	259
Kohinoor Aloo Ki Sabzi, 3.6 oz	83	3	0	0	0	13	3	0	261
Mrs. T's Pierogies									
Potato & Chedder, Mini, 3 oz (7)	130	2	1	0	5	25	1	1	360
Potato & 4 Cheese, Mini, 3 oz (7)	150	5	1	0	5	27	1	1	390
Potato & Onion, 4.3 oz (3)	170	2	0	0	5	34	1	1	420
Potato, Cheddar & Bacon, Mini, 3 oz (7) ..	140	3	1	0	5	25	1	1	450
MEAT AND POULTRY									
DINNERS									
Beef w/gravy, mashed potatoes, 9.1 oz	270	10	4	0	71	19	4	12	742
Veal parmigiana w/tomato sauce, mashed potatoes & peas, 9.1 oz..............	362	19	6	0	26	35	7	15	964
Turkey w/gravy, stuffing, mashed potatoes & corn, 9.4 oz	280	10	3	0	52	34	3	7	1061
Salisbury steak w/mashed potatoes & corn, 9.6 oz...	398	25	9	0	51	28	3	7	1140
Fried chicken w/mashed potatoes & corn, 8.1 oz...	470	27	9	0	89	35	2	3	1500
Meatloaf w/gravy & mashed potaotes, 14 oz..	460	34	10	0	80	39	9	7	1510

Food Food	Cal	Fat	Sat	TFat	Chol	Carb	Fib	Sug	Sod

MEAT AND POULTY - FROZEN DINNERS (CONT'D)

BRANDS . . .

Healthy Choice

Food	Cal	Fat	Sat	TFat	Chol	Carb	Fib	Sug	Sod
Mesquite Chicken BBQ, 10.5 oz	300	5	2	0	45	44	5	14	480
Chicken Broccoli Alfredo, 11.5 oz	300	7	3	0	50	34	2	5	530
Chicken Breast & Vegetables, 10.5 oz	230	5	2	0	25	29	6	3	550
Beef Pot Roast, 11 oz	320	9	3	0	45	39	6	24	550

Lean Cuisine

Food	Cal	Fat	Sat	TFat	Chol	Carb	Fib	Sug	Sod
Chicken a L'Orange, 9 oz	230	2	1	0	35	35	2	10	340
Steak Tips Portobello, 7.5 oz	180	7	2	0	40	13	3	4	460
Chicken w/Basil Cream, 8.5 oz	280	7	3	0	35	34	2	5	470
Glazed Chicken, 8.5 oz	210	4	1	0	40	25	0	5	510
Three Cheese Chicken, 8 oz	230	10	3	0	45	14	2	5	520
On-Cor Chicken & Pasta, 1 cup	150	5	2	0	15	19	1	3	400

Organic Classics

Food	Cal	Fat	Sat	TFat	Chol	Carb	Fib	Sug	Sod
Rice Pilaf & Chicken w/BBQ Sauce, 9 oz	330	4	1	0	50	52	2	6	240
Chicken Cacciatore, 10 oz	340	11	2	0	50	37	3	6	410
Cajun Style ChickenTetrazzini, 10 oz	370	12	5	0	55	43	3	3	470
Chicken Marsala, 9.6 oz	350	15	8	1	70	30	3	3	510

Michelino's Lean Gourmet

Food	Cal	Fat	Sat	TFat	Chol	Carb	Fib	Sug	Sod
Glazed Chicken, 8 oz	260	4	1	0	20	43	2	8	470

Weight Watchers Smart Ones

Food	Cal	Fat	Sat	TFat	Chol	Carb	Fib	Sug	Sod
Apple Glazed Pork Medallions, 10.8 oz	310	6	3	0	35	15	4	15	450
Fiesta Chicken, 8.6 oz	250	2	1	0	25	45	2	3	460
Honey Dijon Chicken, 8.6 oz	220	4	1	0	30	38	2	8	460
Grilled Chicken in Garlic Sauce, 9.1 oz	190	8	2	0	50	10	2	4	490
Chicken Marsala, 9 oz	180	7	1	0	50	10	2	4	530
Chicken Mirabella, 9.3 oz	180	2	1	0	15	33	3	4	550
Roast Turkey Medallions, 9.1 oz	220	2	0	0	55	38	3	1	550
Roast Beef w/Gravy. 9.1 oz	210	9	3	0	45	19	2	1	550
Lean Cuisine Steak Tips Portobello, 7.5 oz	180	7	2	0	40	13	3	4	460

PREPARED ENTREES

Food	Cal	Fat	Sat	TFat	Chol	Carb	Fib	Sug	Sod
Barbecue beef w/sauce, 2.1 oz	130	7	3	0	30	11	0	10	270
Turkey roll, light meat, 2 oz	84	4	1	0	25	0	0	0	279
Chicken roll, light meat, 2 oz	88	4	1	0	29	1	0	0	333
Turkey roll, light and dark meat, 2 oz	85	4	1	0	31	1	0	0	334
Chicken, barbecued w/gravy, 2.1 oz	130	6	2	0	40	11	0	10	340
Chicken breast, oven-roasted, 1.5 oz	33	0	0	0	15	1	0	0	457
Popcorn chicken, 3 oz	190	9	2	0	20	18	1	2	510
Turkey, smoked, cooked, light or dark, 2 oz	95	3	0	0	27	1	0	0	558

DINNERS, ENTREES AND SIDE DISHES
Dinners and Entrees – Frozen/Refrigerated (Meat and Poultry)

Food	Cal	Fat	Sat	TFat	Chol	Carb	Fib	Sug	Sod
MEAT AND POULTRY - FROZEN ENTREES (CONT'D)									
Pot roast, 5 oz	170	5	1	0	55	10	0	3	590
Beef w/gravy, 5 oz	160	7	3	0	55	5	1	3	760
Chicken breast w/broccoli & cheese, 6 oz	240	10	6	0	90	7	1	2	780
Meatloaf, 5 oz	240	12	6	0	55	14	0	7	790
Turkey breast w/gravy, 5.6 oz	130	3	1	0	45	4	0	2	1010
BRANDS . . . *(3 OZ UNLESS NOTED)*									
Most brands are within the generic range, the following are less than the generic:									
Fast Fixin' Chicken Tenders	140	11	2	0	10	4	0	0	160
BBQ Ribz for Sandwiches	120	7	3	0	25	8	1	3	280
Mesquite Grilled Chicken Breast, 2.8 oz	120	5	2	0	55	1	0	1	290
Philly Style Chicken Steak, 3.5 oz	120	5	2	0	35	2	0	1	290
Fajita Grilled Chicken Breast, 2.8 oz	120	6	2	0	55	2	0	1	310
Health Is Wealth Chicken Tenders	150	6	2	0	40	9	0	0	180
Ian's Chicken Nuggets, 8 oz	440	14	2	0	50	60	2	21	320
Tyson's									
Breaded Chicken Breast Tenders	220	13	3	0	35	13	2	13	250
SKILLET MEALS AND DINNER HELPERS									
Birds Eye *Voila!*									
Alfredo Chicken, 7.3 oz	320	17	10	0	60	26	2	5	480
Roasted Garlic Chicken & Veg, 7.9 oz	120	3	1	0	30	13	3	4	520
Lean Cuisine *Skillets*									
Three Cheese Chicken	200	5	2	0	20	25	3	5	420
Chicken Alfredo	190	5	2	0	25	25	3	5	490
Chicken Primavera	180	3	1	0	15	28	3	4	530
PASTA/ITALIAN *(also see Pasta Sauce, pg 100)*									
DINNERS									
Spaghetti w/meat sauce, 10 oz	255	3	1	0	17	43	5	7	473
Fettuccine alfredo, 10 oz	653	39	16	0	64	58	2	4	902
Macaroni & cheese, 12 oz	370	15	8	0	0	38	48	26	1070
Lasagne w/meat sauce, 10.5 oz	370	14	7	0	45	39	4	6	1050
BRANDS . . . *(11 OZ UNLESS NOTED)*									
Amy's Organic, *Lite in Sodium,*									
Veg Lasagna, 9.5 oz	290	8	4	0	15	41	4	8	340
Macaroni & Soy Cheese, 9 oz	370	15	2	0	0	42	4	2	500
Celentano Baked Ziti, 8 oz	460	10	4	0	20	72	6	7	410
Eggplant Parmigiana, 8 oz	380	24	6	0	30	30	6	11	550
Healthy Choice									
Stuffed Pasta Shells, 11.2 oz	290	6	3	0	20	40	5	10	470

Food Food	Cal	Fat	Sat	TFat	Chol	Carb	Fib	Sug	Sod
PASTA/ITALIAN - FROZEN DINNERS (CONT'D)									
Lean Cuisine									
Penne Pasta w/Tomato Basil, 10 oz	270	3	1	0	0	52	4	12	220
Macaroni & Beef, 9.5 oz	250	5	2	0	15	36	4	11	550
Spaghetti w/Meat Sauce, 11.5 oz	280	4	1	0	15	49	4	9	550
Michael Angelo's									
Sausage, Onions & Peppers									
Lasagna, 1 cup	230	7	3	0	10	31	4	9	340
Bowls									
Angel Hair Pomodoro, 7 oz	200	5	1	0	0	34	5	10	390
Chicken Rosemary, 6 oz	250	8	4	0	15	30	3	6	390
Chicken Milano, 7 oz	290	11	6	0	20	30	5	9	430
Angel Hair & Shrimp, 7 oz	200	6	2	0	30	28	3	12	470
Meat Lasagna, 1 cup	290	10	8	0	50	26	4	5	490
Moosewood Pasta e Fagioli, 10 oz	260	4	1	0	0	57	6	8	340
Spicy Penne Puttanesca, 10 oz	300	10	2	0	0	45	2	5	380
Weight Watchers Smart Ones									
Radiatore Romano, 10.5 oz	290	7	3	0	15	43	4	8	490
Lemon Herb Chicken Piccata, 9.1 oz	250	5	2	0	45	36	2	3	510
Penne Pollo, 10.1 oz	280	6	3	0	45	39	3	5	510
Three Cheese Ziti Marinara, 9.1 oz	290	7	3	0	10	44	4	2	430
Angel Hair Marinara, 9.1 oz	230	2	1	0	25	41	2	8	540
Lasagna Bolognese, 9.1 oz	270	4	2	0	15	43	3	3	540
PREPARED ENTREES									
Bernardi Traditional Stuffed Shells,									
2.8 oz	140	6	4	0	40	12	0	1	260
Cedarlane Eggplant Parmesan, 5 oz	160	8	3	0	15	16	3	3	390
Celentano Mini Cheese Ravioli, 4 oz (12)	220	3	2	0	25	36	2	0	190
Light Cheese Ravioli, 4.4 oz (4)	220	2	1	0	20	38	2	2	250
Large Cheese Ravioli, 4.4 oz (4)	230	4	2	0	30	36	2	0	270
Large Beef Ravioli, 3 oz (3)	170	8	4	0	60	17	1	0	360
DiGiorno Lemon Chicken Tortellini	260	5	3	0	30	40	1	2	310
Three Cheese Tortellini, 3 oz	250	5	2	0	25	41	2	3	320
Michael Angelo's Stuffed Shells, 4 oz	210	9	6	0	40	18	1	1	260
Cheese Ravioli, 4 oz	218	8	4	0	35	27	2	7	273
Eggplant Parmesan, 6 oz	280	19	3	0	40	23	4	5	330
Manicotti w/Sauce, 6 oz	230	12	6	0	55	11	5	5	390
Monterey Pasta Co Ravioli, 3.6 oz									
Whole Wheat Chicken/Sun-Dried Tomato	230	5	2	0	40	34	4	2	180
Whole Wheat Tomato/Basil/Mozzarella	250	7	4	0	35	34	4	1	250
Seafood	250	8	4	0	75	30	6	1	270

DINNERS, ENTREES AND SIDE DISHES
Dinners and Entrees – Frozen/Refrigerated (Quiches, Pies and Souffles)

Food	Cal	Fat	Sat	TFat	Chol	Carb	Fib	Sug	Sod
PASTA/ITALIAN - *FROZEN ENTREES (MONTEREY PASTA CO CONT'D)*									
Whole Wheat Classic Italian Cheese	290	6	3	0	35	48	5	1	290
Carb Smart Seafood	220	9	5	0	125	18	5	1	330
Whole Wheat Veg & Cheese	240	6	2	0	25	35	4	1	340
Spinach Ricotta	250	9	4	0	60	30	7	1	350
Putney Pasta									
Sun-Dried Tomato Tortellini, 1 cup	330	7	0	0	45	50	0	0	240
Black Bean Habanero Ravioli, 1 cup	180	0	0	0	0	38	3	4	250
Mushroom Gruyere Tortellini, 1 cup	290	4	0	0	60	42	0	0	250
Butternut Squash Ravioli, 1 cup	200	4	0	0	30	35	0	0	270
Rosetto Toasted Cheese Ravioli, 4 oz	230	10	3	0	10	28	1	2	270
Italian Sausage Ravioli, 4 oz	250	6	3	0	20	38	2	2	280
Cheese Ravioli, square, 4 oz	250	6	4	0	10	37	2	7	290
Chicken Ravioli, 4 oz	230	4	1	0	25	37	2	4	300
Cheese Tortellini, 4 oz	270	6	4	0	40	40	1	2	330
Beef Ravioli, square, 4 oz	270	6	3	0	10	41	2	1	350
Cheese Ravioli, round, 4 oz	260	8	5	0	20	36	1	6	390
SoyBoy Ravioli, all, 3.6 oz (avg)	180	3	1	0	0	30	3	2	130

PIZZA *(see Pizza, pg 102)*

POCKETS *(see Pockets, Sandwiches and Wraps, pg 105)*

QUICHES, PIES AND SOUFFLES

Food	Cal	Fat	Sat	TFat	Chol	Carb	Fib	Sug	Sod
Turkey pot pie, 7 oz	350	18	6	-	32	35	2	-	695
Beef pot pie, 7 oz	449	24	9	-	38	44	2	-	737
Chicken pot pie, 7.8 oz	484	29	10	-	41	43	2	8	857
BRANDS . . .									
Amy's Organic Shepherd's Pie, 8 oz	160	4	0	0	0	27	5	5	490
Fillo Factory Broccoli/Cheese Pie, 1/5	280	15	7	0	30	26	2	2	430
Spinach & Cheese, 1/5	240	11	5	0	20	27	2	1	490
Ian's Shepherd's Pie, 1/2	250	11	2	0	25	23	2	4	350
Shelton's Organic Chicken, 9 oz	260	13	7	0	65	20	2	2	280
Turkey w/white or whole wheat flour, 9 oz	220	10	5	0	50	18	3	0	360
Chicken w/white or whole wheat flour, 9 oz	230	10	5	0	55	18	1	0	370

VEGETARIAN

DINNERS

Food	Cal	Fat	Sat	TFat	Chol	Carb	Fib	Sug	Sod
BRANDS . . . *(10 OZ UNLESS NOTED)*									
Amy's, *Lite in Sodium*, Veggie Loaf	280	7	1	0	0	47	7	6	340
Hain Vegetarian Classics									
Meatless Ravioli in Marinara	220	3	0	-	0	40	8	10	200

Food Food	Cal	Fat	Sat	TFat	Chol	Carb	Fib	Sug	Sod
VEGETARIAN - FROZEN DINNERS (HAIN CONT'D)									
Homestyle Meatloaf	300	6	1	-	0	39	16	8	400
Pepper Steak	310	6	1	-	0	41	9	8	440
Hawaiian Nuggets w/Pineapple	310	5	1	-	0	55	6	14	495
Healthy Choice									
Cheddar Broccoli Potatoes, 10.5 oz	280	7	3	0	25	41	6	8	550
Moosewood Moroccan Stew	160	3	0	0	0	3	04	10	370
Weight Watchers Smart Ones									
Cheddar Broccoli Potatoes	280	7	3	0	25	41	6	8	550

ENTREES AND MEALS -- SHELF-STABLE

Macaroni & cheese, boxed, 1 cup	420	19	5	0	15	50	2	7	750

BRANDS . . .

ASIAN

Thai Kitchen Noodle Cart, Thai Peanut	265	7	1	0	0	47	0	16	200

DINNER MIXES AND HELPERS *(also see Pasta Entrees, pg ??)*

Tuna mix/helper, cheese, 1 cup	290	11	2	-	20	32	1	2	890
Hamburger mix/helper, cheese, 1 cup	310	15	2	-	60	30	1	2	920
Shrimp stir fry, 9.8 oz	200	2	0	-	105	28	5	17	1330

BRANDS . . .
Most brands are within the generic range.

MEAT AND POULTRY
Annie's Homegrown

Cheddar & Herb Chicken, 1 cup	310	2	1	0	5	27	1	3	330

My Own Meal

Chicken Mediterranean, 1 pkg	270	9	2	0	45	28	4	-	320

PASTA *(also see Pasta Entrees, pg 100)*
Annie's Homegrown *Pasta Meal*

Curly Fettucine w/White Cheddar & Broccoli Sauce, 1 cup	250	3	2	0	5	48	1	2	450
DeBoles Rice Shells & Chedder, 1/4 pkg	100	2	1	0	5	19	0	0	100
Near East Basil & Herb Pasta	240	2	1	0	0	38	2	1	430
Road's End Organics									
Dairy-Free Mac & Cheese, Original	230	2	0	0	0	44	8	2	280
Mac & Cheese, Alfredo	300	2	0	0	0	62	5	1	290

FISH AND SEAFOOD ENTREES

(see Fish and Seafood – Frozen/Refrigerated Prepared Entrees, pg 92)

DINNERS, ENTREES AND SIDE DISHES
Pasta Entrees

Food	Cal	Fat	Sat	TFat	Chol	Carb	Fib	Sug	Sod

MEAT AND POULTRY ENTREES

(see Meat and Poultry and Substitutes – Prepared Entrees, pg 95)

PASTA ENTREES

(also see Entrees and Meals – Shelf-Stable, pg 99)

PASTA – DRY *(see Pasta and Noodles, pg 135)*

PASTA SAUCE

Food	Cal	Fat	Sat	TFat	Chol	Carb	Fib	Sug	Sod
Red clam sauce, 1/2 cup	60	1	0	0	10	8	1	4	350
Alfredo sauce, 1/4 cup	110	10	5	0	35	3	0	1	420
White clam sauce, 1/2 cup	140	10	2	0	15	5	0	1	510
Marinara, ready-to-eat, 1/2 cup	93	3	0	0	0	14	1	11	601
Pesto, sun-dried tomato, 1/4 cup	110	8	2	0	5	8	2	4	710
Pesto, basil, 1/4 cup	240	23	4	0	5	5	2	2	730
Spaghetti sauce, mix, prep, 1/2 cup	28	0	0	0	0	6	0	-	848

BRANDS ...
NOTE: Although many of the pasta sauces listed below exceed sodium guidelines, they are less than the generic.

ALFREDO SAUCE

READY-TO-USE *(1/4 CUP UNLESS NOTED)*

Food	Cal	Fat	Sat	TFat	Chol	Carb	Fib	Sug	Sod
Classico Four Cheese Alfredo	80	7	4	0	35	3	0	1	350
Five Brothers Tomato Alfredo	70	4	3	0	0	7	1	6	340
Frank Sinatra Alfredo	160	14	3	0	5	4	0	2	310
Ragu Cheese Creations Classic Alfredo	110	10	4	0	25	3	0	1	340
Walden Farms Calorie Free	0	0	0	0	0	0	0	0	20

CLAM SAUCE

READY-TO-USE *(1/2 CUP UNLESS NOTED)*

Food	Cal	Fat	Sat	TFat	Chol	Carb	Fib	Sug	Sod
Progresso White Clam	130	9	2	0	15	1	0	0	310

MARINARA/PASTA SAUCE

FROZEN/REFRIGERATED *(1/2 CUP UNLESS NOTED)*

Food	Cal	Fat	Sat	TFat	Chol	Carb	Fib	Sug	Sod
Di Giorno Marinara	70	0	0	0	0	15	2	10	220
Plum Tomato/Mushroom	60	0	0	0	0	13	2	10	260
Roasted Garlic	70	2	0	0	0	12	2	8	310

MIX *(1/2 CUP UNLESS NOTED)*

Food	Cal	Fat	Sat	TFat	Chol	Carb	Fib	Sug	Sod
Bernard LS, prep	55	0	0	0	0	14	0	4	140

READY-TO-USE *(1/2 CUP UNLESS NOTED)*

Food	Cal	Fat	Sat	TFat	Chol	Carb	Fib	Sug	Sod
365 Organic Pasta Sauce	70	4	0	0	0	10	1	8	270
Organic FF Pasta Sauce	45	0	0	0	0	10	1	8	270
Amy's LS Marinara	40	1	0	0	0	7	1	5	100
Aunt Millie's Tomato & Herb	70	3	1	0	0	9	2	7	320

Food Food	Cal	Fat	Sat	TFat	Chol	Carb	Fib	Sug	Sod
MARINARA/PASTA SAUCE (CONT'D)									
Carb Fit Portobello Mushroom Pasta	60	3	0	0	0	7	2	2	330
Casa Visco FF	30	0	0	0	0	6	1	3	110
Homestyle	90	3	1	0	0	12	3	0	150
Millenium Marinara	45	2	0	0	0	7	1	4	240
Pepper & Onion	40	3	0	0	0	6	1	3	260
Tomato Basil or Fra Diavolo Hot Sauce .	80	3	1	0	0	13	3	1	260
Filetto di Pomodoro	80	3	1	0	0	13	3	1	260
Classico Roasted Garlic	60	1	0	0	0	11	2	8	220
Sweet Basil Marinara	70	1	0	0	0	13	1	9	280
Spicy Red Pepper	60	2	0	0	0	7	2	5	300
Tomato & Basil	60	1	0	0	0	11	2	6	310
Fire Roasted Tomato & Garlic	50	1	0	0	0	10	2	4	320
Colavita Marinara	70	3	0	0	0	9	2	6	220
Classic Hot	80	3	0	0	0	12	3	6	250
Garden Style	60	3	0	0	0	12	3	0	290
Dei Fratelli All-Purpose Italian Sauce	60	0	0	0	0	12	2	5	255
Eden Organic Spaghetti, NSA	80	3	0	0	0	12	3	6	10
Spaghetti	80	3	0	0	0	12	3	6	320
Enrico's Organic, NSA	45	0	0	0	0	11	1	10	20
All Natural, NSA	53	1	0	0	9	9	1	11	70
Traditional Italian Style, NSA	53	1	0	0	9	9	1	11	70
FF Organic Basil	50	0	0	0	0	8	4	8	220
FF Organic Traditional	45	0	0	0	0	4	6	7	280
Francesco Rinaldi NSA	90	4	0	0	0	11	3	6	25
Full Circle Parmesan Cheese	50	2	0	0	0	8	3	4	330
Manischewitz Pasta, NSA	70	1	0	0	0	12	2	8	45
Med-Diet Spaghetti	20	0	0	0	0	3	-	-	100
Melissa's Chicago Style Veg & Pasta	60	4	1	0	0	8	2	4	300
Michael Angelo's Fire Roasted Tomato	60	3	0	0	0	8	2	4	260
Mom's Spaghetti	60	4	0	0	0	6	-	0	280
Mother Teresa's Pasta	40	1	0	0	0	7	1	3	20
Marinara or Extra Spicy	40	1	0	0	0	7	1	5	20
Muir Glen Garlic Roasted Garlic	50	1	0	0	0	10	0	4	320
Fire Roasted Tomato	70	2	0	0	0	11	2	3	340
Mushroom Marinara	70	2	0	0	0	11	2	3	340
Balsamic Roasted Onion	60	1	0	0	0	11	2	5	350
Chunky Tomato Herb or Italian Herb	60	1	0	0	0	11	2	5	350
Garden Veg or Portabello Mushroom	60	1	0	0	0	10	2	4	350
Patsy's Puttanesca	100	6	1	0	0	8	2	3	315
Rao's Puttanesca	70	5	1	0	0	5	1	3	200
Homemade Marinara	80	6	1	0	0	6	1	3	320

DINNERS, ENTREES AND SIDE DISHES
Pizza

Food	Cal	Fat	Sat	TFat	Chol	Carb	Fib	Sug	Sod
MARINARA/PASTA SAUCE (CONT'D)									
Roselli's Spaghetti Sauce	45	1	0	0	0	9	2	3	35
Tree of Life Classic Tomato, FF	40	0	0	0	0	8	0	6	250
Sweet Pepper, FF	30	0	0	0	0	7	0	6	280
Pasta Sauce Plus, Mushroom/Basil, FF	30	0	0	0	0	7	0	6	300
Walnut Acres Tomato & Basil, LS	40	0	0	0	0	9	1	7	20
Garlic-Garlic..	50	1	0	0	0	10	1	6	280
Roasted Garlic..	60	1	0	0	0	11	1	7	280
Sweet Pepper & Onion	50	1	0	0	0	9	1	6	280
Marinara Zinfandel or Marinara w/Herbs	50	1	0	0	0	9	1	6	330
Tomato & Basil or Zesty Basil	50	1	0	0	0	9	1	7	330
Tomato & Mushroom	50	1	0	0	0	9	1	6	330
PESTO									
FROZEN/REFRIGERATED									
Monterey Pasta Basil	280	28	4	0	10	4	1	1	240
READY-TO-EAT *(1/4 CUP UNLESS NOTED)*									
Candoni Sun Dried Tomato Pesto	190	17	3	0	5	9	2	5	95
Ciba Naturals Sun-Dried Tomato	240	21	2	0	0	8	2	3	140
Basil Pesto	310	31	4	0	5	3	1	1	280
DaVinci Pesto Genovese	400	40	6	0	0	8	2	0	250
Melissa's Basil Pesto	340	34	6	0	10	3	0	1	230
Rising Sun Farms									
Ultimate Classic or Pesto Pronto	200	20	-	0	10	2	-	-	230

PIZZA

Food	Cal	Fat	Sat	TFat	Chol	Carb	Fib	Sug	Sod
Cheese, 12", 1/4	391	18	6	0	20	42	3	5	653
Meat & veg, 12", 1/4	395	21	7	0	23	36	3	5	794
Pepperoni, 12", 1/4	432	22	7	0	22	42	3	5	902
Cheese, meat & veg, 12" rising crust, 1/4 ...	404	18	6	0	28	43	3	5	954
BRANDS . . . *(1 SLICE PIZZA UNLESS NOTED)*									
FROZEN/REFRIGERATED									
A.C. LaRocco Spinach & Artichoke, 1/6 .	128	4	2	0	12	15	8	2	235
Quattro Formaggio, 1/6	140	5	3	0	14	15	8	2	259
Garden Veg, 1/6	216	6	2	0	9	34	3	2	281
Cheese & Garlic, 1/6	216	6	2	0	10	34	3	2	284
Polynesian, 1/6	229	6	2	0	9	35	3	2	288
Tomato & Feta, 1/6	221	6	2	0	10	34	3	2	300
Greek Sesame, 1/6	224	7	2	0	11	33	3	2	304
Shiitake Mushroom, 1/6	228	6	2	0	10	38	3	2	305
Amy's Pesto, 1/3	310	12	4	0	10	39	2	3	480
Roasted Vegetable, 1/3	270	9	2	0	0	42	2	5	490

Food Food	Cal	Fat	Sat	TFat	Chol	Carb	Fib	Sug	Sod
PIZZA (CONT'D)									
California Pizza Kitchen (1/3 pizza)									
Crispy Thin Crust, Margherita	300	13	5	1	20	30	2	3	490
Crispy Thin Crust, Garlic Chicken	290	11	5	1	35	31	2	2	540
Connie's Roasted Veg, 1/3	260	8	4	0	15	37	2	4	430
Cheese, Thin Crust, 1/6	200	10	5	0	25	20	1	3	440
Pepperoni, Thin Crust, 1/6	210	11	5	0	25	21	1	3	440
Roasted Veg, Thin Crust, 1/6	210	11	5	0	25	21	1	3	450
Super, Thin Crust, 1/6	230	11	5	0	25	22	1	3	470
Special, Thin Crust, 1/5	260	12	5	0	30	27	2	4	510
DiGiorno									
Harvest Wheat									
Roasted Veg, Rising Crust, 1/6	230	6	3	0	10	36	4	6	480
Supreme, Thin Crust, 1/5	250	8	4	0	20	32	4	5	520
Thin Crispy Crust									
Grilled Chicken & Spinach, 1/5	260	8	4	0	25	33	2	5	550
Ellio's Cheese, 1 slice	170	4	2	0	10	25	2	6	270
Empire Kosher									
Mushroom Cheese, 1/4	150	3	1	0	5	25	0	1	296
4 Cheese, 1/4	170	4	2	0	10	25	0	1	332
Supreme Cheese, 1/4	181	4	1	0	6	30	0	2	378
Spinach Cheese, 1/4	189	4	2	0	9	29	0	2	420
Giovanni's									
Thin Crust, 3 Cheese, 1/4	350	16	9	0	40	32	3	3	300
Thin Crust, Deluxe, 1/5	300	15	8	0	35	27	2	2	450
Thin Crust, Veggie, 1/5	250	9	5	0	20	30	3	5	480
Ian's Cheese, 2 slices	200	6	4	0	20	28	2	4	400
Cheese Pizza w/side dish, 7 oz	340	7	3	0	25	60	4	23	290
Jack's									
Naturally Rising, Cheese, 12", 1/6	290	10	6	0	25	34	2	11	480
Kid Cuisine									
Primo Pepperoni Pizza, 8 oz	390	7	3	0	5	69	5	30	400
Cheese Pizza Painter, 8 oz	400	8	3	0	10	68	6	23	460
Cheeseburger Builder, 8 oz	390	10	4	0	20	60	4	10	480
Deep Sea Adventure Fish Sticks, 8 oz	390	11	3	0	17	57	5	15	540
Lean Cuisine									
Spinach & Mushroom, 6.1 oz	310	7	4	0	15	46	4	4	430
Roasted Veg, 6 oz	330	5	2	0	10	58	3	7	450
Margherita, 6 oz	320	9	3	0	5	48	4	5	540
Linda McCartney									
Mushroom & Spinach, 1/2	320	10	4	0	20	34	4	5	480
Spicy Tahi Style Vegetarian, 1/2	320	9	3	0	20	36	4	9	540
Mr. P's Cheese, 6.5 oz	410	11	5	0	25	58	5	6	510

DINNERS, ENTREES AND SIDE DISHES
Pizza (Bread Pizza)

Food	Cal	Fat	Sat	TFat	Chol	Carb	Fib	Sug	Sod
PIZZA (CONT'D)									
Mystic Cheese, 1/6	360	15	8	0	30	39	2	2	490
Palermo's Primo Thin, Margherita, 1/6	260	12	5	0	20	26	2	2	520
Schwans Pizza for One									
Margherita-Style Tomato Basil	240	5	2	0	10	36	5	4	490
Tofutti Pizza Pizzaz, 1/3	175	5	2	0	0	24	1	6	320
Tombstone									
Light Vegetable, 1/5	230	6	2	0	10	31	4	5	510
MIX									
Low Carbolicious (sauce & crust									
mix), 1/8 slice	120	8	1	0	0	4	1	1	190
BREAD PIZZA *(also see Pockets, Sandwiches and Wraps, pg 105)*									
Cheese french bread pizza, 6 oz	350	14	5	0	15	42	3	4	660
BRANDS . . .									
FROZEN/REFRIGERATED *(6 OZ UNLESS NOTED)*									
Cedarlane Stuffed Focaccia									
Mediterranean, 1/3 (4 oz)	296	10	6	0	22	37	1	4	485
Roma Tomato & Basil, 1/3 (4 oz)	275	9	4	0	14	33	2	5	528
Lean Cuisine									
Cheese French Bread, 6 oz	320	7	4	0	20	47	3	7	520
Schwan's									
Lasagna & Multi-grain Bread, 1/2 loaf	120	3	0	0	0	20	2	3	320
PIZZA CRUST AND DOUGH									
Pizza crust, mix, 1/4	180	3	3	0	0	33	2	-	264
Refrg, 1/5	150	2	0	0	0	27	1	-	380
BRANDS . . .									
FROZEN/REFRIGERATED									
French Meadow Spelt, 1 slice	90	2	0	0	0	15	2	0	110
Country Sourdough, 1/4	122	2	0	0	0	20	3	0	148
Mama Mary's, 1/2 of 7" or 1/6 of 12"	200	5	1	0	0	32	3	1	135
Gourmet, 1/8 of 12"	148	4	1	0	0	4	2	1	101
MIX *(1 SLICE UNLESS NOTED)*									
Authenic Foods									
Pizza Crust Mix, 1/16	130	2	1	0	0	27	2	1	90
'Cause Your Special, 1 slice	96	0	0	0	0	21	1	2	156
Gluten Free Pantry									
French Bread & Pizza Crust, 1 slice	110	0	0	0	0	25	1	0	115
Martha White									
Deep Dish, 1 slice	110	1	0	0	0	23	0	-	110
Regular, 1 slice	100	2	0	0	0	19	0		125

Food Food	Cal	Fat	Sat	TFat	Chol	Carb	Fib	Sug	Sod
PIZZA CRUST AND DOUGH (CONT'D)									
READY-TO-EAT									
Breadsmith Pizza Dough, 1 oz	79	1	0	0	0	15	1	2	134
Ener-G Rice Shell, 10", 1/8	70	4	0	0	0	9	1	0	70
Yeast-Free Rice Shell, 10", 1/8	90	3	0	0	0	14	1	0	105
Yeast-Free Rice Shell, 6", 1/4	70	3	0	0	0	11	1	0	120
PIZZA SAUCE									
Pizza sauce, ready-to-eat, 1/4 cup	40	2	0	0	0	9	1	3	410
BRANDS . . . *(1/4 CUP UNLESS NOTED)*									
Casa Visco	40	3	1	0	0	6	1	3	110
Cento	30	0	0	0	0	5	1	3	140
Enrico's All Natural	35	2	0	0	0	6	0	5	150
Furmano's Pizza Sauce	25	1	0	0	0	4	1	2	190
Muir Glen	40	0	0	0	0	6	2	3	230

POCKETS, SANDWICHES AND WRAPS

Food Food	Cal	Fat	Sat	TFat	Chol	Carb	Fib	Sug	Sod
Pocket sandwich, cheese, 4.5 oz.................	290	9	4	-	20	38	3	5	450
Croissant w/chicken, broccoli &									
cheese, 4.5 oz	300	11	4	-	35	37	5	5	640
Pocket sandwich, beef & cheese, 4.5 oz	360	18	9	-	50	36	1	5	830
BRANDS . . .									
FROZEN/REFRIGERATED									
Amy's Pocket Sandwich									
Spinach Pizza, 4.5 oz................................	280	9	4	0	15	37	3	3	460
Cheese Pizza, 4.5 oz	300	9	4	0	15	42	4	5	450
Roasted Veg, 4.5 oz	220	8	2	0	0	35	4	5	480
Veg Pie, 5 oz	300	9	2	0	0	45	3	5	490
Aunt Trudy's Fillo Pockets									
Roasted Sweet Potato, 5 oz......................	310	12	2	0	0	45	4	0	270
Roasted Veg, 5 oz	240	11	1	0	0	33	3	1	280
3 Bean Veggie, 5 oz	260	7	1	0	0	42	5	0	300
Eggplant & Roasted Peppers, 5 oz	210	7	1	0	0	34	3	0	310
Mexicali Veg, 5 oz	230	7	1	0	0	38	3	0	350
Samosa, 5 oz	280	10	1	0	0	43	3	1	350
Mushroom & Leek, 5 oz	190	6	1	0	0	32	3	0	380
Spinach & Potato, 5 oz	250	9	1	0	0	40	4	0	380
Cedarlane									
LF Rice & Veg Teriyaki Wrap, 8 oz	320	6	1	0	0	56	2	5	480
LF Pizza Veggie Wrap, 6 oz	220	3	0	0	0	32	2	3	520
Ian's Natural Foods									
Mini Hamburgers, 4.6 oz (2)	360	12	4	0	25	42	1	5	450

DINNERS, ENTREES AND SIDE DISHES
Side Dishes

Food	Cal	Fat	Sat	TFat	Chol	Carb	Fib	Sug	Sod
POCKETS, SANDWICHES AND WRAPS (CONT'D)									
Lean Pockets									
Ultra Supreme Pizza, 9 oz	200	6	3	0	25	19	7	4	540
Lightlife									
Smart Tortilla Wrap, Ranchero	300	6	1	0	0	48	7	6	370
White Castle									
Hamburgers, 2 (3.2 oz)	270	14	6	0	20	23	5	0	270
Cheeseburgers, 2 (3.7 oz)	310	17	9	0	30	23	6	0	480

(SIDE DISHES)

GRAIN SIDES *(see Grain Dishes – Packaged, pg 135)*

KNISHES

Food	Cal	Fat	Sat	TFat	Chol	Carb	Fib	Sug	Sod
Potato, 1 pc	200	4	0	0	0	38	2	0	530

BRANDS . . .

Most brands are within the generic range.

POLENTA

Food	Cal	Fat	Sat	TFat	Chol	Carb	Fib	Sug	Sod
Polenta, ready-to-eat, 4 oz	88	0	0	0	0	20	1	0	376
Mix, prep, 3/8 cup	260	5	2	0	5	48	4	3	550

BRANDS . . .

Food	Cal	Fat	Sat	TFat	Chol	Carb	Fib	Sug	Sod
Bellino Instant Polenta, 1/4 cup	140	0	0	0	0	32	4	0	0

POTATOES

Food	Cal	Fat	Sat	TFat	Chol	Carb	Fib	Sug	Sod
Mashed potatoes, instant, 1/3 cup mix	80	0	0	0	0	18	2	0	20
Hash browns, frozen, 1/2 cup	70	0	0	0	0	17	2	1	70
Mix, 1 oz mix	100	1	0	0	0	22	1	1	570
Gnocci, boxed/packaged, 5.2 oz	250	0	0	0	0	55	1	2	240
Potato pancake, 1 tbsp mix	50	0	0	0	0	12	1	0	270
Fries, seasoned, frozen, 3 oz	120	4	1	0	20	20	2	1	360
Potato dumplings, 1 oz mix	90	0	0	0	0	21	1	0	410
Au gratin potatoes, 1 oz mix	83	1	1	0	0	20	1	1	554
Stuffed potato, cheese, 5 oz	200	9	3	5	0	24	1	9	550
Scalloped potatoes, 1 oz mix	100	1	0	0	0	21	1	1	570
Mashed potatoes, prep, 2/3 cup	190	9	5	0	0	20	3	1	490

BRANDS . . .

BOXED/PACKAGED

NOTE: Most instant mashed potato brands are within the generic range, however, flavored potatoes may contain added sodium.

FROZEN/REFRIGERATED *(1/2 CUP UNLESS NOTED)*

Cascadian Farms Organic

Food	Cal	Fat	Sat	TFat	Chol	Carb	Fib	Sug	Sod
Crinkle or Straight Cut French Fries, 3 oz	130	4	1	0	0	21	2	1	15
Shoe String Fries, 3 oz	140	5	1	0	0	21	2	1	15

Food Food	Cal	Fat	Sat	TFat	Chol	Carb	Fib	Sug	Sod
SIDE DISHES - POTATOES (CASCADIAN FARMS CONT'D)									
Wedge Cut Fries, 3 oz	110	3	1	0	0	21	2	1	15
Country Style, 3/4 cup (3 oz)	50	0	0	0	0	12	1	0	10
Hash Browns, 3 oz	60	0	0	0	0	14	1	0	10
Dr. Praeger's									
Homestyle Potato Pancakes, 1.5 oz	80	3	1	0	15	10	1	1	150
Simply Potatoes									
Red Wedge Potatoes, 1/2 cup	50	0	0	0	0	10	2	2	85
Country Style Mashed Potatoes, 2/3 cup	110	2	2	0	5	20	3	1	105
Mashed Sweet Potatoes, 2/3 cup	160	3	1	1	0	33	2	18	105
Shredded Hash Browns, 1/2 cup	50	0	0	0	0	12	1	0	105
Homestyle Slices, 2/3 cup	70	0	0	0	0	16	1	0	135
Diced Potato w/Onion, 2/3 cup	60	0	0	0	0	13	1	0	220

RICE SIDES *(see Rice and Rice Dishes, pg 136)*

SALADS

	Cal	Fat	Sat	TFat	Chol	Carb	Fib	Sug	Sod
Cole slaw, 3/4 cup	150	8	1	0	5	19	2	15	230
Chicken salad, 1/2 cup	300	26	4	0	45	7	0	1	460
Potato salad, 1/2 cup	230	12	2	0	10	28	3	8	490
Tuna salad, 1/3 cup	220	16	3	0	35	8	1	5	290
3 bean salad, 1/2 cup	113	0	0	0	0	26	3	18	495
Pasta salad, 2/3 cup	120	1	0	0	0	24	0	6	800

BRANDS . . .

Most brands are within the generic range, the following has less than the generic.

	Cal	Fat	Sat	TFat	Chol	Carb	Fib	Sug	Sod
Hanover 3 Bean, 3.1 oz	100	1	0	0	0	22	3	14	120
Vegetable, 3.1 oz	80	0	0	0	0	17	3	15	120

STUFFING AND DRESSING

	Cal	Fat	Sat	TFat	Chol	Carb	Fib	Sug	Sod
Cornbread, 1 oz	110	1	0	0	0	22	4	1	365
Bread, 1 oz	109	1	0	0	0	22	1	2	451

BRANDS . . . *(1 OZ UNLESS NOTED)*

Most brands are within the generic range, the following has less than the generic.

	Cal	Fat	Sat	TFat	Chol	Carb	Fib	Sug	Sod
Stove Top Chicken, lower sodium	110	1	0	0	0	21	0	3	260

VEGETABLE SIDE DISHES

	Cal	Fat	Sat	TFat	Chol	Carb	Fib	Sug	Sod
Succotash, frozen, unprep, 1 cup	145	1	0	0	0	31	6	-	70
Green beans & almonds, 1/2 cup	60	3	0	0	0	5	2	2	95
Corn in butter sauce, 1/2 cup	150	3	1	0	0	28	2	5	260
Corn grits (hominy), instant, 1 oz	100	0	0	0	0	22	2	0	320
Broccoli w/butter sauce, 1/2 cup	50	2	1	0	5	7	2	2	330
Spinach, creamed, 1/2 cup	169	13	4	0	16	9	2	3	335
Peas & onions in sauce, 1/2 cup	60	0	0	0	0	11	3	0	340

DINNERS, ENTREES AND SIDE DISHES
Side Dishes (Vegetables)

Food	Cal	Fat	Sat	TFat	Chol	Carb	Fib	Sug	Sod
VEGETABLE SIDE DISHES (CONT'D)									
Corn grils (hominy) w/cheese, 1 oz	100	1	0	0	0	21	1	-	425
Broccoli & cheese sauce, 1/2 cup	90	5	3	0	5	8	1	4	490

Brands . . .

Most brands are within the generic range, the following has less than the generic.

FROZEN/REFRIGERATED

Food	Cal	Fat	Sat	TFat	Chol	Carb	Fib	Sug	Sod
C&W Cheddar Bacon Corn	130	5	2	0	10	18	3	9	210
Cascadian Farms Chinese-Style or Thai-Style Stirfry Blend, 3/4 cup (3 oz)	25	0	0	0	0	5	2	2	15
California-Style Blend, 3/4 cup	25	0	0	0	0	5	2	2	15
Gardener's Blend, 3/4 cup	25	0	0	0	0	5	2	2	25
Dr. Praeger's									
Broccoli Pancakes, 1.3 oz	60	4	0	0	0	6	1	0	120
Spinach Pancakes, 1.3 oz	60	4	0	0	0	6	1	0	130
Green Giant Green Beans & Almonds, no sauce, 2/3 cup	60	3	0	0	0	5	2	2	95
Melrose									
Zucchini Souffle, 3.6 oz	90	0	0	0	0	19	3	3	160

Food	Cal	Fat	Sat	TFat	Chol	Carb	Fib	Sug	Sod

ETHNIC FOODS

ASIAN

CONDIMENTS, ADDITIVES AND SEASONING MIXES

Food	Cal	Fat	Sat	TFat	Chol	Carb	Fib	Sug	Sod
Wasabi, powder, 1 tsp	0	0	0	0	0	0	0	0	0
Prepared, 1 tsp	15	1	0	0	0	3	0	0	100
Chinese mustard, 1 tsp	10	0	0	0	0	1	0	0	70
Miso/soybean paste, 1 tbsp	28	1	0	0	0	4	1	1	522

BRANDS . . .

Food	Cal	Fat	Sat	TFat	Chol	Carb	Fib	Sug	Sod
Sun Luck Chinese Mustard, 1 tsp	10	0	0	0	0	1	0	0	50
Beef & Broccoli Seasoning, 3/4 tbsp	20	0	0	0	0	5	0	1	140
Westbrae Natural Mellow Barley Miso, 1 tbsp	30	0	0	0	0	3	0	0	300

EGG ROLLS *(see Appetizers and Snacks, pg 89)*

FORTUNE COOKIES

Food	Cal	Fat	Sat	TFat	Chol	Carb	Fib	Sug	Sod
Fortune cookie, 1	30	0	0	0	0	7	0	4	22

BRANDS . . .
Most brands are within the generic range.

FRIED RICE — MIX

Food	Cal	Fat	Sat	TFat	Chol	Carb	Fib	Sug	Sod
Fried rice seasoning mix, 1 1/3 tbsp	30	0	0	0	0	6	0	0	490
Fried rice, mix, prep, 1 cup	260	1	0	0	0	47	1	3	1095

BRANDS . . .
Most brands are within the generic range.

KIM CHEE

Food	Cal	Fat	Sat	TFat	Chol	Carb	Fib	Sug	Sod
Kim chee, 1/4 cup	15	0	0	0	0	2	1	-	340

BRANDS . . .
Most brands are within the generic range.

MEALS — FROZEN AND PACKAGED

(see Dinners and Entrees – Frozen/Refrigerated (Asian), pg 91; Entrees and Meals – Shelf-Stable Asian), pg 99)

NOODLES

Food	Cal	Fat	Sat	TFat	Chol	Carb	Fib	Sug	Sod
Bean threads, 1 cup	190	0	0	0	0	50	0	0	0
Low mein noodles, 1 cup	400	0	0	0	0	2	0	0	2
Chinese, cellophane, or long rice, 1 cup	491	0	0	0	0	121	1	0	14
Chow mein/soba noodles, 1 oz	140	6	1	0	0	19	1	0	220

109

Food	Cal	Fat	Sat	TFat	Chol	Carb	Fib	Sug	Sod
ASIAN FOODS (NOODLES CONT'D)									
Udon noodles, 2 oz	190	2	0	0	0	37	3	5	660
Somen noodles, 2 oz	203	1	0	0	0	42	3	1	1049
BRANDS . . . *(2 OZ UNLESS NOTED)*									
BEAN THREADS, LOW MEIN AND CELLOPHONE/RICE THREADS									
Most brands are within the generic range.									
CHOW MEIN/SOBA NOODLES									
China Boy, 1 oz	130	5	1	0	0	16	1	0	110
Chuka Soba Wel-Pac	210	1	0	0	0	42	1	0	125
Eden 100% Buckwheat Soba	200	1	0	0	0	43	3	2	5
Kamut or Spelt Soba (avg)	200	1	0	0	0	38	3	1	55
Organic Soba	200	2	0	0	0	38	2	3	70
Frieda's Crispy Noodles, 1/2 cup	160	6	0	-	0	17	1	1	160
Ka-Me Buckwheat Noodles (Soba)	200	1	0	0	0	43	2	6	80
Sun Luck Chuka Soba, 3 oz	310	2	0	0	0	61	0	0	140
OTHER NOODLES									
Annie Chun's Rice Noodles, all	210	0	0	0	0	50	0	0	75
Pad Thai Noodles	210	5	0	0	0	50	0	0	75
Eden Kamut Udon	200	2	0	0	0	37	3	0	55
Spelt Udon	200	1	0	0	0	39	2	1	75
Organic or Wheat & Rice Udon	200	2	0	0	0	38	3	1	80
Sun Luck Tomoshiraga Somen, 3 oz	330	15	2	0	0	65	2	0	70
SEAWEED									
Agar, fresh, 1 oz	0	0	0	0	0	2	-	0	3
Nori, fresh, 1 oz	10	0	0	0	0	1	-	0	14
Spirulina, fresh, 1 oz	7	0	0	0	0	1	-	0	28
Spirulina, dried, 1 oz	83	2	1	0	0	7	-	0	309
BRANDS . . .									
Most brands are within the generic range.									
SUSHI									
Vegetable Roll, 9.8 oz	349	7	1	0	0	65	5	9	177
Spicy Tuna Roll, 9.8 oz	449	11	2	0	51	57	2	11	275
Shrimp & Avocado, 7,5 oz	328	5	1	0	44	59	3	6	283
California Roll, 9.8 oz	361	6	1	0	0	66	3	7	637
Crab Roll, 9.8 oz	390	7	1	0	84	60	3	6	865
BRANDS . . .									
Most brands are within the generic range.									

TEMPURA BATTER *(see Batter, Seasoning and Coating Mixes, pg 4)*

Food	Cal	Fat	Sat	TFat	Chol	Carb	Fib	Sug	Sod
ASIAN FOODS (CONT'D)									
VEGETABLES									
Water chestnuts, 1/4 cup	15	0	0	0	0	4	1	1	0
Bamboo shoots, 1/2 cup	12	0	0	0	0	2	1	0	5
Baby corn, 1/2 cup	10	0	0	0	0	6	4	6	20
Bean sprouts, 1/2 cup	11	0	0	0	0	2	1	1	38
Chop suey vegetables, canned, 1/2 cup	110	0	0	0	0	0	2	1	240
Mushrooms, canned, 1/2 cup	20	0	0	0	0	3	2	0	380
Chow mein vegetables, canned, 1/2 cup	200	0	0	0	0	4	1	0	422
BRANDS . . .									
CANNED *(1/2 CUP UNLESS NOTED)*									
Ka-Me Stir Fry Veg	20	0	0	0	0	4	2	0	10
Sun Luck Mushrooms, Straw	10	0	0	0	0	8	0	0	0
Mixed Stir Fry Veg	20	0	0	0	0	4	2	0	10
Bean Sprouts	40	0	0	0	0	6	2	0	20
Mushrooms, Stir Fry	40	0	0	0	0	6	4	0	50
FROZEN/REFRIGERATED									
(see Frozen Vegetables – Mixed Vegetables, pg 163)									
WRAPPERS									
Wonton wrapper, 1	23	0	0	0	1	5	0	0	46
Egg roll wrapper, 1	93	0	0	0	3	19	1	0	183
BRANDS . . .									
Azumaya Wonton, Square, 1	20	0	0	0	1	4	0	0	32
Wonton, Round, 1	16	0	0	0	1	3	0	0	37
Egg Roll, 1	57	0	0	3	0	12	0	0	137
Dynasty Wonton, 1	17	0	0	0	0	4	0	0	18
Egg Roll, 1	57	0	0	0	2	12	0	0	60
Frieda's Wonton, 1	20	0	0	0	0	4	0	0	37
Melissa's Egg Roll Wraps, 1 sheet	75	1	0	0	0	18	0	0	17
Wonton Wrappers, 8 wrappers	150	0	0	0	0	36	1	1	35

ASIAN SAUCES

NOTE: Although some of the following sauces exceed sodium guidelines, they are less than the generic.

BEAN SAUCE

Food	Cal	Fat	Sat	TFat	Chol	Carb	Fib	Sug	Sod
Bean sauce, 1 tbsp	30	0	0	0	0	5	1	4	475

BRANDS . . .
Most brands are within the generic range.

Food	Cal	Fat	Sat	TFat	Chol	Carb	Fib	Sug	Sod
ASIAN SAUCES (CONT'D)									
CHILI/GARLIC SAUCE									
Chili/garlic sauce, 1 tsp	10	0	0	0	0	1	0	1	80
BRANDS ...									
Most brands are within the generic range.									
CURRY PASTE									
Curry Paste, 1 tsp	8	0	0	0	0	1	0	0	190
BRANDS ... *(1 TSP UNLESS NOTED)*									
A Taste of Thai Yellow	3	0	0	0	0	1	1	0	135
HOISIN SAUCE									
Hoisin sauce, 1 tbsp	35	1	0	0	0	7	0	7	258
BRANDS ... *(1 TBSP UNLESS NOTED)*									
Heaven and Earth Raspberry	20	0	0	0	0	4	0	4	140
Polynesian	20	0	0	0	0	5	0	4	80
Ty Ling	20	0	0	0	0	5	0	4	75
LEMON SAUCE									
BRANDS ... *(2 TBSP UNLESS NOTED)*									
Leeann Chin	50	0	0	0	0	12	0	10	35
OYSTER SAUCE									
Oyster sauce, 1 tbsp	9	0	0	0	0	3	0	2	492
BRANDS ... *(1 TBSP UNLESS NOTED)*									
Most brands are within the generic range.									
PEANUT SAUCE									
Peanut sauce, 2 tbsp	90	6	2	0	0	8	0	6	480
BRANDS ... *(2 TBSP UNLESS NOTED)*									
Annie Chun's Thai	120	7	1	0	0	10	1	8	230
A Taste of Thai Satay	80	5	4	0	0	9	1	5	180
Heaven and Earth	200	32	0	0	0	10	0	2	180
Mr. Spice Thai	30	4	0	0	0	8	0	8	0
Thai Kitchen Satay or Spicy Satay	80	5	1	0	0	6	1	4	130
PLUM SAUCE									
Plum sauce, 1 tbsp	35	0	0	0	0	8	0	7	140
BRANDS ... *(1 TBSP UNLESS NOTED)*									
Jok 'n' Al	8	0	0	0	0	2	0	1	42
Wax Orchards	20	0	0	0	0	5	1	5	10

Food	Cal	Fat	Sat	TFat	Chol	Carb	Fib	Sug	Sod
ASIAN SAUCES (CONT'D)									
SOY SAUCE									
Soy sauce, 1 tbsp	8	0	0	0	0	1	0	0	902
Lite, 1 tbsp	10	0	0	0	0	2	0	0	600
BRANDS . . . *(1 TBSP UNLESS NOTED)*									
House of Tsang LS, Ginger	10	0	0	0	0	2	0	0	280
World Harbors Angostura Lite	10	0	0	0	0	1	0	0	390
STIR-FRY SAUCE									
Stir-fry sauce, 1 tbsp	15	0	0	0	0	3	0	3	570
BRANDS . . . *(1 TBSP UNLESS NOTED)*									
Mr. Spice Ginger	15	0	0	0	0	4	0	4	0
The Spice Hunter New Traditions									
Stir-Fry Mix, 1 tsp	15	0	0	0	0	2	1	0	0
Rice Road (avg)	20	0	0	0	0	4	0	3	310
SWEET AND SOUR SAUCE/DUCK SAUCE									
Sweet & sour sauce, 2 tbsp	35	0	0	0	0	9	0	7	190
BRANDS . . . *(2 TBSP UNLESS NOTED)*									
Ah-So Chinese-Style Duck	50	0	0	0	0	13	0	10	15
Contadina w/Pineapple	40	1	0	0		8	0	6	115
Great Impressions Sweet & Sour	80	0	0	0	0	19	0	7	15
Heaven and Earth Tangerine	25	0	0	0	0	6	0	6	5
Ginger Mint	35	0	0	0	0	9	1	9	10
Four Fruit	20	1	0	0	0	9	0	9	10
House of Tsang Sweeet & Sour	70	0	0	0	0	16	0	14	100
Ka-Me w/Ginger	50	0	0	0	0	13	0	7	60
Kraft Sweet 'N Sour	24	0	0	0	0	6	0	5	50
La Choy Sweet & Sour	60	0	0	0	0	14	0	14	120
Mr. Spice Sweet & Sour	18	0	0	0	0	4	0	4	0
Steel's Rocky Mountain	5	0	0	0	0	1	0	0	78
Sun Luck Sweet & Sour	31	0	0	0	0	7	0	6	30
TERIYAKI SAUCE									
Teriyaki sauce, 1 tbsp	15	0	0	0	0	3	0	2	690
Lite, 1 tbsp	15	0	0	0	0	3	0	3	320
BRANDS . . . *(1 TBSP UNLESS NOTED)*									
Billy Bee Honey Teriyaki	25	0	0	0	0	6	0	5	150
Miko Lite	10	0	0	0	0	2	0	3	125
World Harbors Maui Mt Hawaiian	35	0	0	0	0	9	0	8	135

Food	Cal	Fat	Sat	TFat	Chol	Carb	Fib	Sug	Sod
HAWAIIAN									
Poi, 1/3 cup	70	0	0	0	0	18	2	0	30
Lau lau, vegetable, 1	130	0	0	0	0	26	6	0	80
Pork, 1	320	21	9	-	90	5	8	0	980
Chicken, 1	260	21	6	-	75	5	8	0	1010
Kalua pork, 3 oz	260	18	6	-	85	0	0	0	200
Kalua chicken or turkey	205	11	3	-	70	0	0	0	330
Portuguese sausage, 2 oz	180	15	6	-	35	2	0	1	520

BRANDS . . .
Most brands are within the generic range.

Food	Cal	Fat	Sat	TFat	Chol	Carb	Fib	Sug	Sod
HISPANIC									
CHILI PEPPERS									
Whole green chiles, 1.3 oz	15	0	0	0	0	3	1	1	100
Diced green chiles, 2 tbsp	5	0	0	0	0	1	1	0	110
Chipotle peppers in adobo, 2 tbsp	30	1	0	0	0	5	3	1	260
Jalapeños, diced, 2 tbsp	10	0	0	0	0	1	0	0	440
BRANDS . . . *(2 TBSP UNLESS NOTED)*									
Alberto's Sweet Jalapeno Relish									
Sweet and Tangy, all	30	0	0	0	0	7	0	0	0
Cannon *Sweet Hots,* Jalapeno or									
Red Jalapeno	5	0	0	0	0	2	0	2	0
Sweet Hots, Mild	25	0	0	0	0	6	0	6	10
Green Chile, Flame Roasted, Hot or Mild	10	0	0	0	0	2	0	0	0
Green Chile Piccalilli	25	0	0	0	0	6	0	5	30
Casa Fiesta									
Diced or Whole Green Chiles	5	0	0	0	0	1	0	0	85
Chi-Chi's Diced Green Chiles	10	0	0	0	0	2	0	1	60
Whole Green Chiles	10	0	0	0	0	1	0	0	20
Diced Jalapeños, 1.1 oz	10	0	0	0	0	1	0	0	55
El Rio Chopped Green Chiles	5	0	0	0	0	1	0	0	75
Embassa Chipotle Peppers in Adobo	15	1	0	0	0	2	1	1	140
LaPreferida Diced Green Chiles	10	0	0	0	0	2	1	0	75
LaVictoria Diced Green Chiles	5	0	0	0	0	1	0	0	70
Melissa's Fire Roasted Red &									
Green Chiles	10	0	0	0	0	4	2	0	60
Natural Value Whole or Diced	10	0	0	0	0	2	1	1	40
Ortega Diced Jalapeños	10	0	0	0	0	2	0	1	25
Safeway Green Chiles	10	0	0	0	0	2	1	1	40

Food	Cal	Fat	Sat	TFat	Chol	Carb	Fib	Sug	Sod

HISPANIC (CONT'D)

GUACAMOLE *(see Dips and Spreads, pg 142)*

REFRIED BEANS

Food	Cal	Fat	Sat	TFat	Chol	Carb	Fib	Sug	Sod
Canned, 1/2 cup	100	1	0	0	0	17	6	1	530
Mix, prep, 1/2 cup	160	1	0	0	0	29	11	-	610
BRANDS . . . *(1/2 CUP UNLESS NOTED)*									
Bearitos LF, NSA	140	3	0	0	0	23	9	2	5
Casa Fiesta All Natural, NF	130	0	0	0	0	22	7	1	290
All Natural	115	1	0	0	0	20	3	1	330
Eden Refried Beans									
Black Soy & Black Bean	90	3	1	0	0	13	6	1	170
Kidney	80	1	0	0	0	15	6	0	180
Pinto & Spicy Pinto	90	1	0	0	0	19	7	0	180
Black or Spicy Black	110	2	0	0	0	18	7	0	180
La Sierra Refried Pinto	150	5	1	0	0	19	7	2	310
Seneca FF Spicy	120	0	0	0	0	22	8	1	290
Natural Value Refried Black	123	0	0	0	0	22	2	0	259
Refried Pinto	134	0	0	0	0	26	10	0	261
Shari's Organic, Refried Black	110	0	0	0	0	20	4	0	330
Refried Pintos	110	0	0	0	0	20	4	0	330
Refried w/Roasted Garlic	110	0	0	0	0	20	4	0	330

NOTE: Although many of the beans listed above exceed sodium guidelines, they are less than the generic.

SEASONINGS/MIXES

Food	Cal	Fat	Sat	TFat	Chol	Carb	Fib	Sug	Sod
Guacamole seasoning mix, 1/8 pkt	15	0	0	0	0	2	0	0	160
Enchilada sauce mix, 1/6 pkt	20	0	0	0	0	4	0	1	250
Chili seasoning mix, 1/4 pkt	30	1	0	0	0	5	2	1	310
Burrito seasoning mix, 1/6 pkt	15	0	0	0	0	4	0	0	410
Fajita seasoning mix, 1/6 pkt	15	0	0	0	0	3	0	0	450
Taco seasoning mix, 1/6 pkt	20	0	0	0	0	5	0	0	550
BRANDS . . . *(1 TSP UNLESS NOTED)*									
Ancho Mama's Chile	0	0	0	0	0	0	0	0	0
Chipolte Del Sol Southwest	0	0	0	0	0	0	0	0	0
Frontier Taco, 1/4 tsp	10	0	0	0	0	2	0	0	0
Mojave Hot Taco Mix	0	0	0	0	0	0	0	0	0
New Traditions Fajita Mix	8	0	0	0	0	2	0	0	0
Santa Fe Taco Mix	10	0	0	0	0	2	0	0	0
Old El Paso Taco Mix, 40% Less Salt	8	0	0	0	0	2	0	0	165

Food	Cal	Fat	Sat	TFat	Chol	Carb	Fib	Sug	Sod
HISPANIC (CONT'D)									
TOMATILLOS									
Tomatillos, raw, diced, 1/2 cup	21	1	0	0	0	4	1	0	1
Tomatillos, canned, 2.1 oz	15	0	0	0	0	3	2	1	15
BRANDS ...									
Most brands are within the generic range.									
TORTILLAS AND TACO SHELLS									
Corn tortilla, 6" diam, 1	58	1	0	0	0	12	1	0	3
Corn taco shell, shelf-stable, 1	50	2	0	0	0	6	1	0	150
Flour tortilla, 6", 1	94	2	1	0	0	15	1	1	191
10", 1	218	5	1	0	0	36	2	1	445
Whole wheat tortilla, 1	120	2	1	0	0	20	1	0	280
BRANDS ...									
FROZEN/REFRIGERATED *(1 TORTILLA UNLESS NOTED)*									
Azteca Salad Shells	180	11	2	0	0	19	2	2	100
Food for Life Sprouted Grain	150	4	1	0	0	24	5	0	140
French Meadow, 6" Flour	84	2	0	0	0	13	5	0	80
Garden of Eatin'									
Chapati	120	3	0	0	0	20	2	1	110
Whole Wheat	140	3	0	0	0	22	2	1	170
La Tortilla									
Whole Wheat, Low Carb, all	50	2	0	0	0		8	0	180
Manny's Flour	70	1	0	0	0	13	1	0	110
Pinata Flour, 8"	100	2	0	0	0	20	1	0	120
Flour, 10"	150	2	0	0	0	28	1	1	170
Richfood, Flour	70	1	0	0	0	13	1	0	110
Tumaro's									
Low Carb, Multi Grain, Green Onion,									
or Garden Veg, 8"	100	3	0	0	0	13	8	1	115
Low Carb, Salsa, 8"	100	3	0	0	0	13	8	1	125
Premium White Flour, 8"	120	2	0	0	0	23	1	1	130
Chipotle Chili & Peppers, Honey									
Wheat, or Pesto & Garlic, 8"	110	2	0	0	0	23	1	1	135
Jalapeño & Cilantro, Garden Spinach &									
Veg, or Sun-Dried Tomato/Basil, 8"	110	2	0	0	0	23	1	1	140
Low Carb, Green Onion, 10"	140	4	1	0	0	18	11	1	140
Low Carb, Garden Veg, 10"	140	4	1	0	0	19	14	1	140
Low Carb, Multi Grain, 10"	140	4	1	0	0	18	12	1	150
Low Carb, Salsa, 10"	140	4	1	0	0	19	13	1	160

Food	Cal	Fat	Sat	TFat	Chol	Carb	Fib	Sug	Sod
HISPANIC (TORTILLAS AND TACO SHELLS CONT'D)									
SHELF-STABLE *(1 CORN TACO SHELL UNLESS NOTED)*									
Bearitos									
Taco Shells, blue or yellow, 2 shells	140	7	1	0	0	17	1	0	5
Tostada Shells, 2 shells	140	7	1	0	0	17	1	0	5
Casa Fiesta Jumbo Taco Shell	160	7	5	0	5	23	3	0	5
All Natural Taco Shells, 3	150	6	5	0	0	21	2	0	10
Garden of Eatin' Blue or Yellow Corn, 2	140	7	1	0	0	17	1	0	5
La Preferida	55	3	1	0	0	7	1	0	3
Mission Jumbo	90	4	1	0	0	11	1	0	5
Taco Bell, 3	150	6	3	0	0	21	2	0	5

(HISPANIC SAUCES)

Food	Cal	Fat	Sat	TFat	Chol	Carb	Fib	Sug	Sod
CHEESE SAUCE									
Cheese sauce, 2 tbsp	55	4	2	0	9	2	0	0	261
BRANDS . . . *(2 TBSP UNLESS NOTED)*									
Most brands are within the generic range.									
CHILI SAUCE									
Chili sauce, 2 tbsp	35	0	0	0	0	7	2	4	457
BRANDS . . .									
505 Southwestern Hot Green	25	0	0	0	0	5	1	2	40
ENCHILADA SAUCE									
Enchilada sauce, 1/4 cup	25	1	0	0	0	2	1	0	310
BRANDS . . . *(1/4 CUP UNLESS NOTED)*									
La Preferida Green Chili	25	2	0	0	0	2	1	0	250
HOT SAUCE *(also see Hot Pepper Sauce, pg 52)*									
Hot sauce, 1 tsp	0	0	0	0	0	0	0	0	10
BRANDS . . .									
Most brands are within the generic range.									
MOLE									
Mole, 2 tbsp	230	15	2	0	0	12	2	7	460
BRANDS . . .									
Rogelio Bueno, 2 tbsp	150	11	2	0	0	12	1	4	270
SALSA AND TACO SAUCE									
Salsa, canned, 2 tbsp	9	0	0	0	0	2	1	1	198
Salsa, refrg, 2 tbsp	10	0	0	0	0	2	0	1	250

Food	Cal	Fat	Sat	TFat	Chol	Carb	Fib	Sug	Sod

HISPANIC SAUCES (SALSA AND TACO SAUCE CONT'D)

BRANDS . . . *(2 TBSP UNLESS NOTED)*

There are many low-sodium salsas, the following have 80mg or less per serving.

READY-TO-EAT

Food	Cal	Fat	Sat	TFat	Chol	Carb	Fib	Sug	Sod
501 Southwestern Green Chili Sauce, hot, medium, or mild	13	0	0	0	0	2	0	1	20
Alberto's Sweet Jalapeño Relish	3	0	0	0	0	7	0	6	0
American Spoon Corn Salsa	20	1	0	0	0	4	1	1	60
Mango Habanero	35	0	0	0	0	6	1	5	70
Key Lime Salsa Verde	35	0	0	0	0	8	1	6	75
Cannon's Cannon Fire Salsa	5	0	0	0	0	1	0	1	20
Cool Coyote Black Bean & Corn	15	0	0	0	0	4	1	1	80
Dessert Pepper Peach Mango	15	0	0	0	0	4	0	3	25
Diana's Black Bean w/Corn	15	0	0	0	0	3	0	0	20
Three Bean	20	0	0	0	0	3	0	2	45
Enrico's Chunky Style NSA, Mild or Hot	10	0	0	0	0	3	0	2	60
Floribbean Key Lime	15	0	0	0	0	3	0	2	0
Mango	15	0	0	0	0	4	0	3	0
Frontera Chipotle	10	0	0	0	0	2	0	1	70
Habanero	10	0	0	0	0	2	0	1	70
Frog Ranch Hot or Medium	10	0	0	0	0	2	0	0	40
Garlic Survival Co. Tomatillo Garlic	20	0	0	0	0	4	1	0	15
Garlic or XXX Garlic	10	0	0	0	0	2	0	1	70
Gloria's Roasted Garlic & Pineapple	40	0	0	0	0	10	0	9	5
Santiam Ridge Peach Mango	50	0	0	0	0	12	0	10	15
Happy Valley Apple	20	0	0	0	0	4	0	3	45
Goldwater's									
Cochise Corn & Black Bean	30	2	0	0	0	4	1	1	80
Gunther's Black & White Bean	5	0	0	0	0	2	0	0	65
Chesapeake Bay Crab	10	0	0	0	5	1	0	1	70
Marca El Pato Jalapeño	10	0	0	0	0	2	0	1	30
Palmieri, Chunky Hot, Med, or Mild	10	0	0	0	0	2	0	2	65
Salsa Patria Chunky, all heats	5	0	0	0	0	1	0	0	70
Santa Barbara Roasted Garlic	10	0	0	0	0	2	0	0	40
Mango & Peach	15	0	0	0	0	4	0	3	60
Black Bean & Corn, Medium	15	0	0	0	0	3	0	2	80
Singing Pig Sweet Onion	25	0	0	0	0	6	0	5	20
Steel's Caribe Mango	24	0	0	0	0	6	1	4	0
REFRIGERATED									
La Mexicana Mild	10	0	0	0	0	-	0	0	75

Food Food	Cal	Fat	Sat	TFat	Chol	Carb	Fib	Sug	Sod

FISH AND SEAFOOD

ANCHOVY PASTE

	Cal	Fat	Sat	TFat	Chol	Carb	Fib	Sug	Sod
Anchovy paste, 1 tbsp	30	3	2	0	40	0	0	0	1040

BRANDS . . .
Most brands are within the generic range.

CLAM JUICE

	Cal	Fat	Sat	TFat	Chol	Carb	Fib	Sug	Sod
Clam juice, 1/4 cup	1	0	0	0	0	0	0	0	280
BRANDS . . . *(1/4 CUP UNLESS NOTED)*									
Bar Harbor	0	0	0	0	0	0	0	0	120
Blue Crab Bay	0	0	0	0	0	0	0	0	120
Bookbinder's	0	0	0	0	0	0	0	0	135
Look's Atlantic	0	0	0	0	0	0	0	0	120

FISH AND SEAFOOD – CANNED

ANCHOVIES

	Cal	Fat	Sat	TFat	Chol	Carb	Fib	Sug	Sod
Anchovies in oil, 1 oz (6 pieces)	47	2	0	0	19	0	0	0	825

BRANDS . . .
Most brands are within the generic range.

CAVIAR

	Cal	Fat	Sat	TFat	Chol	Carb	Fib	Sug	Sod
Caviar, black or red, 1 oz	71	5	1	0	167	1	0	0	425

BRANDS . . .
Most brands are within the generic range.

CLAMS *(2 OZ UNLESS NOTED)*

	Cal	Fat	Sat	TFat	Chol	Carb	Fib	Sug	Sod
Clams, chopped/minced, 2 oz	30	0	0	0	10	0	0	0	206
BRANDS . . .									
Geisha Fancy Smoked Baby Clams, 1.6 oz	80	9	3	0	20	2	1	0	60
Pacific Pearl Fancy Smoked Clams	130	9	3	0	20	4	1	0	60
Baby Clams	45	2	0	0	30	0	0	0	150

COD

	Cal	Fat	Sat	TFat	Chol	Carb	Fib	Sug	Sod
Cod, 2 oz	60	0	0	0	31	0	0	0	124

BRANDS . . .
Most brands are within the generic range.

CRAB *(2 OZ UNLESS NOTED)*

	Cal	Fat	Sat	TFat	Chol	Carb	Fib	Sug	Sod
Crab, blue, 2 oz	56	1	0	0	50	0	0	0	189

FISH AND SEAFOOD
Fish and Seafood – Canned (Gefilte Fish)

Food	Cal	Fat	Sat	TFat	Chol	Carb	Fib	Sug	Sod
FISH AND SEAFOOD – CANNED (CRAB CONT'D)									
BRANDS . . .									
Miller's Select Jumbo Lump, 3.3 oz	60	1	0	0	75	0	0	0	160
Natural Value Leg & Body Crab Meat	70	1	0	0	30	1	0	0	140
GEFILTE FISH									
Gefilte fish, sweet, 1.5 oz pc	35	1	0	0	13	3	0	3	220
BRANDS . . .									
Dr. Praeger's Gefilte fish, 1.9 oz	85	4	1	0	20	6	0	3	185
Mrs. Adler's No Salt, 1 pc	50	2	1	0	20	3	1	1	-
Ungar's Gefilte, No Sugar Added, 1.9 oz	70	4	1	0	15	3	0	1	180
Gefilte Fish, Lite, 2.5 oz (2 slices)	80	3	0	0	20	5	2	3	190
HERRING AND KIPPER SNACKS *(1 OZ UNLESS NOTED)*									
Herring, pickled, 1 oz	74	5	1	0	4	3	0	2	247
Kippered, boneless, 1 oz	62	4	1	0	23	0	0	0	260
BRANDS . . .									
Alstertor Herring in Dill-Herb Sauce	55	4	0	0	7	1	0	1	26
Herring Fillets in Tomato Sauce	55	4	0	0	7	1	0	1	32
Crown Prince Kipper Snacks, NSA, 1.6 oz	95	7	1	0	30	0	0	0	35
Season Kipper Snacks, NSA	54	3	0	0	20	0	0	0	57
MACKEREL									
Mackerel, jack, 2 oz	88	4	1	0	45	0	0	0	215
BRANDS . . .									
Geisha Jack Mackerel, 1.8 oz	80	3	1	0	40	0	0	0	130
Season Fillet of Mackerel, NSA	90	5	2	0	25	0	0	0	55
MUSSELS *(2 OZ UNLESS NOTED)*									
Mussels, smoked, 2 oz	90	5	2	0	50	3	0	0	250
BRANDS . . .									
Pacific Pearl Smoked	120	7	1	0	13	2	0	1	95
OYSTERS									
Oysters, 2 oz	70	3	1	0	45	3	0	0	140
Smoked, 2 oz	120	7	2	0	35	6	0	0	240
BRANDS . . .									
Most brands are within the generic range.									
SALMON *(2 OZ UNLESS NOTED)*									
Salmon, sockeye, 2 oz	94	4	1	0	25	0	0	0	204
Pink, 2 oz	79	3	1	0	31	0	0	0	314

Food Food	Cal	Fat	Sat	TFat	Chol	Carb	Fib	Sug	Sod
FISH AND SEAFOOD – CANNED (SALMON CONT'D)									
BRANDS . . .									
Bumble Bee Skinless & Boneless Pink	50	1	0	0	20	0	0	0	150
Crown Prince Natural Alaskan Pink	80	5	1	0	15	0	0	0	50
Gefen Fancy Pink	160	9	0	0	75	1	0	0	80
Miramonte	70	3	0	0	30	0	0	0	45
Natural Sea Wild Alaskan Pink	90	5	0	0	40	0	0	0	60
Season Pink, NSA	90	5	1	0	40	0	0	0	40
SARDINES *(2 OZ UNLESS NOTED)*									
Sardines, pacific, in tomato sauce, 1.4 oz (1)	71	4	1	0	23	0	0	0	157
Atlantic, in oil, 1.3 oz (3)	75	4	1	0	51	0	0	0	182
BRANDS . . .									
Crown Prince Brisling in Water, 2.9 oz	210	17	8	0	60	1	1	0	90
Sardines in Spring Water, 1.7 oz	95	6	2	0	28	1	0	0	75
Sardines w/Green Chilies	100	6	1	0	28	0	0	0	85
Sardines in Louisiana Hot Sauce	115	8	3	0	33	0	0	0	95
Brisling in Oil, NSA, 2.9 oz	230	18	6	0	45	0	0	0	125
Dagim Skinless Boneless in Water, 3.2 oz ..	160	9	5	0	75	1	0	0	80
King Oscar Brisling in Water or									
Soya Oil, 3 oz	173	13	5	0	120	0	0	0	70
Reese Skinless/Boneless in Water, LS	60	3	1	0	15	0	0	0	22
Smoked Brisling in Tomato Sauce									
& Sherry	110	9	3	0	40	1	1	1	135
Season Skinless/Boneless in Water, NSA	65	3	1	0	17	0	0	0	25
Norway Sardines in water, NSA	77	5	-	0	58	0	0	0	37
Norway Sardines in oil, NSA	73	5	2	0	55	0	0	0	35
Brisling in Tomato Sauce, NSA	117	9	-	0	58	1	0	0	61
SHRIMP									
Shrimp, 2 oz	57	1	0	0	143	0	0	0	440
BRANDS . . .									
Geisha Tiny Shrimp, 2.1 oz	50	1	0	0	0	182	0	0	240
TUNA (ALBACORE) *(2 OZ UNLESS NOTED)*									
Tuna, packed in oil, 2 oz	105	5	1	0	18	0	0	0	224
Light, packed in water, 2 oz	66	0	0	0	17	0	0	0	192
BRANDS . . .									
Bumble Bee Chunk White Albacore									
in Water, Very LS	70	1	0	0	30	0	0	0	35
Chicken of the Sea									
Chunk White Albacore, Very LS	60	1	0	0	25	0	0	0	35

Food	Cal	Fat	Sat	TFat	Chol	Carb	Fib	Sug	Sod
FISH AND SEAFOOD — CANNED (CHICKEN OF THE SEA TUNA CONT'D)									
Chunk Light in Spring Water, LS	60	1	0	0	30	0	0	0	90
Chunk Light in Spring Water, 50% Less Salt	60	1	0	0	30	0	0	0	125
Crown Prince Albacore in Water, LS	60	0	0	0	20	0	0	0	30
Tongol Light Chunk, NSA	70	0	0	0	35	0	0	0	35
Albacore in Spring Water	60	0	0	0	25	0	0	0	105
Deep Sea Chunk Light Tongol	60	0	0	0	35	0	0	0	50
Miramonte NSA	60	0	0	0	30	0	0	0	5
Natural Sea Chunk, NSA	60	0	0	0	20	0	0	0	120
Natural Value Albacore, NSA	70	1	0	0	30	1	0	0	140
Season Chunk White Albacore, NSA	80	1	0	0	35	0	0	0	50
Chunk Light in Water, NSA	60	1	0	0	25	0	0	0	100
StarKist Chunk White Albacore, LS	60	1	0	0	25	0	0	0	35
Chunk Light, LS	60	1	0	0	25	0	0	0	100
Whole Foods Market 365 Tongol, NSA	60	0	0	0	35	0	0	0	50
Albacore, NSA	65	1	0	0	30	0	0	0	80

FISH AND SEAFOOD – FRESH

(also see Fish and Seafood Substitutes, pg ??)

Food	Cal	Fat	Sat	TFat	Chol	Carb	Fib	Sug	Sod
Monkfish, 3 oz	65	1	0	0	21	0	0	0	15
Trout, rainbow, wild/farmed, 3 oz (avg)	109	4	1	0	50	0	0	0	28
Anchovies, 1 oz	37	1	0	0	17	0	0	0	29
Tuna (albacore), yellowfin, 3 oz	92	1	0	0	38	0	0	0	31
Pike, northern, 3 oz	75	1	0	0	33	0	0	0	33
Catfish, wild, 3 oz	81	2	1	0	49	0	0	0	37
Farmed, 3 oz	115	6	2	0	40	0	0	0	45
Salmon, atlantic, wild, 3 oz	121	5	1	0	47	0	0	0	37
Atlantic, farmed, 3 oz	156	9	2	0	50	0	0	0	50
Chinook or sockeye, 3 oz	152	9	3	0	43	0	0	0	40
Pink, 3 oz	99	3	0	0	44	0	0	0	57
Smoked, 3 oz	99	4	1	0	20	0	0	0	666
Eel, 3 oz	156	10	2	0	107	0	0	0	43
Cod, atlantic, 3 oz	70	1	0	0	37	0	0	0	46
Pacific, 3 oz	70	1	0	0	0	31	0	0	60
Halibut, 3 oz	94	2	0	0	27	0	0	0	46
Sturgeon, 3 oz	89	3	1	0	51	0	0	0	46
Clams, 3 oz	63	1	0	0	29	2	0	0	48
Crayfish, farmed, 3 oz	61	1	0	0	91	0	0	0	53
Perch, 3 oz	77	1	0	0	77	0	0	0	53
Atlantic, 3 oz	80	1	0	0	36	0	0	0	64

Food Food	Cal	Fat	Sat	TFat	Chol	Carb	Fib	Sug	Sod
FISH AND SEAFOOD – FRESH (CONT'D)									
Snapper, 3 oz	85	1	0	0	31	0	0	0	54
Pompano, 3 oz	139	8	3	0	43	0	0	0	55
Haddock, 3 oz	74	1	0	0	48	0	0	0	58
Bass, sea 3 oz	82	2	0	0	35	0	0	0	58
Freshwater, 3 oz	97	3	1	0	58	0	0	0	60
Orange roughy, 3 oz	65	1	0	0	51	0	0	0	61
Sole (flounder), 3 oz	77	1	0	0	41	0	0	0	69
Pollock, atlantic, 3 oz	78	1	0	0	60	0	0	0	73
Walleye, 3 oz	69	1	0	0	60	0	0	0	84
Mackerel, pacific or jack, 3 oz	134	7	2	0	40	0	0	0	73
Atlantic, 3 oz	174	12	3	0	60	0	0	0	77
King, 3 oz	89	2	0	0	45	0	0	0	134
Swordfish, 3 oz	103	3	1	0	33	0	0	0	77
Oysters, pacific, 3 oz	69	2	0	0	43	4	0	0	90
Eastern, farmed, 3 oz	50	1	0	0	21	5	0	0	151
Shrimp, 3 oz	90	1	0	0	129	1	0	0	126
Scallops, 3 oz	75	1	0	0	28	2	0	0	137
Lobster, spiny, 3 oz	95	1	0	0	60	2	0	0	150
Northern, 3 oz	77	1	0	0	81	0	0	0	252
Mussels, 3 oz	73	2	0	0	24	3	0	0	243
Crab, blue or dungeness, 3 oz (avg)	74	1	0	0	68	0	0	0	250
Alaskan king, 3 oz	71	1	0	0	36	0	0	0	711
Abalone, raw , 3 oz	89	1	0	0	72	5	0	0	256
Cuttlefish, 3 oz	67	1	0	0	95	1	0	0	316
SEAFOOD SUBSTITUTES									
Shrimp, imitation, 3 oz	86	1	0	0	31	8	0	-	599
Scallop, imitation, 3 oz	84	0	0	0	18	9	0	-	676
Crab, imitation, 3 oz	87	1	0	0	17	1	0	-	715
BRANDS . . . *(3 OZ PATTY UNLESS NOTED)*									
Louis Kemp Scallop Delights	80	0	0	0	10	12	0	0	385
Lobster Delights	80	0	0	0	10	12	0	4	420
Crab Delights	81	0	0	0	10	11	0	0	470
Veat Vegetarian Fillet (Salmon), 1.8 oz	170	5	1	0	0	19	1	1	90

FISH AND SEAFOOD – FROZEN

NOTE: Frozen fish and seafood have comparable sodium to fresh, however, prepared fish and seafood (i.e. battered or breaded) may contain added sodium.

PREPARED ENTREES *(see Fish and Seafood – Prepared Entrees, pg 92)*

Food	Cal	Fat	Sat	TFat	Chol	Carb	Fib	Sug	Sod

FRUITS

FRUIT JUICE

(see Fruit Juice and Fruit-Flavored Drinks, pg 17)

FRUITS – CANNED

The following fruits are listed alphabetically.

Food	Cal	Fat	Sat	TFat	Chol	Carb	Fib	Sug	Sod
Applesauce, 1 cup	105	0	0	0	0	28	3	25	5
Apples, sliced, 1 cup	137	1	0	0	0	34	4	31	6
Apricot, halves, light syrup, 1 cup	159	0	0	0	0	42	4	38	10
Blackberries, heavy syrup, 1 cup	236	0	0	0	0	59	9	50	8
Blueberries, heavy syrup, 1 cup	225	1	0	0	0	56	4	52	8
Boysenberries, heavy syrup, 1 cup	225	0	0	0	0	57	7	-	8
Cherries, sweet, light syrup, 1 cup	169	0	0	0	0	44	4	40	8
Cherries, sour, light syrup, 1 cup	189	0	0	0	0	49	2	-	18
Figs, light syrup, 1 cup	174	0	0	0	0	45	5	41	3
Fruit cocktail, light syrup, 1 cup	138	0	0	0	0	36	2	34	15
Fruit salad, light syrup, 1 cup	146	0	0	0	0	38	2	-	15
Grapefruit sections, light syrup, 1 cup	152	0	0	0	0	39	1	38	5
Peaches, halves, light syrup, 1 cup	104	0	0	0	0	27	3	-	12
Pears, halves, light syrup, 1 cup	116	0	0	0	0	30	4	31	5
Pineapple, light syrup, 1 cup	131	0	0	0	0	34	2	32	3
Plums, light syrup, 1 cup	159	0	0	0	0	41	2	39	50
Prunes, heavy syrup, 1 cup	246	0	0	0	0	65	9	-	7
Raspberries, heavy syrup, 1 cup	233	0	0	0	0	60	8	51	8
Strawberries, heavy syrup, 1 cup	234	1	0	0	0	60	4	-	10
Mandarin oranges, light syrup, 1 cup	131	0	0	0	0	34	2	32	3

BRANDS . . .
Most brands are within the generic range.

FRUITS – DRIED

The following fruits are listed alphabetically.

Food	Cal	Fat	Sat	TFat	Chol	Carb	Fib	Sug	Sod
Apple, 1 ring	16	0	0	0	0	4	1	4	6
Apricot, 1 half	8	0	0	0	0	2	0	2	0
Currants, 1 cup	408	0	0	0	0	107	10	97	12
Dates, 1	23	0	0	0	0	6	1	5	0
Fig, 1	21	0	0	0	0	5	1	4	1
Peach, 1 half	31	0	0	0	0	8	1	5	1

Food	Cal	Fat	Sat	TFat	Chol	Carb	Fib	Sug	Sod

FRUITS – DRIED (CONT'D)

Food	Cal	Fat	Sat	TFat	Chol	Carb	Fib	Sug	Sod
Pear, 1 half	47	0	0	0	0	13	1	11	1
Prunes, 1	20	0	0	0	0	5	1	3	0

BRANDS . . .
Most brands are within the generic range.

(FRUITS – FRESH)

The following fruits are listed alphabetically.

Food	Cal	Fat	Sat	TFat	Chol	Carb	Fib	Sug	Sod
Apple, 1 med	72	0	0	0	0	19	3	14	1
Apricot, 1	17	0	0	0	0	4	1	3	0
Banana, 1 med	105	0	0	0	0	27	3	14	1
Blackberries, 1 cup	62	0	0	0	0	14	8	7	1
Blueberries, 1 cup	83	0	0	0	0	21	4	14	1
Cantaloupe, med, 1/4	47	0	0	0	0	11	1	11	22
Cherries, sweet with pits, 1 cup	74	0	0	0	0	19	3	15	0
Cranberries, 1 cup	44	0	0	0	0	12	4	4	2
Grapefruit, 1/2	52	0	0	0	0	13	2	9	0
Grapes, 1 cup	110	1	0	0	0	29	1	25	3
Guava	37	1	0	0	0	8	3	5	1
Honeydew, med, 1/4	90	0	0	0	0	23	2	20	45
Kiwi, 1 med	46	0	0	0	0	11	2	7	2
Kumquat	13	0	0	0	0	3	1	2	1
Lemon	17	0	0	0	0	5	2	1	1
Lime	20	0	0	0	0	7	2	1	1
Lychee (litchi), 1	6	0	0	0	0	2	0	1	0
Mango, 1 cup	107	0	0	0	0	28	3	24	3
Nectarine, med	60	0	0	0	0	14	2	11	0
Orange, med	62	0	0	0	0	15	3	12	0
Papaya, 1 cup	55	0	0	0	0	14	2	8	4
Peach, med	38	0	0	0	0	9	2	8	0
Pear, med	96	0	0	0	0	26	5	16	2
Persimmon, japanese, 1	118	0	0	0	0	31	6	21	2
Pineapple, 1 cup	74	0	0	0	0	20	2	14	2
Plum	30	0	0	0	0	8	1	7	0
Pomegranate	105	0	0	0	0	26	1	25	5
Raspberries, 1 cup	64	1	0	0	0	15	8	5	1
Rhubarb, 1 cup	26	0	0	0	0	6	2	1	5
Strawberries, halves, 1 cup	49	0	0	0	0	12	3	7	2
Tangerine, med	45	0	0	0	0	11	2	9	2
Watermelon, 1/16 wedge	86	0	0	0	0	22	1	18	3

Food	Cal	Fat	Sat	TFat	Chol	Carb	Fib	Sug	Sod

FRUITS – FROZEN

The following fruits are listed alphabetically.

Food	Cal	Fat	Sat	TFat	Chol	Carb	Fib	Sug	Sod
Apples, unsweetened slices, 1 cup	83	1	0	0	0	21	3	-	5
Apricots, sweetened, 1 cup	237	0	0	0	0	61	5	-	10
Blackberries, unsweetened, 1 cup	97	1	0	0	0	24	8	16	2
Blueberries, unsweetened, 1 cup	79	1	0	0	0	19	4	13	2
Boysenberries, unsweetened, 1 cup	66	0	0	0	0	16	7	9	1
Cherries, sour, unsweetened, 1 cup	71	1	0	0	0	17	3	14	2
Cherries, sweet, sweetened, 1 cup	231	0	0	0	0	58	5	52	3
Mixed fruit, sweetened, 1 cup	245	0	0	0	0	61	5	-	8
Loganberries, 1 cup	81	0	0	0	0	19	8	11	1
Melon balls, 1 cup	57	0	0	0	0	14	1	-	54
Peaches, sweetened slices, 1 cup	235	0	0	0	0	60	5	55	15
Raspberries, sweetened, 1 cup	258	0	0	0	0	65	11	54	3
Rhubarb, 1 cup	29	0	0	0	0	7	3	2	3
Strawberries, unsweetened, 1 cup	77	0	0	0	0	20	5	10	4

JAMS, JELLIES AND FRUIT SPREADS

(see Jams, Jellies and Fruit Spreads, pg 40)

Food Food	Cal	Fat	Sat	TFat	Chol	Carb	Fib	Sug	Sod

MEAT, POULTRY AND ALTERNATIVES

BREAKFAST MEATS

Pork sausage, links, 1 oz	85	7	2	0	20	0	0	0	178
Heat & serve, 1 oz	106	10	3	0	21	1	0	0	211
Canadian-style bacon, 1 oz	42	2	1	0	14	0	0	0	395
Bacon, turkey, 1 oz	61	4	1	0	16	1	0	0	366
Bacon, pork, 2 slices, uncooked, 1.6 oz	208	20	7	0	31	0	0	0	378
2 slices, cooked	87	7	2	0	18	0	0	0	370

BRANDS . . . *(1 OZ UNLESS NOTED)*

BACON

Bar-S Lower Sodium	75	6	3	0	15	0	0	0	180
Coleman Natural Hickory Smoked, Uncured, 2 slices	70	6	2	0	10	0	0	0	140
Esskay Lower Sodium, 2 slices	60	5	2	0	10	0	0	0	120
Farmland Lower Sodium, 1.3 oz	80	7	3	0	15	0	0	0	190
Godshall's Turkey or Maple Turkey (avg)	40	1	0	0	20	1	0	1	185
Gwaltney Hardwood Smoked, 2 sl cooked	60	5	2	0	10	0	0	0	170
Brown Sugar, 2 slices cooked	60	5	2	0	10	0	0	0	170
Hatfield's Reduced Sodium, 3 sl cooked	70	5	2	0	5	0	0	0	180
Jimmy Dean Fresh Taste Fast! Maple, 3 slices	100	9	4	0	15	1	0	1	140
Kunzler Peppered	45	3	1	0	5	0	0	0	70
Oscar Meyer Lower Sodium, 2 sl cooked	70	5	2	0	15	1	0	0	170
Safeway Select Naturally Smoked, 2 sl	70	6	2	0	10	0	0	0	120
Smithfield's Lower Sodium, 2 sl cooked	80	7	3	0	15	0	0	0	190
Wellshire Farms Uncured Beef Bacon	57	2	1	0	25	0	0	0	114
Sliced Canadian Bacon	40	1	1	0	15	1	0	0	125

NOTE: Many "lower sodium" bacons have as much as 230mg per serving.

BREAKFAST HAM

Wellshire Farms Sunday Breakfast Ham	30	2	1	0	17	1	0	1	125

SAUSAGE

Jones Golden Brown Maple, 0.8 oz	95	9	3	0	18	0	0	0	130
Rapa Scrapple, Beef	55	4	2	0	15	4	0	0	130
Original	60	4	2	0	20	4	0	0	135

BREAKFAST MEAT ALTERNATIVES

Sausage link, meatless, 0.9 oz link	64	5	1	0	0	2	1	0	222
Bacon, meatless, 2 slices cooked	50	5	1	0	0	1	0	0	234

MEAT, POULTRY AND ALTERNATIVES
Beef, Lamb and Veal

Food	Cal	Fat	Sat	TFat	Chol	Carb	Fib	Sug	Sod
BREAKFAST MEAT ALTERNATIVES (CONT'D)									
Sausage patty, meatless, 1.4 oz	98	7	1	0	0	4	1	0	337
BRANDS . . . *(1 OZ UNLESS NOTED)*									
Gardenburger									
Breakfast Sausage, 1.5 oz patty	50	4	0	0	0	2	2	0	120
Lightlife Gimme Lean, Sausage Style	25	0	0	0	0	2	1	1	165
SoyBoy Tofu Breakfast Links	65	3	1	0	0	6	0	1	130

(BEEF, LAMB AND VEAL)

CANNED

Food	Cal	Fat	Sat	TFat	Chol	Carb	Fib	Sug	Sod
Beef Stew, 1 cup	220	12	5	0	37	16	4	2	947
Corned beef hash, canned, 1 cup	380	24	10	0	76	22	3	1	986

BRANDS . . .
Most brands are within the generic range.

DRIED

Food	Cal	Fat	Sat	TFat	Chol	Carb	Fib	Sug	Sod
Beef, dried, 1 oz	43	1	0	0	25	1	0	1	1190

BRANDS . . .
Most brands are within the generic range.

FRESH AND FROZEN

Food	Cal	Fat	Sat	TFat	Chol	Carb	Fib	Sug	Sod
Beef, most cuts, trimmed to 1/8" fat, all									
grades, 4 oz	265	19	8	0	75	0	0	0	66
Ground beef, 30% fat, 4 oz	375	34	13	0	88	0	0	0	76
10% fat, 4 oz	199	11	5	0	73	0	0	0	75
Tongue, 4 oz	253	18	8	0	98	4	0	0	78
Liver, 4 oz	151	4	1	0	308	4	0	0	77
Corned beef brisket, 4 oz	225	17	5	0	61	0	0	0	1380
Lamb, most cuts, trimmed to 1/4" fat, all									
grades, 4 oz	303	24	11	0	82	0	0	0	66
Ground, 4 oz	319	26	12	0	82	0	0	0	67
Veal, most cuts, trimmed to 1/4" fat, all									
grades, 4 oz	127	3	1	0	94	0	0	0	98
Ground, 4 oz	163	8	3	0	93	0	0	0	93

BRANDS . . .
Most brands are within the generic range.

NON-MEAT SUBSTITUTES (GROUND BEEF)

Food	Cal	Fat	Sat	TFat	Chol	Carb	Fib	Sug	Sod
Textured veg protein (TVP), 1/4 cup	80	0	0	-	0	7	4	3	594

Food Food	Cal	Fat	Sat	TFat	Chol	Carb	Fib	Sug	Sod
NON-MEAT SUBSTITUTES (GROUND BEEF CONT'D)									
BRANDS . . .									
FROZEN/REFRIGERATED *(2 OZ UNLESS NOTED)*									
Field Roast Wild Mushroom, 2 oz	87	1	0	0	0	11	1	0	174
Lentil Sage, 2 oz	90	0	0	0	0	8	1	0	240
Lightlife Smart Ground Taco/Burrito	70	0	0	0	0	7	3	1	220
MIX *(1 SERVING UNLESS NOTED)*									
Harvest Direct Soy BBQ	60	0	0	0	0	8	3	2	120
Soy Taco Mix	60	0	0	0	0	8	3	1	135
Seitan Quick Mix	160	1	0	0	0	11	2	0	160
SHELF-STABLE									
Now Naturals TVP Chunks, 1/2 cup	90	1	0	0	0	9	5	0	0

PREPARED ENTREES *(see Meat and Poultry – Prepared Entrees, pg 95)*

BURGERS AND PATTIES

Food	Cal	Fat	Sat	TFat	Chol	Carb	Fib	Sug	Sod
Beef patties, frozen, 4 oz	319	26	11	0	89	0	0	0	77
Turkey Burgers, 4 oz	170	10	3	0	90	0	0	0	110
Seasoned, 4 oz	220	17	4	0	85	0	0	0	240
Turkey, breaded, battered, fried, 3.3 oz	266	17	4	0	58	15	1	0	752
BRANDS . . . *(4 OZ UNLESS NOTED)*									
Wellshire Farms Turkey, frozen	200	2	1	0	30	0	0	0	25
NON-MEAT BURGERS AND PATTIES									
Vegetable burger, garden-style, 2.5 oz	120	3	2	0	10	15	3	2	390
BRANDS . . .									
Boca Burgers Original	70	1	0	0	0	6	4	0	280
Flame Grilled	90	3	1	0	5	4	3	0	280
Grilled Vegetable or Roasted Garlic (avg)	70	1	0	0	5	6	4	0	300
Dr. Praeger's Burgers, all (avg)	110	5	1	0	0	13	3	2	190
Gardenburger Garden Vegan	100	1	0	0	0	12	3	0	230
Black Bean Chipotle	80	3	0	0	0	13	5	1	250
Flame Grilled	120	4	0	0	0	7	4	0	300
Morningstar Farms									
Mushroom Lover's	110	6	1	0	0	8	1	1	220
Grillers Original	130	6	0	0	0	5	2	1	260
Tomato & Basil Pizza Burger	110	5	2	0	10	7	3	2	260
Grillers Vegan	100	3	0	0	0	7	4	1	280
Fajita Burgers	130	7	2	0	5	7	3	1	290

MEAT, POULTRY AND ALTERNATIVES
Chicken and Turkey

Food	Cal	Fat	Sat	TFat	Chol	Carb	Fib	Sug	Sod
NON-MEAT BURGERS AND PATTIES (CONT'D)									
Veggie Patch Garlic Portabella	100	5	0	0	0	4	0	0	270
Chick'n Fillets, 2.3 o	90	4	0	0	0	-	3	-	360
MIX *(1/4 CUP UNLESS NOTED)*									
Authentic Foods Falafel	100	1	0	0	0	17	3	2	240
Dixie Diner Soysage Pattie Mix, 3.1 oz	118	2	0	0	0	12	5	2	343
Fantastic Nature's Burger	170	3	0	0	0	30	5	2	320

CHICKEN AND TURKEY

CANNED

Food	Cal	Fat	Sat	TFat	Chol	Carb	Fib	Sug	Sod
Chicken, canned, 5 oz	230	10	3	0	63	1	0	0	169
Turkey, canned, 5 oz	204	9	3	0	83	0	0	0	584
BRANDS . . .									
Hormel NSA Chicken, 2 oz	50	1	0	0	35	0	0	0	65

FRESH AND FROZEN

Food	Cal	Fat	Sat	TFat	Chol	Carb	Fib	Sug	Sod
Chicken:									
Breast, bone and skin removed, 4 oz	123	1	0	0	65	0	0	0	73
Roasting, skin and meat, 4 oz	242	18	5	0	82	0	0	0	76
Liver, 4 oz	130	5	2	0	386	0	0	0	80
Wing, meat only, 4 oz	141	4	1	0	64	0	0	0	91
Thigh, meat only, 4 oz	133	4	1	0	93	0	0	0	96
Drumstick, meat only, 4 oz	133	4	1	0	86	0	0	0	99
Turkey:									
Light meat, w/o skin, 4 oz	121	1	0	0	74	0	0	0	58
Dark meat, w/o skin, 4 oz	124	4	1	0	91	0	0	0	77
Turkey, ground, 4 oz	170	9	3	0	90	0	0	0	79
Cornish game hen, 1/2	336	24	7	0	170	0	0	0	102

BRANDS . . .

Most brands are within the generic range. NOTE: The amount of sodium in packaged poultry varies within brands and cuts of meat. Some may have as much as 190mg sodium per 4-oz serving.

NON-MEAT SUBSTITUTES

Food	Cal	Fat	Sat	TFat	Chol	Carb	Fib	Sug	Sod
Harvest Direct Soy Chicken, 1 pc	52	0	0	0	0	3	0	3	120

PREPARED ENTREES *(see Meat and Poultry – Prepared Entrees, pg 95)*

GAME MEAT

Food	Cal	Fat	Sat	TFat	Chol	Carb	Fib	Sug	Sod
Rabbit, 3 oz	116	5	1	0	48	0	0	0	35
Deer, 3 oz	102	2	1	0	72	0	0	0	43

Food Food	Cal	Fat	Sat	TFat	Chol	Carb	Fib	Sug	Sod
GAME MEAT (CONT'D)									
Buffalo (bison), top round, 3 oz	145	5	2	0	73	0	0	0	45
Ground, 3 oz	187	13	6	0	59	0	0	0	55
Elk, 3 oz	94	1	0	0	47	0	0	0	49
Duck, meat only, 3 oz	111	5	2	0	65	0	0	0	62
Goose, meat only, 3 oz	135	6	2	0	71	0	0	0	73

BRANDS . . .
Most brands are within the generic range.

(HAM AND PORK)

Pork loin roast, boneless, lean, 3 oz	120	4	2	0	47	0	0	0	38
Pork, whole leg (ham), 3 oz	208	16	6	60	2	0	0	0	40
Pork, ground, 3 oz	223	18	7	0	61	0	0	0	47
Pork ribs, lean, 3 oz	134	7	2	0	54	0	0	0	57
Pork shoulder, lean, 3 oz	126	6	2	0	57	0	0	0	65
Pork, cured ham, canned, 3 oz	162	11	4	0	33	0	0	0	1055
25% less sodium, roasted, 3 oz	140	7	3	0	49	0	0	0	824
Ham, boneless, 3 oz	137	7	2	0	48	3	1	0	1095
Chopped ham, canned, 3 oz	201	16	5	0	41	0	0	0	1147

BRANDS . . . *(2 OZ UNLESS NOTED)*

Boar's Head Ham, 42% Lower Sodium	60	1	0	0	-	0	0	0	460
Schaller & Weber Lower Sodium	50	1	0	0	25	2	0	1	540

PREPARED ENTREES *(see Meat and Poultry – Prepared Entrees, pg 95)*

(HOT DOGS, FRANKFURTERS AND SAUSAGES)

HOT DOGS AND FRANKFURTERS

Corn dog, 2.7 oz	180	10	3	0	35	15	1	1	490
Beef & pork, 1.6 oz	137	12	5	0	23	1	0	0	504
Beef, 1.6 oz	149	13	5	0	24	2	0	2	513
Chicken, 1.6 oz	116	9	3	0	45	3	0	0	617
Turkey, 1.6 oz	102	8	3	0	48	1	0	0	642

BRANDS . . . *(1.6 OZ HOT DOG/FRANKFURTER UNLESS NOTED)*
Many of the hot dogs below exceed sodium guidelines, but are less than the generic.

Aaron's Best Glatt Kosher All Beef	130	11	5	0	25	2	0	1	240
Abeles & Heymann Beef, Reduced Sodium	100	8	3	0	25	0	0	0	195
Applegate Farms Uncured Turkey	80	6	2	0	30	0	0	0	350
Boar's Head Lite Beef, Skinless	90	6	3	0	25	0	0	0	270
Coleman's All NaturalUncured Beef, 2 oz	160	14	6	0	35	1	0	1	320
Hatfield Reduced Sodium	170	15	5	0	35	1	0	1	300

MEAT, POULTRY AND ALTERNATIVES
Luncheon, Deli and Sandwich Meats

Food	Cal	Fat	Sat	TFat	Chol	Carb	Fib	Sug	Sod
HOT DOGS AND FRANKFURTERS (CONT'D)									
Shelton's Uncured Chicken, 1.2 oz	80	7	2	0	35	1	0	0	260
Uncured Turkey, 1.2 oz	60	5	2	0	25	1	0	0	260
Veggie Patch Spiced Apple Sausage, 2 oz									
Simply the Best Veggie Dogs	90	5	2	0	0	3	0	1	310
Wellshire Farms Cheese Franks	110	9	4	0	30	0	0	0	300
NY Style Big Beef or Premium Franks	110	9	4	0	30	0	0	0	300
Chicken Franks	100	8	2	0	30	0	0	0	320
Turkey Franks	110	6	2	0	30	1	0	1	330
CORN DOG									
State Fair LF Turkey Corn Dog, 2.7 oz	140	3	1	1	10	22	1	7	390
NON-MEAT ALTERNATIVES									
Lightlife Tofu Pups, Original	60	3	1	0	0	2	1	0	300
Smart Dogs	45	0	0	0	0	2	1	1	320
SoyBoy Not Dogs	95	3	1	0	0	10	1	1	240
Yves Tofu Dogs, 1.4 oz	45	1	0	0	0	2	0	0	240
Zoglo's Vegetarian Choice, 1.3 oz	145	1	0	0	0	1	1	0	114
SAUSAGES									
Italian sweet sausage, 1 oz	92	2	1	0	8	1	0	0	160
Italian sausage, 1 oz	97	9	3	0	21	0	0	0	205
Bratwurst, pork, 1 oz	93	8	3	0	21	1	0	0	237
Liverwurst, 1 oz	92	8	3	0	44	1	0	0	244
Polish sausage, 1 oz	92	8	3	0	20	0	0	0	248
Knockwurst, 1 oz	87	8	3	0	17	1	0	0	264
Vienna sausage, canned, 1 oz	64	5	2	0	24	1	0	0	271
Kielbasa, turkey and beef, 1 oz	63	5	2	0	20	1	0	0	305
Braunschweiger, 1 oz	92	8	3	0	50	1	0	0	325
Chorizo, 1 oz	127	11	4	0	25	1	0	0	346

BRANDS . . .

Most brands are within the generic range, except for the following:

Bilinski's All Natural Chicken Sausage

Food	Cal	Fat	Sat	TFat	Chol	Carb	Fib	Sug	Sod
Wild Rice Bratwurst, 2 oz	70	2	1	0	25	2	0	0	230
Peppers & Onions, 2 oz	70	4	2	0	60	1	0	0	270
Spinach & Garlic, 2 oz	70	4	1	0	40	1	1	0	270
Sun-Dried Tomato, 2 oz	70	4	2	0	40	2	0	0	280

LUNCHEON, DELI AND SANDWICH MEATS

Food	Cal	Fat	Sat	TFat	Chol	Carb	Fib	Sug	Sod
Pastrami, 1 oz	27	0	0	0	13	0	0	0	283
Turkey pastrami, 1 oz	35	1	1	0	19	1	0	1	278

Food Food	Cal	Fat	Sat	TFat	Chol	Carb	Fib	Sug	Sod
LUNCHEON, DELI AND SANDWICH MEATS (CONT'D)									
Bologna, 1 oz	89	8	3	0	16	1	0	0	302
Turkey bologna, 1 oz	59	4	1	0	21	1	0	1	351
Salami, 1 oz	71	6	2	0	18	1	0	0	302
Turkey salami, 1 oz	43	3	1	0	21	0	0	0	281
Ham, 1 oz	31	1	1	0	13	1	0	0	310
Turkey ham, 1 oz	33	1	0	0	19	0	0	0	291
Turkey, oven-roasted, LF, 1 oz	25	1	0	0	15	0	0	0	350
Beef, 1 oz	42	2	1	0	20	0	0	0	396
BRANDS ... *(1 OZ UNLESS NOTED)*									
BEEF									
Applegate Farms Roast Beef, 2 oz	110	3	1	0	50	0	0	0	230
Boar's Head									
Oven Roasted Top Round, NSA	45	2	1	0	15	0	0	0	20
Deluxe Top Round, LS	40	1	1	0	15	0	0	0	40
Pepper Seasoned Eye Round	45	2	1	0	20	0	0	0	95
Cajun Style Seasoned Eye Round	40	1	0	0	18	0	0	0	130
Dietz & Watson Angus Roast Beef	35	1	1	0	15	0	0	0	95
Sara Lee Roast Beef, 1 slice, 0.8 oz	30	2	1	0	13	0	0	0	130
Steak-umm Sandwich Steaks, 2 oz	190	17	7	0	35	0	0	0	55
BOLOGNA									
Most brands are within the generic range.									
HAM AND PORK									
Boar's Head Ham									
Pesto Parmesan Oven Roasted	45	2	1	0	15	0	0	0	160
Branded Deluxe 42% Lower Sodium	30	1	0	0	13	1	0	1	230
Dietz & Watson									
Roast Sirloin of Pork	30	1	1	0	15	0	0	0	175
PASTRAMI									
Most brands are within the generic range.									
SALAMI									
Best's Beef	85	7	3	0	17	1	0	1	180
Dietz & Watson Genoa Salami	90	2	1	0	5	0	0	0	115
TURKEY AND CHICKEN									
Boar's Head									
Turkey Breast, skinless, Lower Sodium	30	1	0	0	13	0	0	0	170
Dietz & Watson									
Turkey Breast, Gourmet Lite, NSA, 2 oz	70	1	0	0	30	2	0	2	50
OTHER MEATS									
Dietz & Watson									
Prosciutto Classico	25	2	1	0	5	0	0	0	115

MEAT, POULTRY AND ALTERNATIVES
Non-Meat Substitutes

Food	Cal	Fat	Sat	TFat	Chol	Carb	Fib	Sug	Sod

NON-MEAT LUNCHEON MEATS

BRANDS . . . *(1 OZ UNLESS NOTED)*

Lightlife Smart Deli

Food	Cal	Fat	Sat	TFat	Chol	Carb	Fib	Sug	Sod
Old World Bologna (2 slices)	30	0	0	0	0	1	1	0	185
Country Ham Style (2 slices)	45	0	0	0	0	2	1	0	200
Three Peppercorn Pastrami Style (2 slices)	30	0	0	0	0	0	0	0	200

NON-MEAT SUBSTITUTES

(also see Breakfast Meat Substitutes, pg ??; Non-Meat Substitutes (Ground Beef), pg ??; Non-Meat Burgers and Patties, pg ??; Non-Meat Luncheon Meats, above.

TEMPEH

Food	Cal	Fat	Sat	TFat	Chol	Carb	Fib	Sug	Sod
Tempeh, 1/2 cup	160	9	2	0	0	8	4	1	7

BRANDS . . .
Most brands are within the generic range. NOTE: Some seasoned varieties have much more sodium.

TOFU

Food	Cal	Fat	Sat	TFat	Chol	Carb	Fib	Sug	Sod
Tofu, 1/2 cup	88	5	1	0	0	2	1	1	15

BRANDS . . .
Most brands are within the generic range.

PATE

(see Pates and Spreads, pg 43)

SANDWICH SPREADS

(also see Pates and Spreads, pg 43; Dips and Spreads, pg 142)

Food	Cal	Fat	Sat	TFat	Chol	Carb	Fib	Sug	Sod
Chicken, 1 oz	44	5	1	0	16	1	0	0	202
Roast beef, 1 oz	65	5	2	0	20	1	0	0	205
Deviled ham, 1 oz	75	6	2	0	18	0	0	0	230
Ham salad, 1 oz	61	4	1	0	11	3	0	0	259
Pork & beef, 1 oz	67	5	2	0	11	3	0	0	287
Ham & cheese, 1 oz	69	5	2	0	17	1	0	0	339

BRANDS . . .
Most brands are within the generic range.

SAUSAGE

(see Breakfast Meats, pg 127; Sausages, pg 132)

Food Food	Cal	Fat	Sat	TFat	Chol	Carb	Fib	Sug	Sod

PASTA, NOODLES, RICE AND GRAINS

GRAINS

(also see Rice, pg 136)

Food	Cal	Fat	Sat	TFat	Chol	Carb	Fib	Sug	Sod
Wheat bran, 1/2 cup	63	1	0	0	0	19	12	0	1
Oat bran, 1/2 cup	116	3	1	0	0	31	7	1	2
Millet, 1/2 cup	378	4	1	0	0	73	9	-	5
Couscous, dry, 1/2 cup	325	1	0	0	0	67	4	-	9
Barley, pearl, 1/2 cup	352	1	0	0	0	78	16	1	9
Buckwheat groats, roasted, 1/2 cup	284	2	0	0	0	62	8	-	9
Bulgur, 1/2 cup	239	1	0	0	0	53	13	0	12
Quinoa, 1/2 cup	318	5	1	0	0	59	5	0	18

BRANDS . . .
Most brands are within the generic range.

GRAIN DISHES – PACKAGED

Food	Cal	Fat	Sat	TFat	Chol	Carb	Fib	Sug	Sod
Tabouli, mix, prep, 2/3 cup	95	0	0	0	0	22	4	1	340
Couscous w/roasted garlic, mix, prep, 1 cup	200	2	0	0	0	41	2	1	480
Falafel, mix, 1/4 cup	120	2	0	0	0	20	4	3	610

BRANDS . . .

MIX

Nu-World Foods

Food	Cal	Fat	Sat	TFat	Chol	Carb	Fib	Sug	Sod
Garlic Herb, 2 cups	149	2	0	0	0	27	5	0	2
Spanish Tomato Amaranth, 2 cups	151	2	0	0	0	26	4	1	111
Savory Herb, 1 cup	74	1	0	0	0	13	2	0	163

PASTA AND NOODLES

Food	Cal	Fat	Sat	TFat	Chol	Carb	Fib	Sug	Sod
Lasagne, dry, 2 oz	210	1	0	0	0	40	2	0	0
Farfel, matzo, 1 oz	105	0	0	0	0	21	-	-	0
Macaroni & spaghetti, dry, 2 oz	211	1	0	0	0	43	2	1	3
Macaroni & spaghetti, whole wheat, dry, 2 oz	198	1	0	0	0	43	5	0	5
Noodles, egg, dry, 2 oz	219	3	1	0	48	41	2	1	12
Pasta, fresh-refrigerated, 4.5 oz	369	3	0	0	93	70	-	-	33

BRANDS . . .
Most brands are within the generic range.

PASTA, NOODLES, RICE AND GRAINS
Rice and Rice Dishes

Food	Cal	Fat	Sat	TFat	Chol	Carb	Fib	Sug	Sod

PASTA AND NOODLE DISHES *(see Pasta Dinners, pg 96; Pasta Entrees, pg 99)*

PASTA SAUCE *(see Pasta Sauce, pg 100)*

RICE AND RICE DISHES

RICE

Food	Cal	Fat	Sat	TFat	Chol	Carb	Fib	Sug	Sod
White rice, uncooked, 1/2 cup	351	1	0	0	0	77	1	0	1
Brown rice, uncooked, 1/4 cup	344	3	1	0	0	72	3	0	4
Wild rice, uncooked, 1/4 cup	286	1	0	0	0	60	5	2	6
Instant rice, 1/2 cup	190	1	0	0	0	43	1	0	15

BRANDS . . .
Most brands are within the generic range.

RICE DISHES *(also see Fried Rice, pg 109)*

Food	Cal	Fat	Sat	TFat	Chol	Carb	Fib	Sug	Sod
Risotto, mix, 1/4 cup	150	0	0	0	0	34	0	0	420
Rice w/vegetables, frozen, 1 cup	180	4	2	10	0	31	2	2	480
Rice & beans, mix, 1/4 cup	160	0	0	0	0	35	3	1	490
Rice pilaf, mix, prep, 1 cup	210	5	1	0	0	41	1	0	710
Long grain & wild rice, mix, prep, 1 cup	220	5	1	0	0	42	2	0	800
Flavored rice, mix, prep, 1 cup	320	2	0	0	0	51	2	2	1070
1/3 less salt, prep, 1 cup	280	1	0	0	0	53	1	2	640
Spanish rice, mix, prep, 1 cup	300	2	1	0	0	65	2	2	1000
Fried rice, mix, prep, 1 cup	260	1	0	0	0	47	1	3	1095

BRANDS . . .

MIX *(1 CUP PREP UNLESS NOTED)*

Food	Cal	Fat	Sat	TFat	Chol	Carb	Fib	Sug	Sod
Dr. McDougall's Curry Brown & Wild Rice									
Fruited Pilaf	150	2	0	0	0	30	2	1	300
Neera's Northern Indian Biryani	132	1	0	0	0	29	0	0	4
Indian Dal w/Chaunk	140	1	0	0	0	23	0	0	4
Indian Urad & Channa Dal	104	1	0	0	0	18	0	0	4
Jamaican-Style Dirty Rice	175	6	0	0	0	28	0	0	5
Indian Shahi Pilau	286	8	0	0	0	48	0	0	6
Sadaf Basmati Rice									
Aromatic Delight, 1/2 pkg	220	1	0	0	0	67	0	2	20
Roasted Noodle Raisinette, 1/2 pkg	310	3	0	0	0	65	0	3	20
Sabzi Polo, 1/2 pkg	310	3	0	0	0	65	0	3	20
Sweet Harmony, 1/2 pkg	305	2	0	0	0	67	0	13	25
Wild West Favorite, 1/2 pkg	220	1	0	0	0	67	0	2	35
Zatarain's New Orleans Spanish	100	0	0	0	0	21	3	0	280

Food Food	Cal	Fat	Sat	TFat	Chol	Carb	Fib	Sug	Sod

SNACK FOODS

CHIPS AND NIBBLERS

CORN AND TORTILLA CHIPS

Food	Cal	Fat	Sat	TFat	Chol	Carb	Fib	Sug	Sod
Tortilla chips, plain, 1 oz	138	7	1	0	0	19	2	0	110
Ranch, 1 oz	142	7	1	0	0	18	1	1	147
Nacho, 1 oz	144	7	1	0	1	17	1	1	174
Nacho, light, 1 oz	126	4	1	0	1	20	1	0	284
Corn chips, regular, 1 oz	147	8	1	0	0	18	2	0	175
Barbecue, 1 oz	148	9	1	0	0	16	2	0	216
BRANDS . . . *(1 OZ UNLESS NOTED)*									
Bearito's									
Little Bear Corn Chips	150	10	2	0	0	15	1	0	0
Blue Chips, NSA	140	7	1	0	0	18	2	0	10
Blue Chips	140	7	1	0	0	18	2	0	60
Red, White, or Yellow Chips	140	7	1	0	0	18	2	0	65
Blue Farm Blue Corn, NSA	130	5	1	0	0	20	0	0	0
Cucina del Norte									
Yellow Corn Triangles	140	5	1	0	0	20	1	0	70
Garden of Eatin'									
NSA Blue Chips	140	7	1	0	0	18	2	0	10
Blue Chips	140	7	1	0	0	18	2	0	60
Mini Corns, all	140	7	1	0	0	19	2	0	60
Little Soy or Sunny Blues	140	7	1	0	0	17	2	0	70
Black Bean Corn	140	7	1	0	0	18	4	0	70
Red, White, or Yellow Chips (avg)	140	7	1	0	0	18	1	0	70
Sesame Blues	150	8	1	0	0	16	2	0	90
Guiltless Gourmet									
Unsalted Yellow Corn	110	1	0	0	0	22	2	0	26
Naturally Preferred									
Yellow Corn	140	6	1	0	0	19	1	0	40
Nature's Promise									
Natural Blue	140	6	1	0	0	18	1	0	60
Natural Yellow	140	6	1	0	0	18	1	0	65
Que Pasa, all	135	6	1	0	0	19	2	0	42
Rosa Mexicana All Natural	150	6	1	0	0	21	2	0	75
Tostitos Natural									
Blue or Yellow Corn	140	6	1	0	0	19	1	0	80

SNACK FOODS
Chips and Nibblers (Fruit Chips)

Food	Cal	Fat	Sat	TFat	Chol	Carb	Fib	Sug	Sod
FRUIT CHIPS									
Banana chips, 1 oz	147	10	8	0	0	17	2	10	2
BRANDS . . . *(1 OZ UNLESS NOTED)*									
***Seneca* Pear**	150	9	1	0	0	19	2	7	10
Apple	140	7	1	0	0	20	2	11	15
Cinnamon Pear	160	9	1	0	0	20	5	10	15
POTATO CHIPS									
Potato chips, regular, 1 oz	155	11	3	-	0	14	1	1	149
Reduced fat, 1 oz	134	6	1	-	0	19	2	-	139
Sour cream & onion, 1 oz	151	10	3	-	2	15	2	-	177
Barbecue, 1 oz	139	9	2	-	0	15	1	-	213
Cheese, 1 oz	141	8	2	-	1	16	2	-	225
BRANDS . . . *(1 OZ UNLESS NOTED)*									
***Barbara's Bakery* Unsalted**	150	10	1	0	0	15	1	0	20
***Kettle Chips* NS**	150	9	1	0	0	15	1	0	10
Lightly Salted	150	9	1	0	0	15	1	0	110
Michael Seasons									
Unsalted, Reduced Fat	140	7	1	0	0	17	0	1	10
Thick & Crunchy, Unsalted	140	6	1	0	0	18	2	1	75
***Seneca* Cinnamon Sweet Potato**	150	7	1	0	0	18	4	8	30
***Snyder's of Hanover* Unsalted**	140	6	2	0	0	19	2	0	0
***Terra* Sweet Potato, NSA**	140	7	1	0	0	18	1	2	10
Yukon Gold Onion & Garlic	130	5	1	0	0	19	1	1	65
Jalapeno Sweet Potato	140	7	1	0	0	18	1	4	65
Sea Salt White & Russett	140	6	1	0	0	18	1	1	65
Red Bliss Fine Herbs	140	7	1	0	0	18	3	1	70
Original	140	7	1	0	0	18	3	1	70
Yukon Gold, 50% Less Fat	130	5	1	0	0	19	0	0	80
Red Bliss Sun-Dried Tomato	140	7	1	0	0	18	3	1	85
Yukon Gold Barbecue	130	5	1	0	0	19	2	1	90
Sea Salt White, Russet & Blue	140	6	1	0	0	18	1	0	90
***Utz* NS**	150	9	2	0	0	14	1	1	5
Regular, Kettle Classics, or Wavy	150	9	2	0	0	14	1	1	95
Ripple	150	10	3	0	0	14	1	0	95
OTHER CRUNCHIES AND NIBBLERS									
Oriental mix, rice based, 1 oz	143	7	1	0	0	15	4	1	117
Corn nuts, regular, 1 oz	125	4	1	0	0	21	2	0	157
Nacho, 1 oz	124	4	1	0	0	20	2	0	180
Barbecue, 1 oz	124	4	1	0	0	20	2	0	277

Food Food	Cal	Fat	Sat	TFat	Chol	Carb	Fib	Sug	Sod
OTHER CRUNCHIES AND NIBBLERS (CONT'D)									
Chex mix, 1 oz	120	5	2	0	0	18	2	-	288
Cheese puffs, 1 oz	158	10	2	1	0	15	1	1	298
Sesame sticks, 1 oz	153	10	2	0	0	13	1	0	422
Pork skins, plain, 1 oz	155	9	3	0	27	0	0	0	521
Barbecue, 1 oz	153	9	3	0	33	1	0	0	756
BRANDS . . . *(1 oz UNLESS NOTED)*									
Burns & Ricker Garlic Bagel Chips	110	0	0	-	0	22	1	2	30
Party Mix	107	0	0	-	0	23	1	2	38
Kangaroo Baked Pita Chips, Plain	90	2	0	0	0	18	1	1	100
Baked Pita Chips, Crispy Cinnamon	90	2	0	0	0	19	1	2	140
New York Style Bagel Chips, Plain	140	6	3	0	0	17	1	1	70
Bagel Chips, Cinnamon Raisin	130	6	3	0	0	17	1	7	80
Pita Chips, Maple Cinnamon	130	5	3	0	0	18	1	2	90
Mini Bagel Chips, Cinnamon Raisin	130	6	3	0	0	17	1	1	115
Nu-World Foods Amaranth									
Snackers									
Chili Lime	117	2	0	0	0	20	3	1	10
Bar BQ Sweet & Sassy	118	3	0	0	0	20	3	1	36
Bar BQ Hot & Spicy, ...	113	2	0	0	0	20	3	1	47
French Onion	115	2	0	0	0	20	3	1	56
Garden Burst	114	2	0	0	0	20	3	1	69
Mini Ridges									
Sun-Dried Tomato Basil	81	3	0	0	0	17	10	1	65
Rosemary Basil	75	2	0	0	0	19	11	0	77
Old London Cinnamon Raisin Bagel									
Snacks, 0.5 oz	60	1	0	-	0	12	1	2	65
Organic Garden Soynutty Crunchies									
Unsalted, 0.8 oz	113	5	1	0	0	8	6	0	4
Choc Carousel, 0.8 oz	118	6	1	0	0	9	4	3	84
Roberts American Gourmet									
Cocoa Booty	120	2	0	0	0	27	3	15	80
Pirate's Booty w/Caramel	120	2	0	0	0	23	1	12	90
Chaos or Wheat-Free Chaos	140	6	1	0	0	18	2	1	100
Snyder's of Hanover									
Unsalted Nibblers	120	0	0	0	0	25	3	0	50
CheddAirs	135	5	1	0	0	20	3	0	90
Honey Mustard & Onion Nibblers	130	3	2	0	0	23	3	0	95
Weight Watchers									
Cheese Curls, 0.5 oz	70	3	1	-	0	10	0	0	85

Food	Cal	Fat	Sat	TFat	Chol	Carb	Fib	Sug	Sod

(CRACKERS)

Food	Cal	Fat	Sat	TFat	Chol	Carb	Fib	Sug	Sod
Whole wheat, 0.5 oz	63	2	1	-	0	10	2	0	94
Wheat, 0.5 oz	67	3	1	-	0	9	1	2	113
Cheese, 0.5 oz	71	4	1	-	2	8	0	1	141

BRANDS ... *(0.5 OZ UNLESS NOTED)*

There are many low-sodium crackers, the following have less than 100mg per serving.

Food	Cal	Fat	Sat	TFat	Chol	Carb	Fib	Sug	Sod
Bisca Organic Water Crackers (avg)	60	1	0	0	0	11	0	0	85
Casabe Rainforest									
Gluten Free, all (avg)	25	6	1	0	0	14	5	0	17
Dare									
Bremmer LS Wafers	70	2	0	0	0	12	0	0	10
Breton Reduced Fat/Sodium	60	2	1	0	0	9	0	1	55
Cabaret	70	4	2	0	0	9	0	1	70
Ener-G Sesame	160	9	2	0	0	16	4	0	80
Foods Alive Golden Flax, Maple &									
Cinnamon, 1 oz	150	8	1	0	0	12	8	4	15
Health Valley									
Rice Bran	110	3	0	0	0	19	3	4	70
Oat Bran	120	3	0	0	0	22	3	3	80
Bruschetta Vegetable, NSA	60	2	0	0	0	10	1	1	40
Keebler Town House, LS	80	5	1	0	0	10	1	1	80
Kemach									
Snackers, Unsalted, 9	160	8	-	0	0	19	-	-	80
Nabisco									
Ritz Crackers, LS, 1 oz	80	4	1	0	0	10	0	1	35
Triscuits, LS, 1 oz	140	5	1	0	0	22	4	0	75
Wheat Thins, LS, 1 oz	140	6	1	0	0	20	1	3	75
Nairns Stem Ginger Wheat-Free	88	3	1	0	0	15	2	4	60
O'Coco's									
Baked Choc Crisps	90	2	0	0	0	16	1	6	50
Partners, all (avg)	65	3	2	3	0	8	1	2	60
Pepperidge Farm *Goldfish*, Cheddar									
Cheese Baked, Reduced Sodium	75	3	1	-	5	9	1	0	88
Distinctive Butter Thins	70	3	1	-	10	10	0	1	95
Cracker Quartet	70	3	1	-	5	10	1	1	95
Private Harvest									
Spicy Italian Cheese Bruschetta	60	3	2	0	5	6	0	0	65

Food Food	Cal	Fat	Sat	TFat	Chol	Carb	Fib	Sug	Sod
CRACKERS (CONT'D)									
Red Oval Farms Stoned Wheat Thins									
Lower Sodium	60	2	1	0	0	10	1	0	70
Upper Crust									
Sesame Pepper Crostini, 1	35	2	0	-	0	5	0	1	5
Blue Cheese & Walnut, 1	45	3	1	-	0	4	0	0	35
Venus Fat Free									
Cracked Pepper or Garden Veg (avg)	60	0	0	0	0	12	0	1	80
Garlic & Herb	60	0	0	0	0	12	0	1	90
CRISPBREAD AND FLATBREAD									
Crispbread, rye, 0.5 oz	52	0	0	0	0	12	2	0	37
Norweigan flatbread, 0.5 oz	53	0	0	0	0	12	2	0	38
BRANDS . . . (1 OZ UNLESS NOTED)									
Most brands are within the generic range.									
GRAHAM CRACKERS									
Graham crackers, 1 oz	120	3	0	0	0	22	1	9	172
Chocolate, 1 oz	137	7	4	0	0	19	1	12	82
BRANDS . . . (1 OZ UNLESS NOTED)									
Health Valley									
Amaranth	120	3	0	0	0	22	3	4	80
Oat Brand	120	3	0	0	0	22	3	3	80
Keebler									
Cinnamon Crisp	130	4	1	0	0	23	1	9	140
LF Cinnamon Crisp	110	2	0	0	0	23	1	9	140
New Morning									
Mini Bites, Choc	110	3	1	0	0	19	1	7	110
Pepperidge Farm									
Goldfish Choc, 1 pouch (0.7 oz)	100	4	2	0	0	15	2	6	75
Cinnamon, 1 pouch (0.7 oz)	100	3	2	0	5	15	1	5	85
MATZOS									
Matzo, plain, 1 oz	112	0	0	0	0	24	1	0	1
Whole wheat, 1 oz	100	0	0	0	0	22	3	0	1
Egg, 1 oz	111	1	0	0	24	22	1	0	6
Egg & onion, 1 oz	111	1	0	0	13	22	1	0	81
BRANDS . . . (1 OZ UNLESS NOTED)									
Most brands are within the generic range.									
MELBA AND CRISP TOAST									
Melba toast, plain, 0.5 oz	55	0	0	0	0	11	1	0	118

SNACK FOODS
Diet, Energy and Nutritional Bars

Food	Cal	Fat	Sat	TFat	Chol	Carb	Fib	Sug	Sod
MELBA AND CRISP TOAST (CONT'D)									
Whole wheat, 0.5 oz	53	0	0	0	0	11	1	0	119
Rye, 0.5 oz	55	0	0	0	0	11	1	0	128
BRANDS . . . *(0.5 OZ UNLESS NOTED)*									
Devonsheer									
Unsalted, all	50	1	0	-	0	10	2	0	0
Grille'									
Toast No Sodium	68	1	0	0	0	13	1	0	6
Plain	68	1	0	0	0	13	0	1	56
Old London									
Unsalted, most (avg)	50	0	0	-	0	11	2	0	0
Salted, most (avg)	50	0	0	-	0	11	1	0	85
RICE CRACKERS AND OTHER THINS									
Rice crackers, salted, 0.5 oz	55	1	0	0	0	11	1	0	10
Unsalted, 0.5 oz	55	1	0	0	0	11	1	0	0
BRANDS . . .									
Most brands are within the generic range.									
SALTINES									
Saltines, 0.5 oz	62	2	0	0	0	10	0	0	152
Unsalted tops, 0.5 oz	62	2	0	0	0	10	0	0	109
BRANDS . . . *(0.5 OZ UNLESS NOTED)*									
Keebler Zesta Saltines									
Unsalted Tops	60	2	1	1	0	12	1	0	80
Nabisco Premium LS Saltines	60	2	0	0	0	10	0	0	35
SANDWICH CRACKERS									
Sandwich w/cheese filling, 1 pkg	134	6	2	-	1	17	1	1	392
Sandwich w/peanut butter filling, 1 pkg	138	7	1	-	0	16	1	3	201
BRANDS . . . *(1 PKG UNLESS NOTED)*									
Lance									
Peanut Butter on Malt	190	10	2	0	0	18	1	2	130
Peanut Butter with Honey	210	13	2	0	0	19	1	3	170
Toasty, Peanut Butter	180	9	2	0	0	16	1	3	220
Reduced Fat Toastchee	180	7	2	0	0	23	2	2	230

DIET, ENERGY AND NUTRITIONAL BARS

There are many low-sodium diet, energy and nutritional bars, the following have 100mg or less per serving.

Food Food	Cal	Fat	Sat	TFat	Chol	Carb	Fib	Sug	Sod
DIET, ENERGY AND NUTRITIONAL BARS (CONT'D)									
BRANDS . . .									
FROZEN/REFRIGERATED *(3.5 OZ UNLESS NOTED)*									
Cold Fusion									
Protein & Energy Bars (avg)	80	0	0	0	0	21	0	21	0
READY-TO-EAT *(1.8 OZ BAR UNLESS NOTED)*									
Atkins									
Morning Start									
Creamy Cinnamon	150	7	5	0	0	15	9	0	60
Strawberry or Apple Cinn Fruit & Grain	100	2	0	0	15	20	9	1	73
Apple Crisp	180	9	5	0	0	14	7	1	80
Strawberry Crisp	160	9	5	0	0	14	7	1	95
Choc Chip Crisp	160	7	4	0	0	15	5	1	100
Advantage									
Choc Decadence	220	10	7	0	0	26	11	1	80
Caramel Fudge Brownie	160	8	5	0	5	17	9	1	85
Morning Oatmeal Raisin	140	4	1	0	0	15	5	3	95
Choc Coconut	230	10	8	0	0	23	10	1	95
Pralines & Cream	270	12	8	0	0	21	9	0	100
Aunt Candice									
Protein Bars, 2 oz (avg)	240	11	3	0	0	31	3	8	60
Balance *Gold*	210	7	4	0	0	23	1	3	85
Clif Bar Cranberry Apple Cherry	230	3	1	0	0	45	5	21	100
Fi-Bar, 1.2 oz (avg)	120	2	1	0	0	26	3	12	25
Honey Bars, all, 1.4 oz (avg)	180	9	2	0	0	21	2	13	20
Momentum Low Carb Bars									
Chocarnut, 5.6 oz	150	6	3	0	5	-	3	2	110
Nutiva Flax-Raisin, 1.4 oz	200	15	2	0	0	15	4	8	0
Flax-Choc, 1.4 oz	200	12	2	0	0	19	5	10	5
Hempseed, 1.4 oz	210	14	2	0	0	11	5	5	5
Omega Smart most, 2.3 oz (avg)	220	9	0	0	0	33	6	25	0
Power Bar									
Harvest Whole Grain, 2.3 oz (avg)	240	5	1	0	0	42	5	18	140
Pria 110 Plus, 1 bar (avg)	110	4	3	0	0	15	1	9	90
Pria Carb Select									
Cookies 'n Caramel, 1.7 oz	170	7	5	0	5	22	2	1	90
Caramel Nut Brownie, 1.7 oz	170	8	5	0	5	21	2	1	90
Choc Mocha Crisp, 1.7 oz	130	6	4	0	0	16	4	1	115
Performance, 2.3 oz (avg)	230	2	1	0	0	45	2	20	100

Food	Cal	Fat	Sat	TFat	Chol	Carb	Fib	Sug	Sod
DIET, ENERGY AND NUTRITIONAL BARS (CONT'D)									
Slim Fast									
Rich Chewy Caramel	120	4	3	0	5	18	1	9	50
Choc Peanut Nougat	120	4	3	0	5	20	1	9	70
Peanut Butter Crunch	120	4	2	0	0	21	1	12	80
Choc Chip Muffin	140	6	1	0	5	20	1	9	100
Choc Mint Crisp	120	4	3	0	5	19	1	7	100
Peanut Butter Cookie Bar	120	4	2	0	0	19	1	8	105
Choc Chip Cookie Bar	120	4	2	0	0	19	1	9	110
Oatmeal Raisin Cookie Bar	120	4	2	0	0	19	1	8	115
Crispy Peanut Caramel	120	4	3	0	5	20	1	8	120
Tigers Milk									
Peanut Butter Crunch, 1.3 oz	160	8	2	0	0	19	2	16	70
Peanut Butter, 1.3 oz	170	7	2	0	0	19	0	13	80
Original, 1.3 oz	160	6	1	0	0	20	0	13	90
Zoe Foods Nutri Bar									
Choc Delight, 1.7 oz	190	7	3	0	0	27	5	13	70
Heavenly Apple, 1.7 oz	180	5	1	0	0	28	5	10	70
Choc Peanut Butter Bliss, 1.7 oz	200	8	3	0	0	26	5	11	70
Peanut Butter Paradise, 1.7 oz	190	6	1	0	0	27	5	8	70

(DIPS AND SPREADS)

(also see Pates and Spreads, pg 43; Salsa and Taco Sauce, pg 117)

Food	Cal	Fat	Sat	TFat	Chol	Carb	Fib	Sug	Sod
Hummus, 1 oz	46	3	0	0	0	4	1	0	106
Guacamole, 2 tbsp	60	5	1	0	0	3	0	2	140
Bean, 2 tbsp	40	1	0	0	0	5	1	0	170
Creamy herbal, refrigerated, 2 tbsp	100	9	2	0	5	2	1	1	190
Cheese, 2 tbsp	60	4	2	0	5	3	0	0	330
BRANDS ...									
FROZEN/REFRIGERATED *(1 OZ UNLESS NOTED)*									
Cedarlane									
5 Layer Mexican Dip	60	3	2	0	10	4	1	2	100
Cedar's									
Hommus Baba Ghannouj	50	2	0	0	0	5	3	0	80
Oasis Hommus									
Black Bean Dip	11	0	0	0	0	1	1	0	38
Baba Ghannouj	31	2	0	0	0	3	1	0	73
Hommus, Roasted Garlic, Spinach, or Roasted Red Pepper (avg)	32	1	0	0	0	4	1	0	76
Hommus Spread, Original	34	1	0	0	0	4	1	0	81

Food Food	Cal	Fat	Sat	TFat	Chol	Carb	Fib	Sug	Sod
DIPS AND SPREADS (GUILTLESS GOURMET CONT'D)									
Private Harvest									
Italian White Bean	35	2	0	0	0	4	1	1	85
Sabra									
Roasted Red Pepper Hummus	70	5	1	0	0	4	1	0	115
Roasted Garlic Hummus	60	6	1	0	0	4	1	0	130
Classic Hummus	60	6	1	0	0	4	1	0	135
Tribe of Two Shieks									
Hummus, all (avg)	50	3	0	0	0	4	1	0	105
Wild Garden									
Hummus Dip, all	35	2	0	0	0	4	1	1	70
SHELF-STABLE *(1 OZ UNLESS NOTED)*									
Desert Pepper									
Tuscan White Bean	30	1	0	0	0	5	1	1	45
El Paso Chili Co.									
Bean Dips (avg)	25	0	0	0	0	5	2	1	20
Esparrago									
Asparagus Guacamole, all	100	0	0	0	0	2	0	1	95
Garden of Eatin'									
Baja Black Bean	25	0	0	0	0	5	1	1	80
Guiltless Gourmet									
Spicy Black Bean	30	0	0	0	0	5	2	0	110
Mild Black Bean	30	0	0	0	0	5	2	0	115
Hummus, all	35	2	0	0	0	4	1	0	115
Road's End Organics									
Nacho Cheese Dip, Mild or Spicy	11	0	0	0	0	2	1	0	85
Winter Gardens									
Maryland Crab	90	9	5	0	35	1	0	0	140

GRANOLA AND CEREAL BARS

(see Cereal, Granola and Breakfast Bars, pg 33)

JERKY AND MEAT SNACKS

Beef sticks, smoked, 1 oz	156	14	6	-	38	2	0	0	420
Beef jerky, chopped & formed, 1 oz	116	7	3	-	14	3	1	0	627
BRANDS . . .									
Shelton's Turkey, 1 oz	100	1	0	0	50	1	0	0	270
Soy Jerky, 1 oz	90	2	0	0	0	14	2	8	250
Tofurky Jurky Original or Peppered, 1 oz ...	100	2	0	0	0	9	1	3	260

Food	Cal	Fat	Sat	TFat	Chol	Carb	Fib	Sug	Sod

(NUTS AND SEEDS)

Nuts, unsalted:

Food	Cal	Fat	Sat	TFat	Chol	Carb	Fib	Sug	Sod
Almonds, 1 oz	164	14	1	0	0	6	3	0	0
Hazelnuts, 1 oz	178	17	1	0	0	5	3	0	0
Pecans, 1 oz	196	20	2	0	0	4	3	0	0
Pistachios, 1 oz	156	12	2	0	0	8	3	0	0
Macadamia nuts, 1 oz	203	22	3	0	0	4	2	0	1
Pine Nuts, 1 oz	161	14	2	0	0	4	1	0	1
Walnuts, 1 oz	185	19	2	0	0	4	2	0	1
Cashews, 1 oz	163	13	3	0	0	9	1	0	4
Nuts, dry roasted w/salt:									
Macadamia nuts, 1 oz	203	22	3	0	0	4	2	0	75
Almonds, 1 oz	169	15	1	0	0	6	3	0	96
Pecans, 1 oz	201	21	2	0	0	4	3	0	109
Pistachios, 1 oz	161	13	2	0	0	8	3	0	121
Cashews, 1 oz	163	13	3	0	0	9	1	0	181
Mixed nuts, 1 oz	168	15	2	0	0	7	3	0	190
Seeds:									
Sunflower seeds, salted 1 oz	165	14	3	0	0	7	3	1	116
Unsalted, 1 oz	165	14	3	0	0	7	3	1	0
Nuts & Seed Snacks:									
Trail mix, regular, 1 oz	131	8	2	0	0	13	-	-	65
Tropical mix, 1 oz	115	5	2	0	0	19	-	-	3
Mix w/choc chips, 1 oz	137	9	2	1	0	13	-	-	34
Sesame sticks, 1 oz	153	10	2	0	0	13	1	0	422

BRANDS ...

Most brands are within the generic range. NOTE: Nuts that are smoked and/or with added spices (barbecue, chili, etc.) may contain as much as 245mg sodium per 1 oz serving.

PEANUT BARS

Food	Cal	Fat	Sat	TFat	Chol	Carb	Fib	Sug	Sod
Peanut bar, 1.6 oz bar	235	15	2	0	0	21	2	19	70

BRANDS ...

Food	Cal	Fat	Sat	TFat	Chol	Carb	Fib	Sug	Sod
Planters, 1.6 oz	230	14	2	0	0	22	2	13	20

(POPCORN)

Food	Cal	Fat	Sat	TFat	Chol	Carb	Fib	Sug	Sod
Air-popped, 1 oz (2 1/2 cups)	110	1	0	0	0	22	4	0	2
Caramel-coated w/o peanuts, 1 oz	122	4	1	1	0	22	2	15	58
w/peanuts, 1 oz (2/3 cup)	113	2	0	0	0	23	1	13	84
Cheese-flavor, 1 oz (2 1/2 cups)	149	9	2	3	-	15	3	-	252

Food Food	Cal	Fat	Sat	TFat	Chol	Carb	Fib	Sug	Sod
POPCORN (CONT'D)									
Microwaved, 1 oz (2 1/2 cups)	160	12	3	-	0	17	4	0	390
BRANDS . . . *(1 oz or about 2 1/2 cups unless noted)*									
MICROWAVE									
Bearitos									
Organic, NS, 10 cups	110	2	0	0	0	23	5	0	0
Garden of Eatin'									
No Oil Added, 5 cups	110	2	0	0	0	23	4	0	90
Butter, 5 cups	150	6	4	0	0	21	2	0	180
Newman's Own									
LS Butter, 3 1/2 cups	130	5	2	0	0	18	3	0	100
Light Butter	120	4	2	0	0	19	4	0	170
Orville Redenbacher's									
Caramel..	180	10	3	-	0	23	2	12	45
Cinnabon	180	14	3	-	0	15	2	3	90
Honey Butter	180	12	3	-	0	16	3	0	170
Smart Balance LF Low Sodium, 5 cups ..	120	2	0	0	0	24	5	0	80
READY-TO-EAT									
CARAMEL-COATED POPCORN									
Most brands are within the generic range.									
PLAIN AND FLAVORED POPCORN									
Bearitos Organic, Lite, NS, 4 cups	120	2	0	0	0	24	1	0	0
Roberts American Gourmet									
Nude Food	110	1	0	0	0	25	3	0	0
Ya Ya's Herb	160	10	1	0	0	15	2	0	110
Light	130	3	1	0	0	21	1	0	140

PRETZELS

Unsalted pretzel, 1 oz	108	1	0	0	0	22	1	1	82
Choc coated pretzel, 1 oz	130	5	2	0	0	20	1	10	161
Pretzel, plain, 1 oz	108	1	0	0	0	23	1	1	385
Soft pretzel, 1 oz	95	1	0	0	0	19	1	0	393
BRANDS . . . *(1 oz unless noted)*									

Most brands are within the generic range, the following have less than the generic.

Snyder's of Hanover Pretzels									
Milk Choc Mini Dips	130	6	4	0	5	18	2	9	100
White Choc Mini Dips	140	6	3	0	5	19	3	9	110

SNACK FOODS
Rice and Popcorn Snacks

Food	Cal	Fat	Sat	TFat	Chol	Carb	Fib	Sug	Sod

RICE AND POPCORN SNACKS

Food	Cal	Fat	Sat	TFat	Chol	Carb	Fib	Sug	Sod
Rice cakes, 1 cake	35	0	0	0	0	7	0	0	20
Unsalted, 1 cake	35	0	0	0	0	7	0	0	2
Popcorn cakes, 1 cake	38	0	0	0	0	8	0	0	29
Crisped rice bar, choc chip, 1 oz	113	4	1	0	0	20	1	-	78

BRANDS . . . *(0.5 OZ UNLESS NOTED)*
Most brands are within the generic range.

SNACK BARS

(also see Cereal, Granola and Breakfast Bars, pg 33; Diet, Energy and Nutritional Bars, pg 144)

Food Food	Cal	Fat	Sat	TFat	Chol	Carb	Fib	Sug	Sod

SOUPS AND CHILI

BOUILLON, BROTHS AND BASES

Food	Cal	Fat	Sat	TFat	Chol	Carb	Fib	Sug	Sod
Chicken broth, reduced/lower sodium, 1 cup	17	0	0	0	0	1	0	1	554
Chicken broth, 1 cup	39	1	0	0	0	1	0	1	776
Beef broth, 1 cup	17	1	0	0	0	0	0	0	782
Vegetable bouillon, prep, 1 cup	5	0	0	0	0	1	0	0	980
Beef bouillon, prep, 1 cup	20	1	0	0	0	2	0	1	1362
Chicken bouillon, prep, 1 cup	22	1	0	0	0	1	0	1	1484

BRANDS . . .

CANNED *(1 CUP UNLESS NOTED)*

Food	Cal	Fat	Sat	TFat	Chol	Carb	Fib	Sug	Sod
Campbell's Chicken Broth, LS, 1 can	25	1	1	0	5	1	0	1	140
Health Valley Beef Broth, FF, NSA	10	0	0	0	0	0	0	0	120
Chicken Broth, NSA	35	2	1	0	25	0	0	0	130
Nature's Promise Chicken, LS	50	0	0	0	0	0	0	0	140
Pacific Natural Chicken Broth, LS	15	0	0	0	0	1	0	0	70
Shelton's Chicken Broth, FF, LS	10	0	0	0	0	0	0	0	60
Chicken Broth, Organic, FF, LS	20	0	0	0	0	0	0	0	135

CONCENTRATED, CUBED AND POWDERED *(1 CUP PREP UNLESS NOTED)*

Food	Cal	Fat	Sat	TFat	Chol	Carb	Fib	Sug	Sod
Bernard Soup & Gravy Base, Cream of Chicken or Cream of Mushroom	30	1	0	0	0	5	0	1	5
Beef or Chicken	20	1	0	0	0	3	0	1	6
Croyden House LS Instant, Chicken	15	0	0	0	0	3	0	0	5
Frontier Very LS Veg Broth	67	0	0	0	0	13	0	1	26
LS Veg Broth	85	0	0	0	0	6	1	0	60
Herb-Ox Beef or Chicken Bouillon, LS	10	0	0	0	0	2	0	1	5
Home Again SF Beef or Chicken Base	25	1	0	0	0	3	0	0	0
L.B. Jamison's Chicken Soup Base, LS	25	1	0	0	0	3	0	2	48
Minor's LS Base, Beef or Chicken (avg)	15	1	0	0	1	1	0	0	140
Vegetable	13	1	0	0	0	2	0	0	140
More Than Gourmet Veggie Glace Gold, 2 tsp	15	0	0	0	0	3	0	1	60
Rapunzel NSA Veg Bouillon, 1/2 cube	26	1	0	0	0	1	0	0	130
RC/Redi-Base Veg, LS, 1/2 tsp	25	1	0	0	0	3	0	2	5
Beef or Chicken Base, Very LS, 1 tsp	10	0	0	0	0	1	0	0	35
Beef Base, LS, 1/2 tsp	10	1	0	0	0	1	0	0	140
Supreme Chicken or Turkey Base	10	1	0	0	0	1	0	0	140
Supreme Ham Base, LS, 1/2 tsp	10	0	0	0	0	1	0	0	140

149

Food	Cal	Fat	Sat	TFat	Chol	Carb	Fib	Sug	Sod
BOUILLON, BROTHS AND BASES — CONCENTRATED, CUBED AND POWDERED (CONT'D)									
Vogue Cuisine Onion Base, 1 tsp	15	0	0	0	0	2	0	0	136
VegeBase, 1 tsp	15	0	0	0	0	2	0	0	140
Wyler's Chicken or Beef Bouillon SF	10	0	0	0	0	2	0	0	0
FROZEN/REFRIGERATED *(1 CUP UNLESS NOTED)*									
Perfect Addition Veg Stock, NSA	40	1	0	0	0	6	2	4	50
Fish Stock, NSA................................	32	0	0	0	0	2	0	0	100
Chicken or Veal Stock, NSA	40	0	0	0	0	4	0	0	110
Beef Stock, NSA....................................	30	0	0	0	0	4	0	0	130

CHILI

Food	Cal	Fat	Sat	TFat	Chol	Carb	Fib	Sug	Sod
Chili mix, 1/6 pkg	60	2	0	0	0	10	0	0	980
Chili w/o beans, 1 cup.................................	302	18	6	0	54	16	3	3	996
Chili w/beans, 1 cup (avg)	287	14	6	0	44	30	11	3	1336
BRANDS . . . *(1 CUP UNLESS NOTED)*									
CANNED									
Health Valley									
Mild or Spicy Vegetarian, NSA	160	1	0	0	0	30	11	9	65
Mild or Spicy Black Bean or Mild 3 Bean	160	1	0	0	0	28	12	7	320
MIX									
Ass Kickin' Chili Fixin's	180	1	0	0	0	33	0	0	75
Green Chili & Corn Stew	80	1	0	0	0	18	0	0	110
Canterbury Naturals									
White Lightning Chicken Chili Mix	150	1	0	0	0	28	7	5	290
Dixie Diner Dusty Roads Chili Mix	157	2	0	0	0	23	9	4	124
Hurst HamBeens Chili Beans, 1 serv	120	1	0	0	0	22	10	1	170
Slow Cooker Gourmet Chili Mix	5	1	0	0	0	22	-	2	25
CHILI SEASONING									
New Traditions Chili Mix, 1 tsp mix	15	0	0	0	0	3	0	0	0
WhoopAss Chili Mix, 1 oz mix..................	60	1	0	0	0	12	0	0	40
Williams Chili Seasoning, NSA, 1/8 pkt	10	0	0	0	0	2	1	1	0

SOUPS

Food	Cal	Fat	Sat	TFat	Chol	Carb	Fib	Sug	Sod
Clam chowder, manhattan, 1 cup	74	2	0	0	2	12	2	3	558
Tomato, 1 cup	73	1	0	0	0	16	2	10	672
New england, 1 cup	85	2	0	0	5	11	1	1	906
Gazpacho, 1 cup	46	0	0	0	0	4	1	1	739
Vegetable beef, 1 cup	77	2	1	0	5	10	2	1	770
Cream of mushroom, 1 cup	104	7	2	0	0	8	0	2	787

Food Food	Cal	Fat	Sat	TFat	Chol	Carb	Fib	Sug	Sod
SOUPS (CONT'D)									
Chicken w/rice, 1 cup	58	2	0	0	6	7	1	0	793
Cream of chicken, 1 cup	109	7	2	0	10	9	0	1	799
Vegetable, 1 cup	70	2	0	0	0	12	1	4	801
Chicken noodle, 1 cup	63	2	1	0	13	7	0	1	842
Mix, prep, 1 cup	58	1	0	0	10	9	0	1	577
Onion, mix, prep, 1 cup	27	1	0	0	0	5	1	2	847
Minestrone, 1 cup	81	2	1	0	6	11	1	2	887
Cream of celery, 1 cup	88	5	1	0	13	9	1	2	924
Vegetable beef, 1 cup	82	3	1	0	5	9	1	3	926
Chicken gumbo, 1 cup	55	1	0	0	4	8	2	2	928
Beef stew, 1 cup	220	12	5	0	37	16	4	2	947
Oyster stew, 1 cup	57	4	2	0	13	5	4	0	954
Cream of potato, 1 cup	72	2	1	0	6	11	1	2	972
Split pea w/ham, 1 cup	193	4	2	0	8	28	2	1	1027
Black bean, 1 cup	119	2	0	0	0	20	9	0	1271

BRANDS . . . *(1 CUP UNLESS NOTED)*

Although some of the soups listed below exceed sodium guidelines, they are less than the generic.

CANNED

Amy's Light in Sodium									
Minestrone	90	2	0	0	0	17	3	5	290
Butternut Squash	100	3	0	0	0	20	2	4	290
Lentil Veg	150	4	1	0	0	23	6	5	340
Cream of Tomato or Chunky Tomato	120	4	2	0	10	21	2	14	340
Campbell's									
Split Pea, LS, 1 can	240	4	2	0	5	38	6	6	30
Cream Of Mushroom, LS, 1 can	160	8	3	0	10	19	3	6	60
Tomato w/Tomato Pieces, LS, 1 can	150	4	2	0	10	25	4	16	90
Chunky Vegetable, LS, 1 can	160	4	2	0	40	17	6	7	90
Chicken w/Noodles, LS, 1 can	130	5	2	0	25	14	2	3	120
Health Valley Organic Lentil, NSA	115	1	0	0	0	23	7	6	25
Black Bean, NSA	130	1	0	0	0	25	5	7	25
Mushroom Barley, NSA	70	0	0	0	0	17	3	4	25
Potato Leek, NSA	70	0	0	0	0	15	3	5	35
Tomato, NSA	80	0	0	0	0	18	1	14	35
Vegetable, NSA	80	0	0	0	0	14	4	5	40
Minestrone, NSA	70	0	0	0	0	17	3	5	45
Split Pea, NSA	110	0	0	0	0	23	8	5	115
FF Country Corn & Vegetable	70	0	0	0	0	17	7	8	135

Food	Cal	Fat	Sat	TFat	Chol	Carb	Fib	Sug	Sod
SOUPS *(HEALTH VALLEY CONT'D)*									
Split Pea	110	0	0	0	0	23	8	5	160
FF Vegetable Barley	90	0	0	0	0	19	4	4	210
FF Italian Minestrone	90	0	0	0	0	21	8	6	210
Lentil & Carrot, FF	100	0	0	0	0	25	7	7	220
Split Pea & Carrot, FF	110	0	0	0	0	17	4	7	230
Potato & Leek	70	0	0	0	0	15	3	5	230
Tomato, FF or Tomato Veg, FF	80	0	0	0	0	17	5	9	240
Super Broccoli Carotene, FF	70	0	0	0	0	16	7	12	240
14 Garden Veg, FF	80	0	0	0	0	17	4	8	250
5 Bean, FF	140	0	0	0	0	32	10	9	250
Bean & Veg, FF	110	0	0	0	0	24	9	8	280
Manischewitz Borscht, Unsalted	80	0	0	0	0	20	0	20	35
Borscht, Reduced Sodium	80	0	0	0	0	21	0	20	350
Pritikin Ready-to-eat, all (avg)	90	0	0	0	0	18	3	2	290
Rokeach Borscht, Unsalted	80	0	0	0	0	20	0	20	35
ShariAnn's Indian Black Bean	150	1	0	0	0	30	4	0	320
French Green Lentil	130	0	0	0	0	22	1	0	320
Tony Chachere's Cream of Mushroom	25	0	0	0	0	5	0	0	5
FROZEN/REFRIGERATED *(7.5 OZ UNLESS NOTED)*									
Moosewood Tibetan Curried Lentil	130	4	0	0	0	19	7	5	320
Creamy Potato & Corn Chowder	160	5	3	0	15	26	3	5	390
Tabachinack Mushroom, NSA	80	1	0	0	0	17	4	1	40
Vegetable, NSA	90	2	0	0	0	17	4	3	45
Pea, NSA	140	0	0	0	0	34	14	0	50
Cabbage	90	1	0	0	0	21	1	11	160
Wild Rice	80	1	0	0	0	16	1	1	220
Cream of Mushroom	100	5	3	0	15	11	1	3	260
Tomato Rice	110	4	0	0	0	18	3	10	260
Minestrone	100	2	0	0	0	18	4	3	320
Old Fashioned Potato	100	2	0	0	0	21	2	2	330
New England Potato	110	5	3	0	15	17	1	3	330
Yankee Bean	180	2	0	0	0	33	10	2	340
Vegetable	90	2	0	0	0	17	4	3	350
Lentil	160	0	0	0	0	29	8	3	360
Woodstock Organic Creamy Potato or Tomato Rice	110	0	0	0	0	23	3	7	340
MIX *(1 CUP PREP UNLESS NOTED)*									
Ass Kickin' Tortilla & Bean	150	4	0	0	0	23	-	-	290
Aunt Patsy's Navy Bean	130	1	0	0	0	21	10	1	170
Chicken Thyme	100	1	0	0	0	22	4	1	230

Food Food	Cal	Fat	Sat	TFat	Chol	Carb	Fib	Sug	Sod
SOUPS (AUNT PATSY'S CONT'D)									
Many Bean	110	1	0	0	0	25	8	2	240
Red Lentil	90	1	0	0	0	16	4	1	260
Bean Cuisine, most (avg)	100	0	0	0	0	18	6	2	10
Bob's Red Mill 13 Bean	322	2	0	0	0	56	6	2	19
Vegi Soup Mix	330	2	0	0	0	60	8	0	28
Canterbury Naturals									
Black Bean & Pasta Mix	110	1	0	0	0	20	4	0	80
Dixie Diner Creme of Potato & Bacon (Not!)	113	2	0	0	0	19	2	1	103
Creme of Mushroom Soup & Gravy Mix	39	1	0	0	0	6	1	0	133
DDC Creme of Chicken (Not!)	128	2	0	0	0	18	2	2	287
Cheese (Not!) Chicken Enchilada Soup	122	1	0	0	0	19	6	2	304
Carb Counters Cream of Mushroom	51	4	3	0	16	2	0	0	340
Dr. McDougalls Split Pea w/Barley	120	1	0	0	0	21	5	1	300
Tortilla Soup	100	1	0	0	0	17	3	1	310
Ramen, Chicken Flavor	100	1	0	0	0	20	1	1	320
Frontier Carolina Asparagus Almond	77	3	0	0	0	12	2	1	3
PA Woodlands Mushroom Barley	73	0	0	0	0	16	3	0	6
Mississippi Delta Tomato Rice	102	0	0	0	0	23	1	0	7
VA Blue Ridge Cream of Broccoli	72	0	0	0	0	15	2	1	8
South of the Border Tortilla	60	0	0	0	0	12	4	1	10
Connecticut Cottage Chicken Noodle	70	1	0	0	10	14	1	2	25
New Orleans Jambalaya	120	2	0	0	0	24	1	0	30
Georgia Pines Golden Peanut	70	1	0	0	0	24	2	3	35
Goodman's Noodleman Noodle LS	50	1	0	0	10	9	1	2	95
Onion LS	30	1	0	0	0	6	1	3	115
Hurst's HamBeens 15 Bean, 6 oz	120	1	0	0	0	20	9	1	70
Cajun 15 Bean, 6 oz serv	120	1	0	0	0	20	9	1	100
Vegetarian 15 Bean, 6 oz serv	120	1	0	0	0	20	9	1	250
Kedem Veg Mix	120	1	0	0	0	23	7	2	34
Legumes Plus Cajun/Brown Rice Lentil	190	1	0	0	0	-	-	-	170
Zesty Tomato Lentil	180	1	0	0	0	-	-	-	250
Manischewitz Veg w/Mushrooms	120	0	0	0	0	22	3	1	70
Miso-Cup Reduced Sodium, 1 envl	25	1	0	0	0	3	1	1	270
Slow Cooker Gourmet Split Pea	190	1	0	0	0	35	-	5	15
Bean & Pasta	150	0	0	0	0	29	-	3	15
Pot Roast Stew Mix	140	1	0	0	0	25	-	3	15
Hudson River, Am. Pioneer, or 21 Bean	130	1	0	0	0	24	-	2	30
Indiana Chicken Corn Chowder	70	0	0	0	0	13	-	2	85
Streit's Variety Veg	100	0	0	0	0	21	4	0	10
Barley Mushroom	110	0	0	0	0	22	5	1	70

Food	Cal	Fat	Sat	TFat	Chol	Carb	Fib	Sug	Sod

VEGETABLES, BEANS AND LEGUMES

BEANS AND LEGUMES – CANNED

Food	Cal	Fat	Sat	TFat	Chol	Carb	Fib	Sug	Sod
Soybeans, 1/2 cup	149	8	1	0	0	9	5	3	204
50% less salt beans, 1/2 cup (avg)	80	2	0	0	0	23	6	7	220
Lentils, 1/2 cup	115	0	0	0	0	20	8	2	236
Cannellini beans, 1/2 cup	153	0	0	0	0	29	6	0	270
Aduki beans, 1/2 cup	109	0	0	0	0	20	5	0	323
Great northern beans, 1/2 cup	100	1	0	0	0	28	5	0	330
Black-eyed peas, 1/2 cup	120	1	0	0	0	21	6	1	350
Pinto beans, 1/2 cup	103	1	0	0	0	18	6	0	353
Garbanzo beans, 1/2 cup	143	2	0	0	0	27	5	0	359
Lima beans, 1/2 cup	95	0	0	0	0	18	6	0	405
Kidney beans, 1/2 cup	109	0	0	0	0	20	8	0	436
Black beans, 1/2 cup	109	0	0	0	0	20	8	1	461
Fava beans, 1/2 cup	91	0	0	0	0	16	5	0	580
Navy beans, 1/2 cup	148	1	0	0	0	27	7	0	587

BRANDS . . . *(1/2 CUP UNLESS NOTED)*

ADUKI (ADZUKI) BEANS

Food	Cal	Fat	Sat	TFat	Chol	Carb	Fib	Sug	Sod
Eden Organic Aduki	110	0	0	0	0	19	5	0	10

BLACK BEANS (TURTLE BEANS)

Food	Cal	Fat	Sat	TFat	Chol	Carb	Fib	Sug	Sod
365 NSA	110	1	0	0	0	19	7	1	10
Eden Organic	100	0	0	0	0	18	6	0	15
Caribbean Black	90	1	0	0	0	20	7	1	135
Goya LS	100	0	0	0	0	18	8	0	125
Natural Value	100	0	0	0	0	19	5	4	140
Westbrae Natural Organic	100	0	0	0	0	19	5	4	140

BLACK-EYES PEAS

Food	Cal	Fat	Sat	TFat	Chol	Carb	Fib	Sug	Sod
Eden	90	1	0	0	0	16	4	1	25

BROAD BEANS *(see Fava Beans, pg 155)*

BUTTER BEANS *(see Lima Beans, pg 155)*

CANNELLINI BEANS (WHITE BEANS)

Food	Cal	Fat	Sat	TFat	Chol	Carb	Fib	Sug	Sod
Eden Organic	100	1	0	0	0	17	5	1	40

CHICKPEAS *(see Garbanzo Beans, pg 155)*

CHILI BEANS

Food	Cal	Fat	Sat	TFat	Chol	Carb	Fib	Sug	Sod
Kuner's	120	2	0	0	0	21	5	0	15
Westbrae Natural	100	0	0	0	0	19	5	2	150

Food Food	Cal	Fat	Sat	TFat	Chol	Carb	Fib	Sug	Sod
BEANS AND LEGUMES – CANNED (CONT'D)									
FAVA BEANS (BROAD BEANS)									
Most brands are within the generic range.									
GARBANZO BEANS (CHICKPEAS)									
365 NSA	90	2	0	0	0	15	4	1	10
Eden Organic	130	1	0	0	0	23	5	1	30
Goya LS Garbanzo	100	0	0	0	0	20	7	0	120
Natural Value	110	2	0	0	0	18	5	3	140
Westbrae Natural Organic	110	2	0	0	0	18	5	3	140
GREAT NORTHERN BEANS									
Eden Organic	110	1	0	0	0	20	8	1	45
Westbrae Natural Organic	100	0	0	0	0	19	6	2	140
GREEN BEANS *(see Green Beans, pg 158)*									
KIDNEY BEANS (RED BEANS)									
365 NSA	110	1	0	0	0	20	7	1	10
Eden Organic Kidney	100	0	0	0	0	18	10	1	15
Organic Small Red	100	1	0	0	0	17	5	1	25
Goya Red Kidney	110	0	0	0	0	19	8	0	110
Natural Value Kidney or Red (avg)	100	0	0	0	0	18	5	2	140
Westbrae Natural Organic, Red	100	0	0	0	0	19	7	2	140
Kidney	100	0	0	0	0	18	5	2	140
LENTILS									
Westbrae Natural Organic	100	0	0	0	0	17	9	2	150
LIMA BEANS (BUTTER BEANS)									
Eden Organic Butter Beans	100	1	0	0	0	17	4	0	35
Seneca Lima Beans, NSA	90	0	0	0	0	17	4	1	5
Stokely No Salt or Sugar Added	80	0	0	0	0	16	0	0	5
MISC BEANS (INCLUDES MIXED BEANS)									
Eden Organic Rice & Beans									
Rice & Caribbean Black	120	1	0	0	0	23	4	1	100
Rice & Cajun Small Red	110	1	0	0	0	23	3	1	115
Rice & Lentil	120	1	0	0	0	23	2	0	120
Rice & Garbanzo	110	1	0	0	0	23	2	0	135
Rice & Pinto	110	1	0	0	0	24	3	1	140
Westbrae Natural Organic Black Beluga	100	0	0	0	0	16	4	0	120
Jackson Wonder	100	0	0	0	0	19	5	0	135
European Soldier	90	0	0	0	0	16	5	0	140
Scarlet Runner	100	0	0	0	0	20	7	1	140
Trout or Soup Beans (avg)	100	0	0	0	0	18	6	0	140
Salad Beans	100	1	0	0	0	19	5	2	150

Food	Cal	Fat	Sat	TFat	Chol	Carb	Fib	Sug	Sod
BEANS AND LEGUMES – CANNED (CONT'D)									
NAVY BEANS									
Eden Organic	110	0	0	0	0	20	7	0	15
PINTO BEANS (PINK)									
365 NSA	110	0	0	0	0	20	7	1	10
Eden Organic Pinto	100	0	0	0	0	18	6	1	15
Spicy Pinto	120	1	0	0	0	24	7	2	200
Goya Pink	100	0	0	0	0	19	7	0	110
Natural Value Pinto	100	0	0	0	0	19	7	2	140
Westbrae Natural Organic Pinto	100	0	0	0	0	19	7	2	140
SOYBEANS									
Eden Organic Black	120	6	1	0	0	8	7	1	30
Westbrae Natural Organic	150	7	1	0	0	11	3	3	140
WAX BEANS *(see Wax Beans, pg 162)*									
WHITE BEANS *(see Cannellini Beans, pg 154)*									
BAKED BEANS									
Baked beans, 1/2 cup	150	1	0	0	0	29	7	5	550
Pork & beans, 1/2 cup	134	1	0	0	9	25	7	16	524
BRANDS . . . *(1/2 CUP UNLESS NOTED)*									
Eden Baked w/Sorghum & Mustard	150	0	0	0	0	27	7	6	130

BEANS AND LEGUMES – DRIED/RAW

Food	Cal	Fat	Sat	TFat	Chol	Carb	Fib	Sug	Sod
Soybeans, 1/2 cup	387	19	3	0	0	28	9	0	2
Black beans, 1/2 cup	331	1	0	0	0	60	15	2	5
Navy beans, 1/2 cup	350	2	0	0	0	63	25	4	5
Lentils, 1/2 cup	339	1	0	0	0	58	29	2	6
Fava beans (broad beans), 1/2 cup	256	1	0	0	0	44	19	4	10
Kidney beans (red beans), 1/2 cup	310	1	0	0	0	56	14	2	11
Pinto beans, 1/2 cup	335	1	0	0	0	60	15	2	12
Great northern beans, 1/2 cup	310	1	0	0	0	57	19	2	13
Lima beans (butter beans), 1/2 cup	301	1	0	0	0	56	17	8	16
Garbanzo beans (chickpeas), 1/2 cup	364	6	1	0	0	61	17	11	24

BRANDS . . .
Most brands are within the generic range.

BEANS AND LEGUMES – FROZEN

Food	Cal	Fat	Sat	TFat	Chol	Carb	Fib	Sug	Sod
LIMA BEANS									
Baby, 1/2 cup	108	0	0	0	0	21	5	1	43
Fordhook, 1/2 cup	85	0	0	0	0	16	4	1	46

Food Food	Cal	Fat	Sat	TFat	Chol	Carb	Fib	Sug	Sod
BEANS AND LEGUMES – FROZEN (LIMA BEANS CONT'D)									
Speckled, 1/2 cup	100	0	0	0	0	20	4	1	130
w/butter sauce, 1/2 cup	133	3	2	0	5	18	6	1	330
NOTE: Lima beans are often frozen in brine and may contain as much as 213mg sodium per serving.									
BRANDS . . . *(1/2 CUP UNLESS NOTED)*									
Birds Eye Fordhook	100	0	0	0	0	19	5	3	10
Freshlike Fordhook	90	0	0	0	0	17	5	1	10
Seabrook Speckled	145	0	0	0	0	28	2	1	23
Southern Speckled	135	0	0	0	0	25	0	1	30

VEGETABLES – CANNED

ARTICHOKE

Artichoke hearts, marinated, 1 oz	25	2	0	0	0	2	1	0	90
Artichoke hearts, 1/2 cup	35	0	0	0	0	6	4	1	420
BRANDS . . . *(1 OZ UNLESS NOTED)*									
Most brands are within the generic range.									

ASPARAGUS

Asparagus, 1/2 cup	23	1	0	0	0	3	2	1	347
50% less salt, 1/2 cup	15	0	0	0	0	2	1	1	210
BRANDS . . . *(1/2 CUP UNLESS NOTED)*									
Aunt Nellie's	20	0	0	0	0	5	0	3	100
Seneca Cuts, NSA	20	0	0	0	0	3	1	2	40
Stokely Cuts, NSA	20	0	0	0	0	3	0	-	5
*Tillen Farms Pickled Crispy, 3 spears	10	0	0	0	0	1	0	0	75

BEETS

Beets, 1/2 cup	26	0	0	0	0	6	1	5	165
Harvard beets, 1/2 cup	90	0	0	0	0	22	3	0	199
Pickled beets, 1/2 cup	74	0	0	0	0	18	3	12	300
BRANDS . . . *(1/2 CUP UNLESS NOTED)*									
Aunt Nellie's Pickled, Whole, 1.3 oz	20	0	0	0	0	5	1	4	65
Pickled, 4 slices (1.6 oz)	20	0	0	0	0	5	0	3	100
Greenwood Pickled, Sliced, 1 oz	25	0	0	0	0	6	0	5	100
S&W Pickled, 1 oz	15	0	0	0	0		1		50
Seneca, NSA	40	0	0	0	0	8	1	6	25
Stokely NS, No Sugar	40	0	0	0	0	8	0	-	40

CABBAGE

Red cabbage, 1/2 cup	80	0	0	0	0	20	0	16	440

Food	Cal	Fat	Sat	TFat	Chol	Carb	Fib	Sug	Sod
CANNED VEGETABLES (CABBAGE CONT'D)									
BRANDS . . . *(1/2 CUP UNLESS NOTED)*									
Most brands are within the generic range.									
CARROTS									
Carrots, 1/2 cup	18	0	0	0	0	4	1	2	177
BRANDS . . . *(1/2 CUP UNLESS NOTED)*									
Seneca, NSA	30	0	0	0	0	6	2	4	55
Tillen Farms Pickled Crispy, 1 oz	30	0	0	0	0	7	1	6	5
COLLARD GREENS									
Collard greens, 1/2 cup	50	0	0	0	0	7	3	3	300
BRANDS . . .									
Most brands are within the generic range.									
CORN									
Whole kernel corn, 1/2 cup	82	1	0	0	0	20	2	4	273
50% less sodium, 1/2 cup	80	1	0	0	0	17	2	4	180
Creamed corn, 1/2 cup	92	1	0	0	0	23	2	4	365
BRANDS . . . *(1/2 CUP UNLESS NOTED)*									
Del Monte Whole Kernel Sweet, NSA	60	1	0	0	0	11	3	7	10
Cream Style Sweet, NSA	60	1	0	0	0	14	2	7	10
Green Giant Niblets, NSA	90	0	0	0	0	20	3	5	0
Season Cut or Whole Sweet Baby	30	1	0	0	0	4	3	1	35
Seneca Whole Kernel, NSA	60	2	0	0	0	9	2	7	10
Sun Luck Baby Corn, all	10	0	0	0	0	6	4	6	20
GARLIC									
Garlic, crushed or chopped, 1 tsp	10	0	0	0	0	1	0	0	0
BRANDS . . .									
Most brands are within the generic range.									
GREEN BEANS									
Green beans, 1/2 cup	18	0	0	0	0	4	2	2	311
50% less sodium, 1/2 cup	20	0	0	0	0	4	1	2	200
BRANDS . . . *(1/2 CUP UNLESS NOTED)*									
Del Monte Cut Green Beans, NSA	20	0	0	0	0	4	2	2	10
French Style Beans, NSA	20	0	0	0	0	4	2	2	10
Giant Cut, NSA	20	0	0	0	0	4	2	2	15
French Style	20	0	0	0	0	4	2	2	15
Seneca, NSA	20	0	0	0	0	4	2	2	15
Stokely NSA	20	0	0	0	0	4	0	-	5

Food Food	Cal	Fat	Sat	TFat	Chol	Carb	Fib	Sug	Sod

CANNED VEGETABLES (CONT'D)

MIXED VEGETABLES

Food Food	Cal	Fat	Sat	TFat	Chol	Carb	Fib	Sug	Sod
Peas & carrots, 1/2 cup	48	0	0	0	0	11	3	3	332

BRANDS . . . *(1/2 CUP UNLESS NOTED)*

Food	Cal	Fat	Sat	TFat	Chol	Carb	Fib	Sug	Sod
Del Monte Peas & Carrots, NSA	60	0	0	0	0	11	4	6	10
Seneca Mixed Vegetables, NSA	45	0	0	0	0	9	2	2	10
Peas & Carrots, NSA	60	0	0	0	0	10	4	4	15
Veg-All NSA	40	0	0	0	0	8	2	2	25

MUSHROOMS

Food	Cal	Fat	Sat	TFat	Chol	Carb	Fib	Sug	Sod
Mushrooms, 1/2 cup	19	0	0	0	0	4	2	2	332

BRANDS . . . *(1/2 CUP UNLESS NOTED)*

Food	Cal	Fat	Sat	TFat	Chol	Carb	Fib	Sug	Sod
Giorgio Pieces and Stems, NSA	20	0	0	0	0	3	1	0	20
Pennsylvania Dutchman									
Stems and Pieces, NSA	20	0	0	0	0	3	1	0	20
Sun Luck Straw	10	0	0	0	0	8	0	0	0

ONIONS

Food	Cal	Fat	Sat	TFat	Chol	Carb	Fib	Sug	Sod
Onions, 1 oz	5	0	0	0	0	1	0	1	104

BRANDS . . . *(1 OZ UNLESS NOTED)*

Food	Cal	Fat	Sat	TFat	Chol	Carb	Fib	Sug	Sod
Crosse & Blackwell Cocktail	10	0	0	0	0	2	0	0	20

PEAS

Food	Cal	Fat	Sat	TFat	Chol	Carb	Fib	Sug	Sod
Peas, 1/2 cup	66	0	0	0	0	12	4	4	310
50% less sodium, 1/2 cup	60	0	0	0	0	11	3	2	195

BRANDS . . . *(1/2 CUP UNLESS NOTED)*

Food	Cal	Fat	Sat	TFat	Chol	Carb	Fib	Sug	Sod
Del Monte, Fresh Cut, NSA	60	0	0	0	0	11	4	6	10
Seneca, NSA	60	0	0	0	0	10	3	5	15

PEPPERS *See Pickled and Specialty Vegetables, pg 43; Chili Peppers, pg 114)*

POTATOES

Food	Cal	Fat	Sat	TFat	Chol	Carb	Fib	Sug	Sod
Potatoes, 1 cup	88	0	0	0	0	20	3	0	434

BRANDS . . . *(2/3 CUP UNLESS NOTED)*

Food	Cal	Fat	Sat	TFat	Chol	Carb	Fib	Sug	Sod
Giant Whole White, NSA	70	0	0	0	0	15	2	1	15
Seneca, NSA, 2/3 cup	70	0	0	0	0	14	2	1	15

PUMPKIN

Food	Cal	Fat	Sat	TFat	Chol	Carb	Fib	Sug	Sod
100% pumpkin, 1/2 cup	42	0	0	0	0	10	4	4	6
Pumpkin pie filling, 1/2 cup	140	0	0	0	0	36	11	17	281

BRANDS . . .

Most 100% pumpking brands are within the generic range.

Food	Cal	Fat	Sat	TFat	Chol	Carb	Fib	Sug	Sod
CANNED VEGETABLES (PUMPKIN CONT'D)									
PUMPKIN PIE MIX									
Farmer's Market Mix (canned), 1/2 cup ..	102	0	0	0	0	28	2	22	0
SAUERKRAUT									
Sauerkraut, 1/2 cup	22	0	0	0	0	5	3	2	780
BRANDS . . . *(1/2 CUP UNLESS NOTED)*									
Most brands are within the generic range.									
SPINACH									
Spinach, 1/2 cup	22	0	0	0	0	3	2	0	373
BRANDS . . . *(1/2 CUP UNLESS NOTED)*									
Allens Popeye, NSA	40	1	0	0	0	5	2	0	30
Spinach	35	1	0	0	0	4	2	1	135
SWEET POTATOES AND YAMS									
Yam, 1/2 cup....................................	130	1	0	0	0	29	2	23	30
Sweet potato, 1/2 cup	101	0	0	0	0	24	3	18	50
BRANDS . . .									
Most brands are within the generic range.									
TOMATOES									
TOMATO PASTE									
Tomato paste, 2 tbsp	27	0	0	0	0	6	2	4	259
BRANDS . . . *(2 TBSP UNLESS NOTED)*									
Bionaturae	30	0	0	0	0	6	1	4	20
Contadina	30	0	0	0	0	6	1	3	20
Hunt's, NSA	30	0	0	0	0	6	2	4	15
La Squisita	30	0	0	0	0	6	1	3	0
Muir Glen	30	0	0	0	0	6	1	3	20
S&W	30	0	0	0	0	6	1	3	20
Whole Foods Market 365	33	0	0	0	0	6	1	3	20
TOMATO PUREE AND TOMATO SAUCE									
Tomato puree, 1/4 cup	24	0	0	0	0	6	1	3	249
Tomato sauce, 1/4 cup	20	0	0	0	0	5	1	3	321
BRANDS . . . *(1/4 CUP UNLESS NOTED)*									
Contadina Puree	20	0	0	0	0	4	1	1	15
Hunt's, Sauce, NSA	30	0	0	0	0	6	2	4	15
Muir Glen Puree	20	0	0	0	0	5	1	3	20
Sauce, NSA	20	0	0	0	0	5	1	3	30
Progresso Puree	25	0	0	0	0	5	1	3	15
Rokeach Sauce w/Mushrooms, NSA	40	1	0	0	0	7	1	0	25

Food Food	Cal	Fat	Sat	TFat	Chol	Carb	Fib	Sug	Sod

CANNED VEGETABLES (TOMATO PUREE AND TOMATO SAUCE CONT'D)

Food	Cal	Fat	Sat	TFat	Chol	Carb	Fib	Sug	Sod
S&W Puree	30	0	0	0	0	6	2	3	15

TOMATOES - CHOPPED/DICED

Food	Cal	Fat	Sat	TFat	Chol	Carb	Fib	Sug	Sod
Diced & chopped tomatoes, 1/2 cup	25	0	0	0	0	6	2	4	250
Seasoned, 1/2 cup	50	0	0	0	0	11	1	8	650

BRANDS . . . *(1/2 CUP UNLESS NOTED)*

Food	Cal	Fat	Sat	TFat	Chol	Carb	Fib	Sug	Sod
Bionaturae Crushed or Strained	30	0	0	0	0	6	1	4	20
Del Monte Diced	25	0	0	0	0	6	2	4	50
Eden Diced	30	0	0	0	0	6	2	4	5
Diced w/Green Chilies or w/Basil	30	0	0	0	0	5	2	3	35
Diced w/Roasted Onion	30	0	0	0	0	5	2	3	35
Muir Glen Diced, NSA	30	0	0	0	0	6	1	4	15
Pomi Chopped	20	0	0	0	0	4	3	4	10

TOMATOES - CRUSHED/STRAINED

Food	Cal	Fat	Sat	TFat	Chol	Carb	Fib	Sug	Sod
Crushed tomatoes, 1/2 cup	40	0	0	0	0	9	2	3	304

BRANDS . . . *(1/2 CUP UNLESS NOTED)*

Food	Cal	Fat	Sat	TFat	Chol	Carb	Fib	Sug	Sod
Bionaturae Crushed or Strained	30	0	0	0	0	6	1	4	20
Cento	70	0	0	0	0	-	-	-	40
Eden	40	0	0	0	0	6	2	4	0
w/Basil or w/Onion & Garlic	40	0	0	0	0	6	2	4	0
Muir Glen Crushed w/Basil	50	0	0	0	0	10	2	8	190
Ground Peeled	20	0	0	0	0	4	1	4	190
Pomi Strained	60	0	0	0	0	10	6	10	20
Progresso Crushed Fire Roasted	40	0	0	0	0	8	2	4	190
S&W Crushed, Italian Style	40	0	0	0	0	8	2	4	190
Sclafani	70	0	0	0	0	6	2	4	20

TOMATOES - WHOLE/STEWED

Food	Cal	Fat	Sat	TFat	Chol	Carb	Fib	Sug	Sod
Whole tomatoes, 1/2 cup	20	0	0	0	0	5	1	3	154
Stewed tomatoes, 1/2 cup	33	0	0	0	0	8	1	6	282

BRANDS . . . *(1/2 CUP UNLESS NOTED)*

Food	Cal	Fat	Sat	TFat	Chol	Carb	Fib	Sug	Sod
Bel Aria Plum	25	0	0	0	0	6	2	4	0
Del Monte Stewed, NSA	35	0	0	0	0	9	2	7	50
Hunt's Whole	40	0	0	0	0	8	2	6	40
S&W Ready-Cut, NSA	25	0	0	0	0	6	2	4	50
Stewed, NSA	35	0	0	0	0	9	2	7	50
Sclafani Whole	20	0	0	0	0	8	2	4	20

TURNIP GREENS

Food	Cal	Fat	Sat	TFat	Chol	Carb	Fib	Sug	Sod
Turnip greens, 1/2 cup	16	0	0	0	0	3	2	0	324

BRANDS . . . *(1/2 CUP UNLESS NOTED)*
Most brands are within the generic range.

Food	Cal	Fat	Sat	TFat	Chol	Carb	Fib	Sug	Sod

CANNED VEGETABLES (CONT'D)

WAX BEANS

Wax beans, 1/2 cup	23	0	0	0	0	5	2	2	360

BRANDS . . . *(1/2 CUP UNLESS NOTED)*

Seneca NSA	20	0	0	0	0	4	2	2	15

YAM *(see Sweet Potatoes and Yams, pg 160)*

ZUCCHINI

Zucchini, italian style, 1/2 cup	33	0	0	0	0	8	0	1	424

BRANDS . . .
Most brands are within the generic range.

VEGETABLES – DRIED

Mushrooms, shiitake, 4	44	0	0	0	0	11	2	0	2
Peppers, sweet, red or green, 1/4 cup	5	0	0	0	0	1	0	0	3
Tomato halves, 2-3	15	0	0	0	0	3	1	0	5
Seasoned, 2-3	15	0	0	0	0	3	1	0	25

BRANDS . . .
Most brands are within the generic range.

VEGETABLES – FRESH

The following vegetables are listed alphabetically.

Artichoke, globe or french, med, 4.6 oz	60	0	0	0	0	13	7	-	120
Asparagus, 5 spears	16	0	0	0	0	3	2	2	2
Avocado, 1/2	161	15	2	0	0	9	7	1	7
Beets, 1/2 cup	29	0	0	0	0	7	2	5	53
Broccoli, 1/2 cup	15	0	0	0	0	3	1	1	15
Brussel sprouts, 1/2 cup	19	0	0	0	0	4	2	1	11
Cabbage, chopped, 1/2 cup	11	0	0	0	0	3	1	2	8
Carrot, 1 med	25	1	0	0	0	6	2	3	42
Cauliflower, 1/2 cup	13	0	0	0	0	3	1	1	15
Celery, 1 med stalk	6	0	0	0	0	1	1	1	32
Corn, 1/2 cup	66	1	0	0	0	15	2	2	12
Cucumber, 1/2 cup	8	0	0	0	0	2	0	1	1
Eggplant, 1/2 cup	10	0	0	0	0	2	1	1	1
Garlic, 1 clove	4	0	0	0	0	1	0	0	1
Jerusalem artichoke, 1/2 cup	57	0	0	0	0	13	1	8	3
Kale, 1/2 cup	17	0	0	0	0	3	1	-	14
Leeks, 1/2 cup	27	0	0	0	0	6	1	2	9
Lettuce, chopped (avg), 1 cup	8	0	0	0	0	2	1	1	6

Food Food	Cal	Fat	Sat	TFat	Chol	Carb	Fib	Sug	Sod
VEGETABLES – FRESH (CONT'D)									
Mushrooms, 1/2 cup	8	0	0	0	0	1	0	1	2
Mustard greens, 1/2 cup	7	0	0	0	0	1	1	0	7
Onion, 1/2 cup chopped	34	0	0	0	0	8	1	3	2
Peas, green, 1/2 cup	59	0	0	0	0	10	4	4	4
Pepper, jalapeno, 1	4	0	0	0	0	1	0	0	0
Peppers, sweet, 1/2 cup	9	0	0	0	0	2	1	1	1
Potato w/skin, sm (2")	58	0	0	0	0	13	2	1	5
Radish, 1	1	0	0	0	0	0	0	0	2
Rutabaga, 1/2 cup	25	0	0	0	0	6	2	4	14
Shallots, 1 tbsp	7	0	0	0	0	2	0	0	1
Spinach, 1 cup	7	0	0	0	0	1	1	0	24
Squash, summer, 1/2 cup	9	0	0	0	0	2	1	1	1
Squash, winter, 1/2 cup	20	0	0	0	0	5	1	1	2
Sweet potato, 1/2 cup	56	0	0	0	0	13	2	3	36
Tomato, 1 med	22	0	0	0	0	5	2	3	6
Turnips, 1/2 cup	18	0	0	0	0	4	1	3	44
Yam, 1/2 cup	89	0	0	0	0	21	3	0	7
Zucchini, 1/2 cup	10	0	0	0	0	2	1	1	6
SALAD KITS *(2 CUPS PREP WITH DRESSING UNLESS NOTED)*									
Caesar Kit	150	13	2	0	10	8	2	2	370
Asian Kit	170	10	2	0	0	17	2	8	380
BRANDS . . .									
Dole Sunflower Ranch Kit	160	16	2	0	5	5	2	3	220
Fall Harvest Kit	150	11	2	0	0	10	0	9	220
Asian Crunch Kit	120	6	1	0	0	12	2	5	230
Et Tu Oriental Kit	70	2	0	0	0	13	0	8	95
Spinach Kit	100	8	1	1	0	6	1	4	190
Italian Kit	100	8	1	0	0	6	0	1	210
Caesar Kit	120	12	1	0	10	4	0	0	260
Fresh Express Coleslaw Kit	120	8	1	0	5	12	2	10	135

(VEGETABLES – FROZEN)

Food	Cal	Fat	Sat	TFat	Chol	Carb	Fib	Sug	Sod
Artichoke hearts, 3 oz	32	0	0	0	0	7	3	0	40
Broccoli, 3 oz	22	0	0	0	0	4	3	1	20
Brussel sprouts, 3 oz	35	0	0	0	0	7	3	0	9
Carrots, 3 oz	31	0	0	0	0	7	3	4	58
Cauliflower, 3 oz	20	0	0	0	0	4	2	2	20
Corn, 3 oz	75	0	0	0	0	18	2	3	3

VEGETABLES, BEANS AND LEGUMES
Vegetables – Frozen

Food	Cal	Fat	Sat	TFat	Chol	Carb	Fib	Sug	Sod
VEGETABLES – FROZEN (CONT'D)									
Mixed vegetables, 3 oz	54	0	0	0	0	11	3	-	40
Peas & onions, 3 oz	60	0	0	0	0	11	3	-	52
Peas & carrots, 3 oz	45	0	0	0	0	9	3		67
Succotash, 3 oz	79	1	0	0	0	17	3	-	38
Onions, 3 oz	30	0	0	0	0	7	1	3	9
Onion rings, 3 oz	217	12	4	-	0	26	2	-	207
Peas, 3 oz	65	0	0	0	0	12	4	5	95
Potatoes, whole, 3 oz	66	0	0	0	0	15	1	1	21
Hashed brown, 3 oz	70	1	0	0	0	15	1	0	19
French fried, 3 oz	125	4	1	-	0	21	2	0	282
Spinach, 3 oz	26	1	0	0	0	4	3	1	63

BRANDS ... *(1/2 CUP UNLESS NOTED)*

Most frozen unprepared vegetables have minimal sodium and are within the generic range. Those packaged with sauces or for convenience may have added sodium.

PREPARED VEGETABLE SIDE DISHES *(see Vegetable Side Dishes, pg 107)*

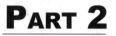

PART 2

QUICK-SERVE RESTAURANT CHAINS

QUICK-SERVE RESTAURANTS

Menu Item	Cal	Fat	Sat	TFat	Chol	Carb	Fib	Sug	Sod

(ARBY'S)

Contact Arby's or their website (www.arbys.com) for nutritional info.

BREAKFAST ITEMS

100-150MG SODIUM
  Chocolate Twist
150-200MG SODIUM
  Croissant • Cinnamon Twist
350-400MG SODIUM
  Original Gourmet Cinnamon Roll®
400-450MG SODIUM
  Pecan Sticky Bun
450-500MG SODIUM
  French Toastix • Blueberry Muffin
Other breakfast items exceed 650mg sodium.

SANDWICHES AND WRAPS

700-750MG SODIUM
  Junior Roast Beef (Kids Meal)
Other sandwiches and wraps exceed 750mg sodium.

SUBS — *exceed 1800mg sodium.*

CHICKEN TENDERS

Three pieces exceed 1350mg sodium.

SALADS *(W/O DRESSING)*
450-500MG SODIUM
  Martha's Vineyard™
Other salads exceed 600mg.

SALAD DRESSINGS
350-400MG SODIUM
  Raspberry Vinaigrette
  Other dressings exceed 450mg sodium.

POTATOES

0-50MG SODIUM
  Sour Cream Baked Potato
150-200MG SODIUM
  Butter & Sour Cream Baked Potato
300-350MG SODIUM
  Deluxe Baked Potato
Other potatoes exceed 750mg sodium.

AU BON PAIN

Menu Item	Cal	Fat	Sat	TFat	Chol	Carb	Fib	Sug	Sod

ARBY'S (CONT'D)

SIDE ITEMS

300-350MG SODIUM

Onion Petals, regular

Other sides exceed 350mg sodium.

CONDIMENTS

0-50MG SODIUM

Bronco Berry® Dipping Sauce

50-100MG SODIUM

Mayonnaise

Other condiments exceed 125mg sodium.

DESSERTS

200-250MG SODIUM

Apple or Cherry Turnover, w/ or w/o icing • Choc Chip Cookie

SHAKES

350-400MG SODIUM

Shakes, regular, all varieties

Other shakes exceed 400mg sodium.

(AU BON PAIN)

BAKED GOODS

BAGELS *(1 BAGEL)*

Menu Item	Cal	Fat	Sat	TFat	Chol	Carb	Fib	Sug	Sod
Cinnamon Raisin	290	1	0	0	0	62	3	4	420
French Toast	400	7	2	0	0	72	3	14	420
Cinnamon Crisp	400	6	1	0	0	88	3	16	440
Plain	280	1	0	0	0	57	2	4	440
Sesame Seed	320	5	1	0	0	59	3	4	440

CROISSANTS *(1 CROISSANT)*

Menu Item	Cal	Fat	Sat	TFat	Chol	Carb	Fib	Sug	Sod
Choc	340	17	10	0	30	42	3	17	190
Plain	270	15	8	0	40	28	1	4	200
Apple	230	10	6	0	25	31	2	11	230
Raspberry	340	18	10	1	55	39	1	16	270
Sweet Cheese	350	20	12	1	70	36	1	11	290
Spinach & Cheese	260	14	8	0	40	25	2	3	290

MUFFINS, PASTRIES AND OTHER BAKED GOODS *(1 BAKED GOOD)*

Menu Item	Cal	Fat	Sat	TFat	Chol	Carb	Fib	Sug	Sod
Danish Pretzel	603	24	12	-	53	92	1	63	104
Cherry Strudel	390	19	0	0	0	49	1	5	135
Apple Strudel	410	18	0	0	0	56	1	19	140
Almond Artisan Pastry	464	30	14	-	123	41	2	12	143
Strawberry Puff Pastry	242	13	6	-	42	30	1	20	143

Menu Item	Cal	Fat	Sat	TFat	Chol	Carb	Fib	Sug	Sod
AU BON PAIN (BAKED GOODS CONT'D)									
Hurricanes	622	12	3	-	2	130	4	80	146
Blueberry Sweet Cheese Artisan Pastry	408	23	13	-	105	44	1	14	151
Dutch Apple Nuns	307	12	3	-	24	49	3	19	162
Cinnamon Roll	300	13	7	0	30	39	2	8	250
Pecan Roll	520	28	9	2	30	61	2	29	270
Choc Caramel Creme Puff	536	25	9	-	43	72	4	33	277
LF Triple Berry Muffin	290	2	1	0	25	61	2	31	310
Cherry Danish	410	19	11	-	65	52	1	20	330
Cinnamon Scone	420	23	11	3	120	50	2	15	340
Orange Scone	380	19	11	0	130	48	2	10	360
BREAKFAST									
Oatmeal	150	3	1	0	0	27	4	1	0
Museli	340	7	2	0	5	64	6	26	40
Chol and FF Eggs, 1 egg (1/4 cup)	25	0	0	0	0	1	0	0	70
Arugula and Tomato Frittata	290	13	7	0	260	27	2	3	210
Other breakfast items exceed 700mg sodium.									
SANDWICHES									
Classic Grilled Cheese	560	22	14	-	64	68	3	3	374
Grilled Chicken	394	24	4	-	55	28	1	0	494
Mozzarella, Tomato & Pesto	381	3	0	-	17	66	6	4	555
Caprese	337	15	4	-	15	31	4	2	607
Classic Tuna	975	15	3	-	0	157	9	7	615
CREATE-A-SANDWICH – *The amount of sodium in possible ingredient combinations exceed the featured sandwiches above.*									
WRAPS									
Riviera Chopped	227	14	4	-	21	21	2	16	431
Riviera Tuna	244	16	4	-	16	11	2	8	562
Chicken Caesar Asiago	276	21	5	-	60	5	1	3	665
SALADS *(W/O DRESSING)*									
Garden, small	50	1	0	0	0	10	3	2	10
Fresh Fruit & Yogurt	115	0	0	0	3	26	2	20	83
Garden, large	110	2	0	0	0	19	5	3	300
Caesar	240	11	6	0	25	23	4	4	310
Steak w/Cranberries & Mandarin Oranges	290	7	4	0	40	46	7	27	400
SALAD DRESSINGS *(2 TBSP)*									
Orange Citrus Vinaigrette	120	10	2	0	0	7	0	7	90
FF Raspberry	80	0	0	0	0	18	0	16	190
Other salad dressings exceed 450mg sodium.									

AUNTIE ANNE'S

Menu Item	Cal	Fat	Sat	TFat	Chol	Carb	Fib	Sug	Sod
AU BON PAIN (CONT'D)									
SOUPS (*1 CUP*)									
Old Fashioned Tomato Rice, LS	80	1	0	0	0	16	2	4	230
Southwest Vegetable, LS	70	2	0	0	0	11	2	2	250
Jamaican Black Bean, LS.............................	112	1	0	0	0	30	17	3	310
Tomato Basil Bisque, LS	140	5	4	0	20	20	4	12	330
Mediterranean Pepper, LS	70	2	0	0	0	12	4	2	390
CREAM CHEESE (*2 OZ*)									
Honey Walnut	140	9	6	-	30	12	0	12	150
Plain	120	11	7	-	35	4	0	4	180
DESSERTS									
Choc Covered Strawberry	31	2	0	0	0	4	1	4	6
Fruit Cup, small, 6 oz	70	0	0	0	0	16	1	15	10
Fruit Cup, large, 12 oz	140	1	0	0	0	32	2	30	20
Plain Yogurt, LF, small, 7 oz	190	2	2	-	10	36	0	31	95
Yogurt w/Granola and Fruit, small	310	6	2	-	10	56	2	36	130

SPECIALTY DRINKS

0-50MG SODIUM

Fresh Orange Juice • Caramel Mocha Blast (med) • Homestyle Lemonade •
Passion Fruit Pina Colada (lrg and sm) • Vanilla Mocha Blast (sm) •
Peach & Cream Blast (med & lrg) • Peach Iced Tea • Strawberry Blast (reg & lrg)

50-100MG SODIUM

Cafe Au Lait (sm) • Caramel Mocha Blast (lrg) • Frozen Mocha Blast (reg & lrg) •
Hot Cappuccino (sm) • Vanilla Mocha Blast

(AUNTIE ANNE'S)

Menu Item	Cal	Fat	Sat	TFat	Chol	Carb	Fib	Sug	Sod
PRETZELS (*1 PRETZEL*)									
Stix - Cinnamon Sugar w/o Butter	233	1	0	-	0	49	1	11	273
Stix - Cinnamon Sugar	300	6	3	-	17	55	2	17	287
Almond w/o Butter	350	2	1	-	0	72	2	15	390
Almond w/Butter	400	8	5	-	20	72	2	15	400
Cinnamon Sugar w/o Butter	350	2	0	-	0	74	2	16	410
Cinnamon Sugar	450	9	5	-	25	83	3	26	430
Other pretzels exceed 450mg sodium.									
SPREADS AND DIPPING SAUCES									
Choc Flavored Dip	130	4	2	-	2	24	1	12	65
Strawberry Cream Cheese	110	10	6	-	35	4	0	3	105
Caramel Dip..	135	3	2	-	5	27	0	21	110
Sweet Mustard	60	2	1	-	40	8	0	8	120
Light Cream Cheese	70	6	4	-	25	1	0	1	140

170

Menu Item	Cal	Fat	Sat	TFat	Chol	Carb	Fib	Sug	Sod

AUNTIE ANNE'S (CONT'D)

BEVERAGES

DUTCH ICE™
0-50MG SODIUM
  Most varieties and sizes except Mocha Dutch.

DUTCH LATTE™ (14 OZ)
100-150MG SODIUM
  Coffee Dutch Latte™ • Mocha Dutch Latte™

DUTCH SHAKES
Exceed 300mg sodium.

DUTCH SMOOTHIES (14 OZ)
50-100MG SODIUM
  Grape • Kiwi-Banana • Orange Creme • Lemonade • Pina Colada •
  Blue Raspberry • Strawberry • Wild Cherry

BAJA FRESH MEXICAN GRILL

Contact Baja Fresh or their website (www.bajafresh.com) for nutritional info.

TACOS
200-250MG SODIUM
  Baja Style, Charbroiled Steak • Baja Style, Chicken
250-300MG SODIUM
  Baja Style, Charbroiled Shrimp • Baja Style, Savory Pork Carnitas
400-450MG SODIUM
  Grilled MahiMahi • Baja Fish Taco

SPECIALTIES
NACHOS – *exceed 2500mg sodium.*
QUESADILLAS – *exceed 2100mg sodium.*
TACQUITOS – *exceed 1700mg sodium.*
BURRITOS – *exceed 1800mg sodium.*
FAJITAS – *exceed 2400mg sodium.*

SALADS (W/O DRESSING)
200-250MG SODIUM
  Side Salad
Other salads exceed 950mg sodium.

SALAD DRESSINGS
250-300MG SODIUM
  Olive Oil Vinaigrette
  Other salad dressings exceed 350mg sodium.

BIG APPLE BAGELS

Menu Item	Cal	Fat	Sat	TFat	Chol	Carb	Fib	Sug	Sod

BAJA FRESH MEXICAN GRILL (CONT'D)

SIDE ITEMS
250-300MG SODIUM
 Guacamole, small
300-350MG SODIUM
 Pronto Guacamole!™
Other sides exceed 750mg sodium.

BIG APPLE BAGELS

Contact Big Apple Bagels or their website (www.bigapplebagels.com) for nutritional info.

BAGELS *(1 BAGEL)*
250-300MG SODIUM
 Quiche Lorraine • Spinach
Other bagels exceed 400mg sodium.

CREAM CHEESE
50-100MG SODIUM
 Honey Cinnamon • Nutty Honey • Very Berry
100-150MG SODIUM
 Plain Lite • Soft/Plain • Onion Chive • Santa Fe Vegetable Lite • Strawberry Lite

SANDWICHES
800-850MG SODIUM
 Mediterranean Veg-Out • Pizzah Bagel
Other sandwiches exceed 850mg sodium.

BREAKFAST SANDWICHES
850-900MG SODIUM
 Morning Classic
Other breakfast sandwiches exceed 1150mg sodium.

SALADS *(W/O DRESSING)*
550-600MG SODIUM
 Classic Caesar Cafe Salad
650-700MG SODIUM
 Garden Mix Cafe Salad, with or w/o egg • Tuna Salad Plate (low carb)
Other salads exceed 1000mg sodium.

SALAD DRESSINGS – *exceed 400mg sodium.*

SOUPS – *exceed 750mg sodium.*

SPECIALTY DRINKS
0-50MG SODIUM
 Americano • Black Forest Coffee • Cafe Caramello

Menu Item	Cal	Fat	Sat	TFat	Chol	Carb	Fib	Sug	Sod

BIG APPLE BAGEL (SPECIALTY DRINKS CONT'D)

100-150MG SODIUM

Italiano w/FF or 2% milk (16 oz) • Oregon Chai® Tea Latte w/FF or 2% milk (16 oz)

150-200MG SODIUM

Cappuccino w/FF milk, 16 oz • Cinnamon Toast Latte w/FF milk, 16 oz •
Creme Caramel Latte w/FF milk, 16 oz • Italiano w/FF or 2% milk, 20 oz •
Oregon Chai® Tea Latte w/FF or 2% milk, 20 oz •
Raspberry Cheesecake Latte w/FF milk, 16 oz

Other specialty drinks exceed 200mg sodium.

(BLIMPIE)

Contact Blimpie® or their website (www.blimpie.com) for nutritional info.

SUBS *(6" WHITE SUB ROLL)*

800-850MG SODIUM

Hot Grilled Chicken

Other subs exceed 850mg sodium.

CAFE SANDWICHES

450-500MG SODIUM

BCC It! Union Square Ultimate Veggie (low-carb)

700-750MG SODIUM

Union Square Ultimate Veggie

Other sandwiches exceed 1000mg sodium.

WRAPS – *exceed 1600mg sodium.*

TOPPINGS AND SAUCES

0-50MG SODIUM

Oil and Vinegar (for 6" Subs) • Honey Mustard • Swiss Cheese

50-100MG SODIUM

GourMayo Wasabi Horseradish, Sun-Dried Tomato, or Chipotle Chili

Other toppings and sauces exceed 200mg sodium.

SALADS *(W/O DRESSING)*

400-450MG SODIUM

Seafood

Other salads exceed 850mg sodium.

SALAD DRESSINGS – *nutritional info unavailable*

SOUPS

600-650MG SODIUM

Garden Vegetable

Other soups exceed 700mg sodium.

BOJANGLES

Menu Item	Cal	Fat	Sat	TFat	Chol	Carb	Fib	Sug	Sod

BLIMPIE (CONT'D)

SIDE ITEMS

150-200MG SODIUM
BLIMPIE Chips, Regular Flavor

200-250MG SODIUM
BLIMPIE Chips, Cheddar & Sour Cream, Jalapeño, Sour Cream & Onion, or Romano & Garlic • Cole Slaw
Other sides exceed 550mg sodium.

COOKIES

100-150MG SODIUM
Macadamia White Chunk
Other cookies exceed 200mg sodium.

BOJANGLES

BREAKFAST

Menu Item	Cal	Fat	Sat	TFat	Chol	Carb	Fib	Sug	Sod
Bo Berry™ Sweet Biscuit	220	10	3	-	1	29	1	-	410
Cinnamon Sweet Biscuit	320	18	4	-	1	37	1	-	560
Egg Biscuit Sandwich	400	30	6	-	120	26	1	-	630

CHICKEN (1 PIECE UNLESS NOTED)

Menu Item	Cal	Fat	Sat	TFat	Chol	Carb	Fib	Sug	Sod
Leg, Southern Style	254	15	-	-	94	11	1	-	446
Thigh, Cajun Spiced	310	23	-	-	67	11	1	-	465
Leg, Cajun Spiced	264	16	-	-	96	11	1	-	530
Breast, Cajun Spiced	278	17	-	-	75	12	1	-	565

SANDWICHES

Menu Item	Cal	Fat	Sat	TFat	Chol	Carb	Fib	Sug	Sod
Cajun Filet w/o Mayo	337	11	5	-	45	41	3	-	401
w/Mayo	437	22	7	-	55	41	3	-	506
Grilled Filet w/o Mayo	235	5	3	-	51	25	2	-	540

SIDE ITEMS

Menu Item	Cal	Fat	Sat	TFat	Chol	Carb	Fib	Sug	Sod
Corn on the Cob, 1	140	2	0	-	0	34	2	-	20
Potato Rounds	235	11	4	-	13	31	3	-	328

BOSTON MARKET

Contact Boston Market or their website (www.bostonmarket.com) for nutritional info.

ENTREES

250-300MG SODIUM
Roasted Sirloin (5 oz) • 1/4 Dark Original Rotisserie Chicken, no skin (5 oz)

400-450MG SODIUM
1/4 White Original Rotisserie Chicken, no skin (5 oz)

Menu Item	Cal	Fat	Sat	TFat	Chol	Carb	Fib	Sug	Sod

BOSTON MARKET (CONT'D)

SOUPS AND SIDES

0-50MG SODIUM
Cranberry Walnut Relish • Fresh Fruit Salad • Cinnamon Apples •
Fresh Steamed Vegetables

100-150MG SODIUM
Sweet Corn • Garlic Dill New Potatoes

150-200MG SODIUM
Garden Fresh Coleslaw • Chicken Noodle Soup (6 oz)

200-250MG SODIUM
Sweet Potato Casserole • Cornbread
Other sides exceed 250mg sodium.

SALADS

250-300MG SODIUM
Caesar Salad w/o dressing

300-350MG SODIUM
Market Chopped Salad w/o dressing

SALAD DRESSINGS – *exceed 900mg sodium.*

SANDWICHES

750-800MG SODIUM OR LESS
Beef Au Jus
Other sandwiches exceed 1400mg sodium.

DESSERTS

150-200MG SODIUM
Strawberry Bliss

200-250MG SODIUM
Choc Fudge Bliss • Choc Cake
Other desserts exceed 300mg sodium.

(**BRUEGGER'S**)

Contact Bruegger's® or their website (www.brueggers.com) for nutritional info.

BAGELS

500-550MG SODIUM
Blueberry • Choc Chip • Cranberry Orange • Cinnamon Sugar •
Cinnamon Raisin • Fortified • Honey Grain • Rosemary Olive Oil

CREAM CHEESE

100-150MG SODIUM
Garden Veggie Light • Honey Walnut • Herb and Garlic Light • Strawberry •
Wild Berry

BURGER KING

Menu Item	Cal	Fat	Sat	TFat	Chol	Carb	Fib	Sug	Sod

BRUEGGER'S (CONT'D)

MUFFINS
250-300MG SODIUM
   Blueberry

BREAKFAST SANDWICHES – *exceed 1000mg sodium.*

SANDWICHES
600-650MG SODIUM
   Garden Veggie Bagel
650-700MG SODIUM
   Leonardo da Veggie Bagel
Other sandwiches exceed 750mg sodium.

WRAPS
300-350MG SODIUM
   Wheat w/o ingredients

SOUPS
300-350MG SODIUM
   Moroccan Stew
Other soups exceed 550mg sodium.

SALADS *(W/O DRESSING)*
650-700MG SODIUM
   Mandarin Medley w/Asian Dressing
Other salads exceed 700mg sodium.

SALAD DRESSINGS
150-200MG SODIUM
   Asian
Other salad dressings exceed 300mg sodium.

DESSERTS
100-150MG SODIUM
   Luscious Lemon Bar • Pecan Choc Chunks • Raspberry Sammies •
   Choc Chunk Brownie

BURGER KING

Contact Burger King® or their website (www.burgerking.com) for nutritional info.

BREAKFAST ITEMS
400-450MG SODIUM
   French Toast Sticks, 5 sticks • Hash Brown Rounds, small
700-750MG SODIUM
   Croissan'wich® w/Egg and Cheese
Other breakfast items exceed 950mg sodium.

176

Menu Item	Cal	Fat	Sat	TFat	Chol	Carb	Fib	Sug	Sod

BURGER KING (CONT'D)

BURGERS AND SANDWICHES

450-500MG SODIUM

Whopper Jr.® w/o pickles • Whopper Jr.® w/o mayo •
The Angus Steak Burger, Low Carb

550-600MG SODIUM

Whopper Jr.® • Hamburger • Double Hamburger

Other burgers and sandwiches (including chicken, fish, and veggie) exceed 750mg sodium.

CHICKEN ENTREES

450-500MG SODIUM

Chicken Tenders, 4 pc

DIPPING SAUCES

0-50MG SODIUM

Honey Flavored

50-100MG SODIUM

Sweet and Sour • Ranch

100-150MG SODIUM

Ketchup

Other dipping sauces exceed 200mg sodium.

SALADS *(W/O DRESSING OR TOAST)*

0-50MG SODIUM

Side Garden Salad

700-750MG SODIUM

Tendergrill® Chicken Caesar Salad • Tendergrill® Chicken Garden Salad

SALAD DRESSINGS AND TOPPINGS

100-150MG SODIUM

Garlic Parmesan Toast

400-450MG SODIUM

Light Italian Dressing

Other salad dressings exceed 500mg sodium.

SIDE ITEMS

0-50MG SODIUM

Strawberry-Flavored Applesauce

200-250MG SODIUM

French Fries, small, unsalted

250-300MG SODIUM

Onion Rings, small

Other side items exceed 350mg sodium.

Menu Item	Cal	Fat	Sat	TFat	Chol	Carb	Fib	Sug	Sod

BURGER KING (CONT'D)

DESSERTS AND SHAKES
150-200MG SODIUM
Hershey's® Sundae Pie • Vanilla or Strawberry Shake (kids)
200-250MG SODIUM
Vanilla or Strawberry Shake (small)
Other desserts and shakes exceed 250mg sodium.

CARL'S JR.

Contact Carl's Jr.® or their website (www.carlsjr.com) for nutritional info.

BREAKFAST
450-500MG SODIUM
French Toast Dips® w/Jam
600-650MG SODIUM
Croissant Sunrise Sandwich™ w/Bacon
Other breakfast items exceed 900mg sodium.
BREAKFAST SIDES – *exceed 450mg sodium.*

BURGERS AND SANDWICHES
450-500MG SODIUM
Sourdough Bacon Cheeseburger
Other burgers and sandwiches (including chicken and fish) exceed 950mg sodium.

SALADS *(W/O DRESSING)*
50-100MG SODIUM
Side Salad
850-900MG SODIUM
Charbroiled Chicken Salad

SALAD DRESSINGS
350-400MG SODIUM
Blue Cheese
Other salad dressings exceed 400mg sodium.

SIDE ITEMS
150-200MG SODIUM
French Fries (kids or small)
250-300MG SODIUM
French Fries (med)
300-350MG SODIUM
Chicken Stars (4 pcs)
Other side items exceed 350mg sodium.

Menu Item	Cal	Fat	Sat	TFat	Chol	Carb	Fib	Sug	Sod

CARL'S JR (CONT'D)

DESSERTS AND SHAKES

200-250MG SODIUM

Strawberry Swirl Cheesecake • Vanilla or Strawberry Shake (16 oz)

250-300MG SODIUM OR LESS

Chocolate Shake (16 oz)

Other desserts and shakes exceed 300mg sodium.

⌈ CHICK-FIL-A ⌉

BREAKFAST

Menu Item	Cal	Fat	Sat	TFat	Chol	Carb	Fib	Sug	Sod
Egg, 1	90	6	2	0	240	1	0	1	70
Cinnamon Cluster	370	12	5	2	35	60	1	30	260
Sunflower Multigrain Bagel	220	3	0	0	0	41	2	6	350
Hashbrowns	260	17	4	1	5	25	3	0	380

Other breakfast items exceed 600mg sodium.

SANDWICHES AND CHICKEN

Menu Item	Cal	Fat	Sat	TFat	Chol	Carb	Fib	Sug	Sod
Chicken Nuggets, 4 pc (kids)	130	6	1	0	35	6	0	1	550
Chargrilled Chicken, w/o bun & pickles	100	2	0	0	65	1	0	2	610

Other sandwiches and chicken exceed 850mg sodium.

WRAPS

Menu Item	Cal	Fat	Sat	TFat	Chol	Carb	Fib	Sug	Sod
Chargrilled Chicken Cool Wrap®	390	7	3	0	65	54	3	7	1020
Spicy Chicken Cool Wrap®	380	6	3	0	60	52	3	5	1090

SALADS *(W/O DRESSING)*

Menu Item	Cal	Fat	Sat	TFat	Chol	Carb	Fib	Sug	Sod
Side Salad	60	3	2	0	10	4	2	2	75
Chargrilled Chicken Garden Salad	180	6	3	0	65	9	3	6	620
Southwest Chargrilled Salad	240	8	4	0	60	1	5	6	770

SALAD DRESSINGS *(2 TBSP)*

Menu Item	Cal	Fat	Sat	TFat	Chol	Carb	Fib	Sug	Sod
Spicy	140	14	2	0	5	2	0	1	130
Reduce Fat Raspberry Vinaigrette	80	2	0	0	0	15	0	11	190
FF Honey Mustard	60	0	0	0	0	14	0	11	200

TOPPINGS *(1 PACKET)*

Menu Item	Cal	Fat	Sat	TFat	Chol	Carb	Fib	Sug	Sod
Honey Roasted Sunflower Kernels	80	7	1	0	0	3	1	2	38
Tortilla Strips	70	4	1	0	0	9	1	1	53
Garlic and Butter Croutons	50	3	0	0	0	6	0	0	90

SIDE ITEMS *(1 CUP UNLESS NOTED)*

Menu Item	Cal	Fat	Sat	TFat	Chol	Carb	Fib	Sug	Sod
Fruit Cup	60	0	0	0	0	16	2	13	0
Carrot and Raisin Salad	170	6	1	0	10	28	2	18	110
Waffle Potato Fries (small)	270	13	3	2	0	34	4	0	115
Cole Slaw	260	21	4	0	25	17	2	11	220

CHURCH'S CHICKEN

Menu Item	Cal	Fat	Sat	TFat	Chol	Carb	Fib	Sug	Sod
CHICK-FIL-A (CONT'D)									
DIPPINGS SAUCES (1 PACKET)									
Honey Roasted BBQ Sauce	60	6	1	0	5	2	0	1	90
Honey Mustard Sauce	45	0	0	0	0	10	0	10	150
Barbecue Sauce..	45	0	0	0	0	11	0	9	180
DESSERTS AND SHAKES									
Icedream® Cone	160	4	2	0	15	28	0	24	80
Icedream® Cup	240	6	4	0	25	41	0	42	105
Fudge Nut Brownie	330	15	4	3	20	45	2	29	210
All shakes exceed 500mg sodium.									

(CHURCH'S CHICKEN)

Contact Church's Chicken or their website (www.churchs.com) for nutritional info.

CHICKEN (1 PIECE OR SERVING)

250-300MG SODIUM
Original Leg
400-450MG SODIUM
Original Breast • Original Tender Strips
Other chicken exceeds 450mg sodium.

DIPPING SAUCES

0-50MG SODIUM
Purple Pepper • Honey
100-150MG SODIUM
Sweet and Sour • Honey Mustard • Creamy Jalapeño
Other sauces exceed 150mg sodium.

SIDE ITEMS

0-50MG SODIUM
Corn on the Cob
150-200MG SODIUM
Cole Slaw • Collard Greens
250-300MG SODIUM
Cajun Rice
Other sides exceed 250mg sodium.

DESSERTS

100-150MG SODIUM
Strawberry Cream Cheese Pie
150-200MG SODIUM
Double Lemon Pie
200-250MG SODIUM
Apple Pie

Menu Item	Cal	Fat	Sat	TFat	Chol	Carb	Fib	Sug	Sod

COUSINS SUBS

Contact Cousins Subs® or their website (www.cousinssubs.com) for nutritional info.

SUBS (ON ITALIAN BREAD)

4" MINI SUBS

500-550MG SODIUM
Seafood w/Crab • Tuna

550-600MG SODIUM
Lower Fat Ham

Other mini subs exceed 650mg sodium.

7 1/2" SUBS

350-400MG SODIUM
Lower Fat Garden Veggie

450-500MG SODIUM
Lower Fat Roast Beef

550-600MG SODIUM
Lower Fat Steak • Lower Fat Hot Veggie

650-700MG SODIUM
Garden Veggie

Other subs exceed 800mg.

BREADS AND WRAPS

550-600MG SODIUM
Ciabatta Bread

600-650MG SODIUM
Low-Carb Wraps

Other breads exceed 700mg sodium.

SOUPS

700-750MG SODIUM
Tomato Basil w/Ravioli (regular)

Other soups exceed 850mg sodium sodium.

SALADS (W/O DRESSING)

300-350MG SODIUM
Side Salad

400-450MG SODIUM
Garden Salad

Other salads exceed 650mg sodium.

SALAD DRESSINGS - *nutritional info unavailable*

SIDE ITEMS

200-250MG SODIUM
French Fries (small)

181

CULVER'S

Menu Item	Cal	Fat	Sat	TFat	Chol	Carb	Fib	Sug	Sod

COUSINS SUBS (CONT'D)

DESSERTS
100-150MG SODIUM
Choc Chip Cookie

CULVER'S

Contact Culver's or their website (www.culvers.com) for nutritional info.

BURGERS, SANDWICHES AND OTHER ENTREES
500-550MG SODIUM
Corn Dog (kids' meal)
550-600MG SODIUM
Chicken Tenders, Breaded, 2 pcs (kids' meal)
600-650MG SODIUM
Wisconsin Swiss Melt
650-700MG SODIUM
ButterBurger, Single • Wisconsin Swiss Melt, Jumbo • Mushroom & Swiss Burger
Other burgers, sandwiches, and other entrees exceed 700mg sodium.

SALADS
100-150MG SODIUM
Side Salad
150-200MG SODIUM
Side Caesar
350-400MG SODIUM
Garden Fresco
Other salads exceed 1000mg sodium.

SALAD DRESSINGS
150-200MG SODIUM
Raspberry Vinaigrette • Ranch, Reduced Calorie

SOUPS *– exceed 1050mg sodium.*

SIDE ITEMS
0-50MG SODIUM
Fries, Junior • Seasoned Green Beans
150-200MG SODIUM
Fries, Regular or Large • Dinner Roll
200-250MG SODIUM
Mashed Potatoes

DESSERTS
0-50MG SODIUM
Turtle Custard Cake

Menu Item	Cal	Fat	Sat	TFat	Chol	Carb	Fib	Sug	Sod

CULVER'S (DESSERTS CONT'D)

50-100MG

Candy Bars & Cream Custard Cake • Cookies & Cream Custard Cake •
Baby Scoop Choc or Vanilla Cake Cone • Caramel Swirl, No Sugar Added •
Brownies • Vanilla Cake or Waffle Cone, 1 scoop • Vanilla Dish, 1 scoop

MALTS, SHAKES, CONCRETE

150-200MG SODIUM

Vanilla Concrete Shake, short • Vanilla Shake, short

200-250MG SODIUM

Vanilla Concrete Malt, short • Vanilla Shake or Concrete Shake, med •
Vanilla Malt, short

(DAIRY QUEEN / BRAZIER)

Contact Dairy Queen® or their website (www.dairyqueen.com) for nutritional info.

BURGERS, SANDWICHES AND OTHER ENTREES

600-650MG SODIUM

DQ Homestyle® Hamburger

Other burgers, sandwiches, and other entrees (including chicken) exceed 700mg sodium.

SALADS *(W/O DRESSING)*

50-100MG SODIUM

Side Salad

600-650MG SODIUM

Crispy Chicken Salad

Other salads exceed 900mg sodium.

SALAD DRESSINGS

350-400MG SODIUM

Honey Mustard • Ranch • FF Italian

Other salad dressings exceed 750mg sodium.

SIDE ITEMS – *exceed 600mg sodium.*

DESSERTS

50-100MG SODIUM

Vanilla or Choc Soft Serve Cup, 1/2 cup

100-150MG SODIUM

Vanilla or Choc Cone (small) • Dipped Cone (small)

SPECIALTY DRINKS

250-300MG SODIUM

Choc Shake (small)

Other specialty drinks exceed 300mg sodium.

D'ANGELO

D'ANGELO

Contact D'Angelo's® or their website (www.dangelos.com) for nutritional info.

SUBS (SMALL SUB ON HONEY WHEAT)

350-400MG SODIUM
Turkey D'Lite (Kidz Meal)

450-500MG SODIUM
Steak • Cheeseburger Sub (Kidz Meal)

500-550MG SODIUM
Hamburger • Salad • Turkey

600-650MG SODIUM
Tuna Sub (Kidz Meal)

650-700MG SODIUM
Roast Beef • Turkey Club
Other subs exceed 750mg sodium.

SANDWICHES (SMALL SUB ON WHITE ROLL)

600-650MG SODIUM
Turkey • Turkey Cranberry

650-700MG SODIUM
Fresh Veggie
Other sandwiches exceed 800mg sodium.

POKKET SANDWICHES (HONEY WHEAT POKKET)

400-450MG SODIUM
Classic Veggie No Cheese • Hamburger • Steak

450-500MG SODIUM
Salad • Turkey
Other pokket sandwiches exceed 700mg sodium.

WRAPS (WHITE WRAP)

300-350MG SODIUM
Steak • Salad • Hamburger

350-400MG SODIUM
Turkey

500-550MG SODIUM
Roast Beef
Other wraps exceed 550mg sodium.

SOUPS

250-300MG SODIUM
Hearty Vegetable, small

Menu Item	Cal	Fat	Sat	TFat	Chol	Carb	Fib	Sug	Sod

D'ANGELO (SOUPS CONT'D)

400-450MG SODIUM

Hearty Vegetable, large

Other soups exceed 650mg sodium.

SALADS *(W/O DRESSING)*

0-50MG SODIUM

Tossed

50-100MG SODIUM

Turkey

200-250MG SODIUM

Roast Beef

Other salads exceed 550mg sodium.

SALAD DRESSINGS

200-250MG SODIUM

Honey Mustard

250-300MG SODIUM

Bleu Cheese

Other dressings exceed 300mg sodium.

BREADS AND TOPPINGS

150-200MG SODIUM

Plain Wrap

250-300MG SODIUM

Honey Wheat Pokket Bread

300-350MG SODIUM

White Pokket Bread

350-400MG SODIUM

Honey Wheat Sub

Other breads and wraps exceed 450mg sodium.

TOPPINGS

0-50MG SODIUM

Cucumber • Lettuce • Olive Oil Blend • Onions • Sweet Peppers • Tomato • Vinegar

50-100MG SODIUM

FF Mayonnaise • Swiss Cheese

100-150MG SODIUM

Mushrooms • Mayonnaise

150-200MG SODIUM

Honey Dijon Mustard • Pickles

Other toppings exceed 200mg sodium.

DEL TACO

Menu Item	Cal	Fat	Sat	TFat	Chol	Carb	Fib	Sug	Sod

(DEL TACO)

Contact Del Taco® or their website (www.deltaco.com) for nutritional info.

BREAKFAST
500-550MG SODIUM
  Breakfast Burrito
Other breakfast items exceed 700mg sodium.

BREAKFAST SIDES
150-200MG SODIUM
  5-Piece Hash Brown Sticks • Side of Bacon, 2 slices
300-350MG SODIUM
  8-Piece Hash Brown Sticks

TACOS
150-200MG SODIUM
  Taco
300-350MG SODIUM
  Soft Taco
450-500MG SODIUM
  Carne Asada Taco • Crispy Fish Taco
500-550MG SODIUM
  Chicken Soft Taco • Chicken Del Taco Carbon
Other tacos exceed 650mg sodium.

BURRITOS – *exceed 1000mg sodium.*

QUESADILLAS
850-900MG SODIUM
  Cheddar Quesadilla
Other quesadillas exceed 900mg sodium.

COMBO MEALS – *exceed 1100mg sodium.*

BURGERS
650-700MG SODIUM
  Hamburger
Other burgers exceed 700mg sodium.

SALADS
350-400MG SODIUM
  Taco Salad
Other salads exceed 2200mg sodium.

SIDE ITEMS
150-200MG SODIUM
  Fries (kids)

186

Menu Item	Cal	Fat	Sat	TFat	Chol	Carb	Fib	Sug	Sod

250-300MG SODIUM
Fries (small) • Chips & Salsa (small)
Other sides exceed 350mg sodium.

SHAKES

250-300MG SODIUM
Strawberry (small)
Other shakes exceed 300mg sodium.

(DENNY'S)

Contact Denny's® or their website (www.dennys.com) for nutritional info.

BREAKFAST ITEMS

0-50MG SODIUM
Grapefruit, Banana, or Grapes • Applesauce
100-150MG SODIUM
One Egg
150-200MG SODIUM
Egg Beaters® Egg Substitute • Oatmeal • Toast, dry, 1 slice • English Muffin, dry
250-300MG SODIUM
Kellogg's® Dry Cereal (avg)
Other breakfast items exceed 400mg sodium.

SENIORS

600-650MG SODIUM
Senior Starter™
650-700MG SODIUM
Senior French Toast Slam
Other senior breakfast items exceed 750mg sodium.

ENTREES

200-250MG SODIUM
Carb-Watch Grilled Tilapia
600-650MG SODIUM
Steakhouse Strip Dinner
Other entrees exceed 650mg sodium.
NOTE: Entree values do not include side dishes and bread.

SENIORS

150-200MG SODIUM
Senior Grilled Tilapia
600-650MG SODIUM
Senior Bacon Cheddar Burger
Other senior entrees exceed 650mg sodium.

DENNY'S

| --- | --- | --- | --- | --- | --- | --- | --- | --- | --- |

DENNY'S (CONT'D)

SANDWICHES

650-700MG SODIUM

Carb-Watch Bacon-Cheddar Burger

Other sandwiches exceed 750mg sodium.

SENIORS

600-650MG SODIUM

Senior Bacon Cheddar Burger

Other senior sandwiches exceed 1300mg sodium.

SOUPS – *exceed 800mg sodium.*

SALADS *(W/O DRESSING)*

100-150MG SODIUM

Side Salad

Other salads exceed 700mg sodium.

SALAD DRESSINGS

100-150MG SODIUM

Honey Mustard Dressing

150-200MG SODIUM

Thousand Island Dressing • Ranch Dressing

Other salad dressings exceed 300mg sodium.

SIDE ITEMS AND APPETIZERS

0-50MG SODIUM

Sliced Tomatoes, 3 slices • Plain Baked Potato • Green Beans • Applesauce

150-200MG SODIUM

Corn

200-250MG SODIUM

French Fries, unsalted

Other sides and appetizers exceed 500mg sodium.

CONDIMENTS AND TOPPINGS

0-50MG SODIUM

Whipped Cream • Cherry Topping • Blueberry Topping • Strawberry Topping •
Maple-Flavored Syrup • Sour Cream

50-100MG SODIUM

Maple-Flavored Syrup, Sugar-Free • Fudge Topping • Cream Cheese •
Country Gravy • Cinnamon Apple Filling

DESSERTS AND SHAKES

0-50MG SODIUM

Single Scoop Sundae

50-100MG SODIUM

Hot Fudge Brownie a la mode • Double Scoop Sundae

Menu Item	Cal	Fat	Sat	TFat	Chol	Carb	Fib	Sug	Sod

DENNY'S (DESSERTS CONT'D)

150-200MG SODIUM

Banana Split

200-250MG SODIUM

French Silk Pie

250-300MG SODIUM

Vanilla or Choc Milkshake • Vanilla or Choc Malted Milkshake

Other desserts and shakes exceed 300mg sodium.

DOMINO'S PIZZA

FEAST PIZZAS *(1/8 SLICE UNLESS NOTED)*

Crunchy Thin Crust:

Menu Item	Cal	Fat	Sat	TFat	Chol	Carb	Fib	Sug	Sod
Vegi Feast®, 12"	160	10	4	0	15	16	2	2	355
Barbecue Feast, 12"	210	12	5	0	20	20	1	5	375
Philly Cheese Steak, 12"	180	11	6	0	20	13	1	1	375
Deluxe Feast®, 12"	180	12	4	0	15	16	2	2	395
Bacon Cheeseburger®, 12"	220	15	6	0	30	15	2	2	405
Hawaiian Feast®, 12"	170	10	4	0	15	17	2	3	405

Classic Hand-Tossed:

Menu Item	Cal	Fat	Sat	TFat	Chol	Carb	Fib	Sug	Sod
Vegi Feast®, 14"	240	9	4	0	15	32	2	4	450

BUILD A PIZZA *(1/8 SLICE UNLESS NOTED)*

CRUSTS

Menu Item	Cal	Fat	Sat	TFat	Chol	Carb	Fib	Sug	Sod
Crunchy Thin, 12"	80	4	1	0	0	12	1	1	15
Crunchy Thin, 14"	110	5	1	0	0	16	1	1	20
Ultimate Deep Dish, 12"	160	3	1	0	0	28	1	3	110
Ultimate Deep Dish, 14"	220	4	1	0	0	38	2	3	150

TOPPINGS

Onions, Mushrooms, Bell Peppers, Pineapple, Green Chili Peppers,

Menu Item	Cal	Fat	Sat	TFat	Chol	Carb	Fib	Sug	Sod
Garlic & Tomatoes (avg)	3	0	0	0	0	3	0	1	1
Anchovies	0	0	0	0	0	0	0	0	35
Cheddar Cheese (avg)	32	3	2	0	7	0	0	0	50
Black Olives (avg)	10	1	0	0	0	1	0	0	63
Philly Steak (avg)	13	1	0	0	5	0	0	0	73
Beef (avg)	45	4	2	0	10	0	0	0	85

SALADS *(W/O DRESSING)*

Menu Item	Cal	Fat	Sat	TFat	Chol	Carb	Fib	Sug	Sod
Garden Fresh Salad	70	4	2	0	10	6	1	3	85
Grilled Chicken Caesar	105	4	2	0	25	6	1	3	320

SALAD DRESSINGS – *exceed 350mg sodium.*

DONATOS PIZZERIA

Menu Item	Cal	Fat	Sat	TFat	Chol	Carb	Fib	Sug	Sod
DOMINO'S PIZZA (CONT'D)									
BUFFALO WINGS *(1 PIECE)*									
Barbeque	50	2	1	0	26	2	0	1	175
Hot Wings	85	5	2	0	50	2	0	1	250
SIDE ITEMS									
Breadstick, 1	130	7	2	0	0	14	1	1	90
Cheesy Bread	140	7	2	0	5	14	1	1	140
Pizza Chicken Kickers®	45	2	0	0	10	3	0	0	160
Other sides exceed 200mg sodium.									
DESSERTS									
CinnaStix, 1	140	7	2	0	0	17	1	4	80

DONATOS PIZZERIA

Contact Donato's or their website (www.donatos.com) for nutritional info.

PIZZAS *(7" INDIVIDUAL OR 1/4 OF 14" PIZZA)*
1000-1050MG SODIUM
  White, Individual NoDough
  Other pizzas exceed 1100mg sodium

SUBS *(WHOLE SUB)* – *exceed 1700mg sodium.*

TORTILLA SUBS – *exceed 1450mg sodium.*

SALADS *(W/O DRESSING)*
150-200MG SODIUM
  Side Tuscan Caesar
350-400MG SODIUM
  Side Italian
  Other salads exceed 700mg sodium.

  SALAD DRESSINGS
  250-300MG SODIUM
    Dijon Honey Mustard
    Other salad dressings exceed 300mg sodium.

SIDE ITEMS – *exceed 350mg sodium.*

DESSERTS
150-200MG SODIUM
  Choc Chunk Cookie • Oatmeal Raisin Cookie

Menu Item	Cal	Fat	Sat	TFat	Chol	Carb	Fib	Sug	Sod

(DUNKIN' DONUTS)

Contact Dunkin' Donuts® or their website (www.dunkindonuts.com) for nutritional info.

BREAKFAST SANDWICHES – *exceed 700mg sodium.*

DONUTS

100-150MG SODIUM

French Cruller

150-200MG SODIUM

Glazed Lemon Cake • Frosted Lemon Cake

250-300MG SODIUM

Glazed • Sugar Raised • Jelly Filled • Marble Frosted • Strawberry • Strawberry Frosted • Maple Frosted • Apple Crumb • Apple N'Spice • Bavarian Kreme • Black Raspberry • Blueberry Crumb • Boston Kreme • Choc Frosted • Choc or Vanilla Kreme Filled

MUNCHKINS

150-200MG SODIUM

Lemon Filled • Glazed Cake

200-250MG SODIUM

Glazed • Plain, Powdered, or Cinnamon Cake • Jelly Filled • Glazed Choc Cake

STICKS

300-350MG SODIUM

Plain Cake • Glazed Cake • Jelly Stick • Powdered Cake • Cinnamon Cake

DANISHES, FRITTERS AND OTHER PASTRIES

250-300MG SODIUM

Eclair • Choc Iced Bismark • Apple, Cheese, or Strawberry Cheese Danish

300-350MG SODIUM

Coffee Roll • Glazed Fritter • Maple Frosted Coffee Roll • Vanilla Frosted Coffee Roll • Choc Frosted Coffee Roll

MUFFINS

300-350MG SODIUM

English Muffin

450-500MG SODIUM

Blueberry • Reduced Fat Blueberry • Honey Bran Raisin

BAGELS AND CROISSANTS

250-300MG SODIUM

Croissant, plain

400-450MG SODIUM

Cinnamon Raisin Bagel

Other bagels exceed 600mg sodium.

191

EL POLLO LOCO

Menu Item	Cal	Fat	Sat	TFat	Chol	Carb	Fib	Sug	Sod

DUNKIN' DONUTS (CONT'D)

CREAM CHEESE
100-150MG SODIUM
   Shedd's Buttermatch Blend • Strawberry
150-200MG SODIUM
   Salmon • Plain
200-250MG SODIUM
   Chive • Lite
   Other cream cheese exceeds 300mg sodium.

COOKIES
100-150MG SODIUM
   All cookies

(EL POLLO LOCO)

Contact El Pollo Loco or their website (www.elpolloloco.com) for nutritional info.

TACOS
200-250MG SODIUM
   Taco Al Carbon
500-550MG SODIUM
   Chicken Soft Taco

FLAME-BROILED CHICKEN
200-250MG SODIUM
   Leg • Thigh • Drumstick Chicken (Kids Meal)
300-350MG SODIUM
   Wing
   Other chicken exceed 500mg sodium.

BURRITOS – *exceed 1350mg sodium.*

SALADS *(W/O DRESSING)*
250-300MG SODIUM
   Garden Salad
   Other salads exceed 800mg sodium.

POLLO BOWLS – *exceed 1400mg sodium.*

SALAD DRESSINGS
250-300MG SODIUM
   Creamy Cilantro Dressing
   Other salad dressings exceed 350mg sodium.

SIDE ITEMS
0-50MG SODIUM
   3" Corn Cobbette

Menu Item	Cal	Fat	Sat	TFat	Chol	Carb	Fib	Sug	Sod

EL POLLO LOCO (SIDE ITEMS CONT'D)

50-100MG SODIUM

  Fresh Vegetables

100-150MG SODIUM

  3 Corn Tortillas

250-300MG SODIUM

  Guacamole

300-350MG SODIUM

  French Fries (Kid's Meal)

Other side items exceed 350mg sodium.

SAUCES AND TOPPINGS

0-50MG SODIUM

  Sour Cream • Fried Serrano Pepper

50-100MG SODIUM

  House Salsa • Ketchup

100-150MG SODIUM

  Pico de Gallo Salsa • Jalapeño Hot Sauce

Other sauces and toppings exceed 150mg sodium.

DESSERTS

100-150MG SODIUM

  Foster's Freeze Soft Serve Cup

150-200MG SODIUM

  Caramel Flan

200-250MG SODIUM

  Churros

(FAZOLI'S)

BUILD YOUR OWN PASTA

Choose a Pasta:

Menu Item	Cal	Fat	Sat	TFat	Chol	Carb	Fib	Sug	Sod
All pasta, small serving (avg)	370	2	0	0	0	73	4	4	20
All pasta, regular serving (avg)	560	3	0	0	0	109	5	5	30

Choose a Sauce:

Menu Item	Cal	Fat	Sat	TFat	Chol	Carb	Fib	Sug	Sod
Spicy Marinara, small	60	2	0	0	0	11	3	8	640
Parmesan Alfredo Tomato, small	80	3	1	0	0	10	2	4	670

Choose a Topping:

Menu Item	Cal	Fat	Sat	TFat	Chol	Carb	Fib	Sug	Sod
Garlic Shrimp	80	0	0	0	70	1	0	0	260
Broccoli	45	2	0	0	0	5	3	2	280
Broccoli & Tomatoes	50	2	2	0	0	7	3	2	280
Zesty Peppers & Onions	80	5	1	0	0	8	1	3	290

FLAMERS

Menu Item	Cal	Fat	Sat	TFat	Chol	Carb	Fib	Sug	Sod
FAZOLI'S (CONT'D)									
CLASSIC PASTAS – *exceed 1300mg sodium.*									
KID'S MEALS									
Spaghetti w/Marinara Sauce	260	2	0	0	0	51	3	4	290
Spaghetti w/Hearty Meat Sauce	270	3	0	0	0	51	4	4	370
Fettuccine Alfredo	290	5	2	0	5	50	2	4	420
PIZZAS – *exceed 1200mg sodium.*									
SUBS AND PANINIS – *exceed 1000mg sodium.*									
SALADS *(W/O DRESSING)*									
Garden Side	25	0	0	0	6	4	3	2	30
Caesar Side	110	5	1	0	5	12	2	1	180
Grilled Chicken Salad	100	2	0	0	50	6	4	2	410
SALAD DRESSINGS – *nutritional information unavailable*									
BREADSTICKS AND EXTRAS									
Breadstick, dry, 1	100	2	0	0	0	20	0	1	160
Other breadsticks and extras exceed 200mg sodium.									
DESSERTS									
Lemon Ice, regular	180	0	0	0	0	45	0	45	15
Lemon Ice, large	280	0	0	0	0	73	0	73	20
Freezi's, Strawberry Banana Twist	380	4	4	0	0	91	1	80	85
Freezi's, Very Strawberry	390	4	4	0	0	93	0	83	120

(FLAMERS)

Contact Flamers Grill or their website (www.flamersgrill.com) for nutritional info.

BURGERS AND SANDWICHES

300-350MG SODIUM

Charbroiled or Lemon Pepper Chicken w/o pickles • Cajun Chicken w/o pickles

400-450MG SODIUM

Hamburger, 4 oz or 6 oz w/o pickles • BBQ Chicken w/o pickles

Other burgers and sandwiches exceed 500mg sodium.

(GODFATHER'S PIZZA)

Contact Godfather or their website (www.godfathers.com) for nutritional info.

PIZZAS

Mini, Original Crust, 1/4

200-250MG SODIUM

Cheese

Menu Item	Cal	Fat	Sat	TFat	Chol	Carb	Fib	Sug	Sod

GODFATHER'S PIZZA (1/4 MINI, ORIGINAL CRUST PIZZA CONT'D)

 250-300MG SODIUM

  Hawaiian • Pepperoni • Super Hawaiian • Veggie

Medium, Thin Crust, 1/8

 200-250MG SODIUM

  Pepperoni

 250-300MG SODIUM

  Cheese

 300-350MG SODIUM

  Veggie • Hawaiian • Super Hawaiian

Large, Thin Crust, 1/10

 300-350MG SODIUM

  Cheese

 350-400MG SODIUM

  Veggie

DESSERTS

 100-150MG SODIUM

  Alum Pan Desserts, 1/6

HÄAGEN-DAZS

Häagen-Dazs products are low sodium, the following have the least in each category.

SORBET *(1/2 CUP UNLESS NOTED)*

Menu Item	Cal	Fat	Sat	TFat	Chol	Carb	Fib	Sug	Sod
Strawberry or Raspberry	120	0	0	0	0	30	2	26	0
Orchard Peach	130	0	0	0	0	33	1	29	0
Strawberry	120	0	0	0	0	30	1	30	10
Mango	120	0	0	0	0	37	0	36	10

FROZEN YOGURT *(1/2 CUP UNLESS NOTED)*

Menu Item	Cal	Fat	Sat	TFat	Chol	Carb	Fib	Sug	Sod
Vanilla Raspberry Swirl	170	3	2	0	25	32	0	24	35
Strawberry	140	0	0	0	5	31	0	20	40
Coffee	200	5	3	0	65	31	0	20	50
Vanilla	200	5	3	0	65	31	0	21	55

LIGHT ICE CREAM *(1/2 CUP UNLESS NOTED)*

Menu Item	Cal	Fat	Sat	TFat	Chol	Carb	Fib	Sug	Sod
Cherry Fudge Truffle	230	7	4	0	50	37	0	33	40
Vanilla Bean	200	7	4	0	65	29	0	26	55
Mint Chip	230	8	5	0	55	34	0	30	65

ICE CREAM *(1/2 CUP UNLESS NOTED)*

Menu Item	Cal	Fat	Sat	TFat	Chol	Carb	Fib	Sug	Sod
Mango	250	14	8	0	85	28	1	27	50
Choc Choc Chip or Black Raspberry Chip	290	19	12	1	103	25	2	24	55

HARDEE'S

Menu Item	Cal	Fat	Sat	TFat	Chol	Carb	Fib	Sug	Sod
HAAGEN DAZ (CONT'D)									
Peaches & Cream	240	12	7	0	75	29	0	27	55
Pineapple Coconut	230	13	8	1	90	25	0	24	55
Mayan Choc	310	19	11	1	90	29	1	26	55
Cherry Vanilla	240	15	9	1	100	23	0	22	60
Choc or Rum Raisin (avg)	270	18	10	1	113	22	1	21	60

(HARDEE'S)

Contact Hardee's® or their website (www.hardees.com) for nutritional info.

BREAKFAST
50-100MG SODIUM
  Folded Egg • Scrambled Egg
600-650MG SODIUM
  Loaded Omelet
Other breakfasts exceed 750mg sodium.

BREAKFAST SIDES
  200-250MG SODIUM
    Sunrise Croissant • Bacon, 2 1/2 strips
    Other breakfast sides exceed 350mg sodium.

BURGERS
550-600MG SODIUM
  Hamburger
Other burgers exceed 650mg sodium.

SANDWICHES – *exceed 850mg sodium.*

CHICKEN – *exceed 550mg sodium.*

SIDE ITEMS
100-150MG SODIUM
  Cole Slaw, small • French Fries, kids
200-250MG SODIUM
  French Fries, small
Other sides exceed 300mg sodium.

CONDIMENTS
0-50MG SODIUM
  Horseradish
50-100MG SODIUM
  Sweet N Sour Dipping Sauce • Mayonnaise
100-150MG SODIUM
  BBQ Dipping Sauce • Ketchup

Menu Item	Cal	Fat	Sat	TFat	Chol	Carb	Fib	Sug	Sod

HARDEE'S (CONT'D)

DESSERTS AND SHAKES
50-100MG SODIUM
   Single Scoop Ice Cream Bowl
100-150MG SODIUM
   Single Scoop Ice Ceam Cup
200-250MG SODIUM
   Peach Cobbler • Vanilla or Strawberry Shake, regular

(HUNGRY HOWIES PIZZA) —————————————————————————

Contact Hungry Howies or their website (www.hungryhowies.com) for nutritional info.

PIZZAS
Thin Crust
   250-300MG SODIUM
      Cheese, medium, 1/8 slice
   300-350MG SODIUM
      Cheese, large, 1/10 slice
Regular Crust
   350-400MG SODIUM
      Cheese, small, 1/6 slice
ADD TOPPINGS *(PER MEDIUM PIZZA SLICE)*
   0-50MG SODIUM
      Mushrooms • Pineapple • Onions • Green Peppers • Bacon • Olives
   50-100MG SODIUM
      Pepperoni • Ham • Beef
   100-150MG SODIUM
      Sausage
Other toppings exceed 150mg sodium.
CALZONE SUBS – *exceed 850mg sodium.*

CHICKEN
450-500MG SODIUM
   Chicken Tenders
Other chicken exceeds 750mg sodium.
   DIPPING SAUCE – *exceed 200mg sodium.*
SALADS *(W/O DRESSING)*
0-50MG SODIUM
   Large or Small Garden
300-350MG SODIUM
   Large Chef, 1/4

IN-N-OUT BURGERS

Menu Item	Cal	Fat	Sat	TFat	Chol	Carb	Fib	Sug	Sod
HUNGRY HOWIE'S PIZZA (SALADS CONT'D)									
350-400MG SODIUM									
Small Chef, 1/2									
450-500MG SODIUM									
Large Antipasto, 1/4									
Other salads exceeds 500mg sodium.									
SALAD DRESSINGS									
50-100MG SODIUM									
Greek									
150-200MG SODIUM									
French Style									
200-250MG SODIUM									
Creamy Italian • Thousand Island • Ranch									
Other salad dressings exceed 250mg sodium.									

IN-N-OUT BURGER

BURGERS

Menu Item	Cal	Fat	Sat	TFat	Chol	Carb	Fib	Sug	Sod
Hamburger, Protein Style *(bun replaced with lettuce)*	240	17	4	-	40	11	3	7	370
Hamburger	390	19	5	-	40	39	3	10	650

SIDES

Menu Item	Cal	Fat	Sat	TFat	Chol	Carb	Fib	Sug	Sod
French Fries	400	18	5	-	0	54	2	0	245

SHAKES *(15 oz)*

Menu Item	Cal	Fat	Sat	TFat	Chol	Carb	Fib	Sug	Sod
Strawberry	690	33	22	-	85	91	0	75	280
Chocolate	690	36	24	-	95	83	0	62	350
Vanilla	680	37	25	-	90	78	0	57	390

JACK IN THE BOX

BREAKFAST

Menu Item	Cal	Fat	Sat	TFat	Chol	Carb	Fib	Sug	Sod
Original French Toast Sticks	470	23	5	5	25	58	4	14	450
Blueberry French Toast Sticks	450	20	5	5	0	59	3	15	550
Other breakfasts exceed 750mg sodium.									

BREAKFAST SIDES

Menu Item	Cal	Fat	Sat	TFat	Chol	Carb	Fib	Sug	Sod
Hashbrowns	150	10	3	3	0	13	2	0	230

BURGERS

Menu Item	Cal	Fat	Sat	TFat	Chol	Carb	Fib	Sug	Sod
Hamburger Deluxe	370	21	7	1	45	31	2	6	560
Hamburger	310	14	6	1	45	30	1	6	600
To reduce sodium, omit pickles, ketchup, and/or mustard.									

CHICKEN AND MORE

Menu Item	Cal	Fat	Sat	TFat	Chol	Carb	Fib	Sug	Sod
Chicken Breast Strips, 2 (kids)	250	12	3	3	40	18	2	1	630

Menu Item	Cal	Fat	Sat	TFat	Chol	Carb	Fib	Sug	Sod
JACK IN THE BOX (CHICKEN AND MORE CONT'D)									
Chicken Sandwich	400	21	5	3	35	38	2	4	730
Southwest Chicken Pita, no salsa	230	4	1	0	40	34	3	3	790
DIPPING SAUCES									
Sweet & Sour Dipping Sauce	45	0	0	0	0	11	0	6	160
TACO									
Regular Beef Taco	160	8	3	1	15	15	2	4	270
Beef Monster Taco®	240	14	5	2	20	20	3	4	390
SALADS *(W/O DRESSING)*									
Side Salad	60	3	2	0	10	5	2	3	65
Asian Chicken Salad	140	1	0	0	25	19	5	13	470
SALAD DRESSINGS – *exceed 550mg sodium*									
TOPPINGS									
Roasted Slivered Almonds	110	9	1	0	0	4	2	1	5
Wonton Strips	110	6	2	0	0	13	2	1	45
Country Ranch Sliced Almonds	100	9	1	0	0	3	2	1	130
SIDE ITEMS									
Applesauce	100	0	0	0	0	25	1	23	0
Egg Roll, 1	130	6	2	1	5	15	2	1	310
Natural Cut Fries (kids)	210	10	3	3	0	28	2	0	350
Other sides exceed 400mg sodium.									
CONDIMENTS *(1 OZ UNLESS NOTED)*									
Grape Jelly, 0.5 oz	35	0	0	0	0	9	0	9	10
Sour Cream	60	5	3	0	15	2	1	1	25
Log Cabin® Syrup, 1.5 oz	190	0	0	0	0	49	0	18	35
Country Crock Spread®	25	3	1	1	0	0	0	0	45
Mustard, 0.2 oz	5	0	0	0	0	1	0	0	50
Taco Sauce, 0.3 oz	0	0	0	0	0	0	0	0	80
Mayo-Onion Sauce, 0.5 oz	90	10	2	0	5	1	0	0	85
Ketchup, 0.3 oz	10	0	0	0	0	2	0	2	105
Salsa, Fire Roasted	5	0	0	0	0	1	0	1	105
DESSERTS AND SHAKES									
Cheesecake	310	16	9	1	55	34	0	23	220
Vanilla Shake, small	570	29	18	1	115	65	0	54	220
Strawberry Shake, small	640	28	18	1	110	84	0	71	220

Menu Item	Cal	Fat	Sat	TFat	Chol	Carb	Fib	Sug	Sod

KFC

Contact KFC® or their website (www.kfc.com) for nutritional info.

CHICKEN *(1 PIECE)*

350-400MG SODIUM

Whole Wing, Original or Extra Crispy

400-450MG SODIUM

Breast, Original Recipe (w/o skin or breading) •

Drumstick, Original or Extra Crispy

Other chicken exceeds 700mg sodium.

SANDWICHES

450-500MG SODIUM

Honey BBQ KFC® Snacker

Other sandwiches exceed 600mg sodium.

SALADS *(W/O DRESSING)*

0-50MG SODIUM

House Side

100-150MG SODIUM

Caesar Side

Other salads exceed 850mg sodium.

SALAD DRESSINGS – *exceed 400mg sodium.*

TOPPINGS

150-200MG SODIUM

Parmesan Garlic Croutons Pouch

SIDE ITEMS

0-50MG SODIUM

Corn on the Cob, 3" or 5.5"

200-250MG SODIUM

Baked! Cheetos®

300-350MG SODIUM

Cole Slaw • Mashed Potatoes w/o Gravy

Other sides exceed 350mg sodium.

DESSERTS

50-100MG SODIUM

Quaker Chewy® S'mores Granola Bar

100-150MG SODIUM

Lil' Bucket™ Strawberry Short Cake

150-200MG SODIUM

Lil' Bucket™ Fudge Brownie • Lil' Bucket™ Choc Cream

Menu Item	Cal	Fat	Sat	TFat	Chol	Carb	Fib	Sug	Sod

KOO-KOO-ROO

Contact Koo-Koo-Roo or their website (www.kookooroo.com) for nutritional info.

ENTREES

50-199MG SODIUM
  Fresh Roasted Turkey, Sliced Breast
500-550MG SODIUM
  Rotisserie Chicken, Leg and Thigh

SANDWICHES – *exceed 1100mg sodium.*

WRAPS – *exceed 1850mg sodium.*

BURRITOS – *exceed 2150mg sodium.*

CHICKEN BOWLS – *exceed 800mg sodium.*

SOUPS

400-450MG SODIUM
  Chicken Noodle • Ten Vegetable

SALADS *(W/O DRESSING)*

200-250MG SODIUM
  House Salad
Other salads exceed 850mg sodium.

SALAD DRESSINGS

200-250MG SODIUM
  Ranch • Caesar

SIDE ITEMS

0-50MG SODIUM
  Sticky Rice • Butternut Squash • Tossed Salad w/o Dressing • Baked Yams •
  Cantaloupe and Honeydew • Celery Sticks, 6 • Steamed Vegetables
50-100MG SODIUM
  Lahvash, 1 pc
100-150MG SODIUM
  Italian Vegetable
150-200MG SODIUM
  Cucumber Salad • Tangy Tomato Salad • Kernel Corn • Green Beans
Other sides exceed 200mg sodium.

SAUCES AND CONDIMENTS *(1 OZ UNLESS NOTED)*

0-50MG SODIUM
  Cranberry Sauce • Sour Cream
50-100MG SODIUM
  Pico De Gallo • Salsa • Chipotle Sauce
Other sauces and condiments exceed 200mg sodium.

KRISPY KREME DOUGHNUTS

Menu Item	Cal	Fat	Sat	TFat	Chol	Carb	Fib	Sug	Sod

KRISPY KREME DOUGHNUTS

DOUGHNUTS

Menu Item	Cal	Fat	Sat	TFat	Chol	Carb	Fib	Sug	Sod
Cinnamon Twist	230	9	3	0	5	33	1	19	85
Sugar	200	12	3	4	5	21	0	10	95
Original Glazed	200	12	3	4	5	33	1	21	95
Original Glazed Doughnut Holes	200	11	3	4	5	24	1	13	95
Choc Iced Glazed	250	12	3	4	5	33	1	21	100
Choc Iced w/Sprinkles	260	12	3	4	5	38	1	24	100
Glazed Cinnamon	210	12	3	4	5	24	1	12	100
Maple Iced Glazed	240	12	3	4	5	32	1	20	100
Glazed Raspberry Filled	300	16	4	5	5	38	1	22	130
Cinnamon Bun	260	16	4	5	5	28	1	13	125
Glazed Lemon Filled	290	16	4	5	5	35	1	18	135
Powdered Strawberry Filled	290	16	4	5	5	33	1	13	135
Choc Iced Kreme Filled	350	20	5	6	5	38	1	23	140
Choc Iced Custard Filled	300	17	4	5	5	35	1	19	140
Glazed Kreme Filled	340	20	5	6	5	38	1	23	140
Powdered Blueberry Filled	290	16	4	5	5	33	1	14	140
Cinnamon Apple Filled	290	16	4	5	5	32	1	14	150
Key Lime Pie	320	17	5	5	5	40	1	24	150
Dulce De Leche	290	18	5	5	5	30	1	12	160
Caramel Kreme Crunch	350	19	5	5	5	43	1	25	170
New York Cheesecake	320	19	5	6	10	35	1	17	190

FROZEN BLENDS

Menu Item	Cal	Fat	Sat	TFat	Chol	Carb	Fib	Sug	Sod
Reduced Calorie Double Choc, 12 oz	99	1	0	0	2	38	1	8	104
Reduced Calorie Latte Blend, 12 oz	99	1	0	0	2	34	0	11	117
Raspberry, 12 oz	430	13	10	-	25	74	0	56	160
Original Kreme, 12 oz	440	15	12	-	25	70	0	41	200
Original Kreme w/Coffee, 12 oz	440	15	12	-	25	70	0	39	210
Latte, 12 oz	440	16	13	-	25	69	0	41	210
Double Choc, 12 oz	440	16	11	-	25	69	0	46	210
Double Choc w/Coffee, 12 oz	440	16	10	-	25	69	0	46	210

KRYSTAL

BREAKFAST

Menu Item	Cal	Fat	Sat	TFat	Chol	Carb	Fib	Sug	Sod
Krystal Sunriser	240	14	5	-	255	14	2	1	460

BREAKFAST SIDES

Menu Item	Cal	Fat	Sat	TFat	Chol	Carb	Fib	Sug	Sod
Kryspers	190	13	5	-	10	17	2	0	340

Menu Item	Cal	Fat	Sat	TFat	Chol	Carb	Fib	Sug	Sod
KRYSTAL (CONT'D)									
SANDWICHES									
Krystal Sandwich	160	7	3	-	20	17	1	1	260
Cheese Krystal	180	9	4	-	25	17	2	1	430
Bacon Cheese Krystal	190	10	5	-	25	16	2	2	430
Corn Pup	260	19	8	-	50	19	1	5	480
Plain Pup	170	9	4	-	25	15	1	-	500
Chili Cheese Pup	210	12	5	-	40	17	2	2	510
SALADS									
Chik'n Bites Salad	290	20	11	-	65	12	4	1	490
SIDE ITEMS									
Fries, regular	470	20	8	-	20	53	7	0	90
DESSERTS									
Lemon Ice Box Pie, 1 slice	260	9	2	-	25	41	2	37	180

(LA SALSA FRESH MEXICAN GRILL)

Contact LaSalsa or their website (www.lasalsa.com) for nutritional info.

TACOS *(1 TACO)*
  250-300MG SODIUM
   Taco La Salsa® w/Chicken (w/o chips)
  300-350MG SODIUM
   Taco La Salsa® w/Steak (w/o chips)
  350-400MG SODIUM
   Baja Fish Taco (w/o chips) • Taco La Salsa® w/Carnitas (w/o chips)
  450-500MG SODIUM
   Baja Style Shrimp (w/o chips)
  500-550MG SODIUM
   Sonora Fish Taco (w/o chips)
BURRITOS *– exceed 1000mg sodium.*

QUESADILLAS *– exceed 1000mg sodium.*

SALADS *– exceed 1200mg sodium.*

KID'S PLATES *– exceed 1000mg sodium.*

SIDES AND APPETIZERS
  150-200MG SODIUM
   Chips and Salsa
  Other sides and appetizers exceed 500mg sodium.

LITTLE CAESAR'S

LITTLE CAESAR'S

Contact Little Caesar's® or their website (www.littlecaesars.com) for nutritional info.

PIZZA
150-200MG SODIUM
  Cheese, thin crust, 12", 1/8 slice
200-250MG SODIUM
  Cheese, 14" thin crust, 1/10 slice
250-300MG SODIUM
  Cheese, 12", 1/8 slice • Pepperoni, 14" thin crust
300-350MG SODIUM
  Cheese, 14", 1/10 slice • Cheese, 16", 1/12 slice • Cheese, 18", 1/14 slice • Cheese, deep dish, medium, 1/8 slice

ADD TOPPINGS *(PER SLICE)*
0-50MG SODIUM
  Mushrooms • Pineapple • Onions • Green Peppers • Tomato • Black Olives
50-100MG SODIUM
  Sausage • Ham • Beef • Hot Peppers
100-150MG SODIUM
  Pepperoni • Bacon
Other toppings exceed 150mg sodium.

SANDWICHES – *exceed 950mg sodium.*

SALADS *(W/O DRESSING)*
150-200MG SODIUM
  Tossed • Caesar
550-600MG SODIUM
  Antipasto • Greek

SALAD DRESSINGS
200-250MG SODIUM
  Greek
Other salad dressings exceed 350mg sodium.

SIDES
50-100MG SODIUM
  Cinnamon Crazy Bread, 2 sticks
100-150MG SODIUM
  Crazy Bread, 1 stick
200-250MG SODIUM
  Chicken Wing, 1
Other sides exceed 350mg sodium.

Menu Item	Cal	Fat	Sat	TFat	Chol	Carb	Fib	Sug	Sod

LONG JOHN SILVER'S

Contact Long John Silver's or their website (www.ljsilvers.com) for nutritional info.

ENTREES *(1 PIECE)*
150-200MG SODIUM
  Battered Shrimp
200-250MG SODIUM
  Baked Cod
450-500MG SODIUM
  Chicken Plank
Other entrees exceed 550mg sodium.

SANDWICHES *– exceed 900mg sodium.*

SALADS *(W/O DRESSING) – exceed 800mg sodium.*

SIDE ITEMS
0-50MG SODIUM
  Corn Cobbette
200-250MG SODIUM
  Hushpuppie • Cocktail Sauce • Tartar Sauce
300-350MG SODIUM
  Cheesestick • Cole Slaw • Fries (regular)

DESSERTS
150-200MG SODIUM
  Choc Cream Pie • Pecan Pie
200-250MG SODIUM
  Pineapple Creme Pie

MCDONALD'S

Contact McDonald's® or their website (www.mcdonalds.com) for nutritional info.

BREAKFAST
200-250MG SODIUM
  Scrambled Eggs, 2
400-450MG SODIUM
  Warm Cinnamon Roll
600-650MG SODIUM
  Hotcakes w/2 pats margarine & syrup
Other breakfast items exceed 650mg sodium.

BREAKFAST SIDES
250-300MG SODIUM
  Hash Browns • English Muffin
  Other sides exceed 300mg sodium.

MCDONALD'S

Menu Item	Cal	Fat	Sat	TFat	Chol	Carb	Fib	Sug	Sod

MCDONALD'S (CONT'D)

SANDWICHES
500-550MG SODIUM
Hamburger
600-650MG SODIUM
Filet-O-Fish®
Other sandwiches exceed 700mg sodium.

CHICKEN
450-500MG SODIUM OR LESS
Chicken McNuggets, 4 piece
Other chicken exceeds 650mg sodium.

DIPPING SAUCES
0-50MG SODIUM
Honey
150-200MG SODIUM
Sweet 'N Sour • Tangy Honey Mustard
Other dipping sauces exceed 250mg sodium.

SALADS *(W/O DRESSING)*
0-50MG SODIUM
Side Salad • Asian Salad w/o chicken
50-100MG SODIUM
Fruit & Walnut Salad
150-200MG SODIUM
Caesar Salad w/o Chicken
250-300MG SODIUM
Bacon Ranch w/o Chicken
400-450MG SODIUM
California Cobb w/o Chicken
Other salads exceed 850mg sodium.

SALAD DRESSINGS AND TOPPINGS
150-200MG SODIUM
Butter Garlic Croutons
Salad dressings exceed 400mg sodium.

SIDE ITEMS
100-150MG SODIUM
French Fries (small)

DESSERTS AND SHAKES
0-50MG SODIUM
Apple Dippers (w/ or w/o Caramel Sauce) • Kiddie Cone

Menu Item	Cal	Fat	Sat	TFat	Chol	Carb	Fib	Sug	Sod

MCDONALD'S (DESSERTS CONT'D)

50-100MG SODIUM
Fruit 'n Yogurt Parfait (w/ or w/o Granola) • Vanilla Reduce Fat Ice Cream Cone •
Strawberry Sundae • Choc Chip Cookie

100-150MG SODIUM
Hot Caramel Sundae • Oatmeal Raisin Cookie • Sugar Cookie •
Baked Apple Pie • Strawberry Triple Thick® Shake (12 oz) •
Vanilla Triple Thick® Shake (12 oz)

150-200MG SODIUM
Hot Fudge Sundae (w/ or w/o nuts) • McFlurry® w/M&M's® (12 oz) •
McDonaldLand® Cookies • Choc Triple Thick® Shake (12 oz) •
Strawberry Triple Thick® Shake (16 oz) • Vanilla Triple Thick® Shake (16 oz)
Other desserts and shakes exceed 300mg sodium.

MRS. FIELDS COOKIES

Contact Mrs. Fields or their website (www.mrsfields.com) for nutritional info.

COOKIES *(1 COOKIE)*

100-150MG SODIUM
Oatmeal Choc Chip • Triple Choc

150-200MG SODIUM
Debra's Special • Milk Choc and Walnuts • Milk Choc w/o Nuts •
Milk Choc Macadamia • Oatmeal Raisin • Semi-sweet Choc •
Semi-sweet Choc and Walnuts • White Chunk Macadamia

BITE-SIZED NIBBLERS *(2 COOKIES)*

50-100MG SODIUM
White Chunk Macadamia • Semi-Sweet Choc • Triple Choc • Peanut Butter •
Debra's Special • Cinnamon Sugar

BROWNIES AND BARS

0-50MG SODIUM
Butterscotch • Special Walnut Fudge Blondie • Raspberry Bark

50-100MG SODIUM
Pecan Pie • Pecan Fudge • Double Fudge • Mint Fudge • Walnut Fudge •
Pecan Pie Choc Chip

100-150MG SODIUM
Peanut Butter Krunch Bar

150-200MG SODIUM
Caramel Oat Bar • Raspberry Oat Bar

CAKES

250-300MG SODIUM
Carrot • Choc • Cinnamon Sugar Pecan • Lemon Bundt • Raspberry Choc Chip

207

MY FAVORITE MUFFIN

Menu Item	Cal	Fat	Sat	TFat	Chol	Carb	Fib	Sug	Sod

(MY FAVORITE MUFFIN)

Contact My Favorite Muffin® or their website (www.bigapplebagels.com) for nutritional info. See Big Apple Bagels, pg 172, for sandwiches, salads, and other items.

MUFFINS
100-150MG SODIUM
All regular muffins except Lemon Poppyseed
150-200MG SODIUM
Lemon Poppyseed • FF Cinnamon Bun • FF Raspberry Amaretto • FF Cherry Pie • FF Blueberry

BAGELS
300-350MG SODIUM
Honey Grain
450-500MG SODIUM
Whole Wheat • Cinnamon Raisin • Russian Black Bread
Other bagels exceed 500mg sodium.

CREAM CHEESE
50-100MG SODIUM
Honey Cinnamon • Nutty Honey • Very Berry
100-150MG SODIUM
Plain Lite • Soft/Plain • Onion Chive • Santa Fe Vegetable Lite • Strawberry Lite

(NATHAN'S FAMOUS)

Contact Nathan's Famous or their website (www.nathansfamous.com) for nutritional info.

HOT DOGS, BURGERS AND SANDWICHES
400-450MG SODIUM
Hot Dog Nuggets, 6
Other hot dogs, burgers and sandwiches exceed 650mg sodium.

SIDES
200-250MG SODIUM
French Fries • Corn Muffin
300-350MG SODIUM
Cole Slaw

(PANDA EXPRESS)

APPETIZERS

Menu Item	Cal	Fat	Sat	TFat	Chol	Carb	Fib	Sug	Sod
Veggie Spring Roll, 1	80	4	1	0	0	11	2	1	270
Chicken Egg Roll, 1	170	8	2	0	25	17	2	2	410

Menu Item	Cal	Fat	Sat	TFat	Chol	Carb	Fib	Sug	Sod
PANDA EXPRESS (CONT'D)									
ENTREES									
Sweet and Sour Pork	400	23	5	0	30	35	2	15	360
Mixed Vegetables	50	2	0	0	0	7	3	3	370
Beef w/Broccoli	150	7	2	0	25	11	4	3	510
Chicken w/Mushrooms	130	6	2	0	45	8	3	4	520
Kung Pao Chicken	240	15	3	0	65	12	5	3	540
Chicken Breast w/Garlic Black Bean Sauce	140	8	2	0	25	8	3	3	540
Chicken w/String Beans	160	8	2	0	25	10	4	3	550
Tangy Shrimp w/Pineapple	150	5	1	0	85	16	2	11	550
RICE									
Steamed Rice	380	3	1	0	0	81	4	0	30
SAUCES									
Sweet and Sour Sauce	80	0	0	0	0	19	0	17	135

(PAPA JOHN'S PIZZA)

PIZZAS (*1/8 SLICE UNLESS NOTED*)

Menu Item	Cal	Fat	Sat	TFat	Chol	Carb	Fib	Sug	Sod
Spinach Alfredo, 14" thin crust	220	14	5	0	20	19	1	1	370
Spinach Alfredo Chicken Tomato, 14" thin crust	230	13	5	0	25	21	1	1	430
Garden Fresh, 14" thin crust	210	11	3	0	15	23	2	3	430
Spinach Alfredo, 12" original	200	8	3	0	15	26	1	3	450
Grilled Chicken Alfredo, 14" thin crust	240	13	5	0	30	20	1	1	470
Spinach Alfredo Chicken Tomato, 12" original	210	8	3	0	20	27	2	3	490
Garden Fresh, 12" orginal	200	7	2	0	10	28	2	4	490
Cheese, 14" thin crust	240	13	4	0	20	22	1	2	500
Cheese, 12" original	210	8	3	0	15	27	1	3	510
Grilled Chicken Alfredo, 12" original	220	9	4	0	28	26	1	3	520

SIDE ITEMS – *exceed 250mg sodium.*

DIPPING SAUCES

Menu Item	Cal	Fat	Sat	TFat	Chol	Carb	Fib	Sug	Sod
Honey Mustard, 2 tbsp	150	15	2	0	10	5	0	4	120
Pizza Sauce, 2 tbsp	20	0	0	0	0	3	0	2	140
Cheese, 2 tbsp	70	6	2	0	0	1	0	0	150

(PAPA MURPHY'S)

PIZZAS

Thin Crust:, 1/10 slice

Menu Item	Cal	Fat	Sat	TFat	Chol	Carb	Fib	Sug	Sod
Cheese deLITE	140	7	4	0	20	13	1	2	270
Veggie deLITE	150	8	4	0	20	13	1	1	275

PIZZA HUT

Menu Item	Cal	Fat	Sat	TFat	Chol	Carb	Fib	Sug	Sod
PAPA MURPHY'S (PIZZA CONT'D)									
Gourmet Vegetarian	160	9	4	0	21	13	1	1	290
Veggie Mediterranean	165	9	4	0	20	15	2	3	325
Hawaiian deLITE	150	7	4	0	22	15	1	4	335
Gourmet Chicken Garlic	170	9	5	0	27	13	1	1	360
Vegetarian Combo	150	8	4	0	20	14	1	1	360
Pepperoni deLITE	160	9	5	0	26	13	1	2	365
Herb Chicken Mediterranean	180	9	4	0	23	16	2	3	380
Barbecue Chicken	180	8	4	0	30	17	1	4	430
Gourmet Classic Italian	180	10	5	0	24	13	1	1	430
Rancher	175	9	5	0	29	13	1	1	440
Specialty of the House	170	9	5	0	20	13	1	1	450

Other pizzas exceed 450mg sodium per slice.

CALZONES AND STUFFED PIZZAS *(1/6 SLICE)* – *exceed 850mg sodium.*

SALADS *(INDIVIDUAL SALAD W/O DRESSING)*

Menu Item	Cal	Fat	Sat	TFat	Chol	Carb	Fib	Sug	Sod
Caesar Salad	85	4	3	0	10	6	4	3	240
Garden Salad	160	11	6	0	23	10	5	3	380
Italian Salad	220	16	8	0	38	9	4	3	590

Other salads exceed 650mg sodium.

SALAD DRESSINGS – *nutritional information unavailable*

(PIZZA HUT)

Contact Pizza Hut® or their website (www.pizzahut.com) for nutritional info.

PIZZAS *(1 SLICE)*

Fit n' Delicious Pizza™

350-400MG SODIUM

Green Pepper, Red Onion & Diced Red Tomato, 14"

400-450MG SODIUM

Green Pepper, Red Onion & Diced Red Tomato, 12"

450-500MG SODIUM

Diced Chicken, Red Onion & Green Pepper, 14"

500-550MG SODIUM

Diced Chicken, Red Onion & Green Pepper, 12" •

Ham, Red Onion & Mushroom, 14" • Ham, Pineapple & Diced Tomato, 14"

Pan Pizza

450-500MG SODIUM

Veggie Lover's®, 12" or 14"

500-550MG SODIUM

Cheese Only, 14" • Chicken Supreme, 14"

Menu Item	Cal	Fat	Sat	TFat	Chol	Carb	Fib	Sug	Sod

PAPA JOHN'S PIZZA (PIZZA CONT'D)

Thin 'N Crispy Pizza

500-550MG SODIUM

Veggie Lover's®, 12" or 14" • Cheese Only, 14" • Chicken Supreme, 14"

SIDE ITEMS

200-250MG SODIUM

Breadsticks, 1

300-350MG SODIUM

Mild Wings, 2 pieces • Cheese Breadsticks, 1

DIPPING SAUCES – *exceed 300mg sodium.*

DESSERTS

150-200MG SODIUM

Cinnamon Sticks, 2 pcs

200-250MG SODIUM

Apple or Cherry Dessert Pizza, 1 slice

(**POPEYES**)

Contact Popeyes or their website (www.popeyes.com) for nutritional info.

CHICKEN

250-300MG SODIUM

Leg, Spicy (skin & breading removed)

300-350MG SODIUM

Wing, Spicy (skin & breading removed)

350-400MG SODIUM

Leg, Mild (skin & breading removed) • Wing, Spicy

SANDWICHES – *exceed 1300mg sodium.*

SEAFOOD – *exceed 700mg sodium.*

LOUISIANA LEGENDS™

350-400MG SODIUM

Chicken Sausage Jambalaya

400-450MG SODIUM

Chicken Étouffée

500-550MG SODIUM

Crawfish Étouffée

SIDES

0-50MG SODIUM

Corn on the Cob

250-300MG SODIUM

Coleslaw

Menu Item	Cal	Fat	Sat	TFat	Chol	Carb	Fib	Sug	Sod

POPEYES (CONT'D)

DESSERTS
250-300MG SODIUM
  Cinnamon Apple Turnover

(**ROUND TABLE PIZZA**)

Contact Round Table or their website (www.roundtablepizza.com) for nutritional info.

PIZZAS
  Skinny Crust, 14", 1/12 slice
  400-450MG SODIUM
    Gourmet Veggie™
  450-500MG SODIUM
    Cheese • Guinevere's Garden Delight® • Chicken & Garlic Gourmet™
  Original Crust, 14", 1/12 slice
  450-500MG SODIUM
    Gourmet Veggie™

CHICKEN – *exceed 700mg sodium.*

SANDWICHES – *exceed 1600mg sodium.*

SALADS *(W/O DRESSING)*
  200-250MG SODIUM
  Garden Salad
  350-400MG SODIUM
  Caesar Salad
  Adding chicken to salad increases the sodium by more than 450mg.
    SALAD DRESSING – *nutritional information unavailable*

(**RUBIOS FRESH MEXICAN GRILL**)

Contact Rubios or their website (www.rubios.com) for nutritional info.

TACOS AND TAQUITOS *(W/CORN TORTILLAS; IF ORDERING W/FLOUR, ADD 270MG SODIUM)*
  150-200MG SODIUM
  HealthMex MahiMahi Taco
  200-250MG SODIUM
  MahiMahi Taco • Chicken Street Taco • Fish Taco Original
  250-300MG SODIUM
  Carnitas Street Taco • Chicken Taquitos, 3
  300-350MG SODIUM
  Fish Taco Especial
  350-400MG SODIUM
  Carne Asada Street Taco • HealthMex Chicken Taco

Menu Item	Cal	Fat	Sat	TFat	Chol	Carb	Fib	Sug	Sod

RUBIO'S FRESH MEXICAN GRILL (CONT'D)

KID'S MEALS
100-150MG SODIUM
Fish Taco Original
200-250MG SODIUM
Taquitos, 2
Other kid's meals exceed 650mg sodium.

ADD SIDES
50-100MG SODIUM
Mini Churro
100-150MG SODIUM
Rice
200-250MG SODIUM
Chips

BURRITOS – *exceed 1000mg sodium.*

NACHOS AND QUESADILLAS – *exceed 1350mg sodium.*

BOWLS AND SALADS – *exceed 1000mg sodium.*

SIDES
100-150MG SODIUM
Guacamole • Churro
200-250MG SODIUM
Rice w/Health Mex meals
Other sides exceed 250mg sodium.

(SCHLOTZSKY'S DELI)

Contact Schlotzsky's or their website (www.schlotzskys.com) for nutritional info.

SANDWICHES AND PANINIS
500-550MG SODIUM
Classic Swiss & Tomato Panini
800-850MG SODIUM
Fresh Veggie, small
850-900MG SODIUM
Mozzarella & Portobello Panini
Other sandwiches and paninis exceed 900mg sodium.

BUNS AND TORTILLA
300-350MG SODIUM
LF Wheat Tortilla
550-600MG SODIUM
Dark Rye Bun, small • Sourdough Bun, small

Menu Item	Cal	Fat	Sat	TFat	Chol	Carb	Fib	Sug	Sod

SCHLOTZSKY'S DELI (CONT'D)

WRAPS

900-950MG SODIUM
Mediterranean Tuna
Other wraps exceed 1000mg sodium.

PIZZAS – *exceed 1300mg sodium.*

SALADS *(W/O DRESSING)*

0-50MG SODIUM
Fruit Salad
300-350MG SODIUM
Caesar
450-500MG SODIUM
Garden
600-650MG SODIUM
Baby Spinach & Feta
Other salads exceed 800mg sodium.

SALAD DRESSINGS – *nutritional information unavailable*

BAKED POTATOES

250-300MG SODIUM
Bacon & Cheddar
Other baked potatoes exceed 700mg sodium.

SIDE ITEMS

150-200MG SODIUM
Regular (Plain) Chips
200-250MG SODIUM
Side Salad • Pasta Salad • Jalapeño or Sour Cream & Onion Chips

DESSERTS

0-50MG SODIUM
Sugar Cookie
50-100MG SODIUM
Oatmeal Raisin Cookie • White Choc Macadamia Cookie • Choc Chip Cookie •
Fudge Choc Chip Cookie • Peanut Butter Cookie
200-250MG SODIUM
Cheesecake

SKIPPER'S

Contact Skipper's® or their website (www.skippers.net) for nutritional info.

FISH ONLY

50-100MG SODIUM
Grilled Salmon Fillet • Grilled Chicken Breast • Grilled Halibut Fillet

Menu Item	Cal	Fat	Sat	TFat	Chol	Carb	Fib	Sug	Sod

SKIPPER'S (CONT'D)

FISH AND CHICKEN MEALS – *exceed 1200mg sodium.*

KIDS MEALS – *exceed 1000mg sodium.*

SANDWICHES *(W/CHIPS AND SLAW) – exceed 1500mg sodium.*

SALADS

0-50MG SODIUM
　Green Salad w/o dressing, large or small
300-350MG SODIUM
　Caesar, small
350-400MG SODIUM
　Caesar w/Chicken or Salmon, small
Other salads exceed 550mg sodium.

SIDES

0-50MG SODIUM
　Plain Baked Potato • Grilled Veggies
150-200MG SODIUM
　Coleslaw, small
200-250MG SODIUM
　Coleslaw, cup
Other sides exceed 450mg sodium.

SONIC DRIVE-IN

Contact Sonic Drive-in® or their website (www.sonicdrivein.com) for nutritional info.

BREAKFAST

250-300MG SODIUM
　French Toast Sticks, 2
550-600MG SODIUM
　French Toast Sticks, 4
Other breakfast items exceed 1000mg sodium.

SMOOTHIES

100-150MG SODIUM
　Sunshine, regular
150-200MG SODIUM
　Strawberry, regular • Strawberry-Banana, regular • Tropical Fruit

BURGERS AND SANDWICHES

400-450MG SODIUM
　Breaded Chicken Sandwich
750-800MG SODIUM
　Sonic® Burger w/mayonnaise or mustard
Other burgers and sandwiches exceed 800mg sodium.

SOUP PLANTATION / SWEET TOMATOES

Menu Item	Cal	Fat	Sat	TFat	Chol	Carb	Fib	Sug	Sod

SONIC DRIVE-IN (CONT'D)

CHICKEN

500-550MG SODIUM

   Chicken Strips, 2 (kid's meal)

Other chicken entrees items exceed 750mg sodium.

CONEYS

450-500MG SODIUM

   Corn Dog

Other Coneys exceed 1100mg sodium.

WRAPS

800-850MG SODIUM

   Grilled Chicken w/o Ranch Dressing

850-900MG SODIUM

   Chicken Strip w/o Ranch Dressing

Other wraps exceed 1000mg sodium.

SALADS *(W/O DRESSING) – exceed 800mg sodium.*

SIDE ITEMS

300-350MG SODIUM

   Onion Rings, regular

Other sides exceed 450mg sodium.

FROZEN DESSERTS

200-250MG SODIUM

   Dish of Vanilla • Strawberry Sundae • Ice Cream Cone • Banana Split •
Pineapple Sundae • Strawberry, Cherry, or Orange Slush Float, regular •
Coca-Cola Float or Blended Float Drink, regular

(SOUPLANTATION / SWEET TOMATOES)

PASTAS *(1 CUP UNLESS NOTED)*

Menu Item	Cal	Fat	Sat	TFat	Chol	Carb	Fib	Sug	Sod
Carbonara w/Bacon	280	8	4	-	20	43	2	3	250
Creamy Pepper Jack	290	15	6	-	50	35	2	6	360
Creamy Herb Chicken	310	17	8	-	80	32	2	7	360
Italian Sausage w/Red Pepper Puree	250	10	4	-	45	35	2	7	380
Smoked Salmon and Dill	380	16	8	-	45	41	2	2	390
Nutty Mushroom	390	20	9	-	45	42	2	4	410
Southwestern Alfredo	350	16	9	-	50	42	1	3	420
Bruschetta	260	4	2	-	10	41	3	3	450
Garden Veg w/Meatballs	270	7	3	-	10	42	3	2	460
Italian Veg Beef	270	6	2	-	10	43	4	3	470
Lemon Cream and Asparagus	230	9	2	-	0	34	1	4	470
Vegetable Ragu	250	5	2	-	10	41	3	4	480

Menu Item	Cal	Fat	Sat	TFat	Chol	Carb	Fib	Sug	Sod

SOUP PLANTATION / SWEET TOMATOES (CONT'D)

SALADS

TOSSED SALADS

Menu Item	Cal	Fat	Sat	TFat	Chol	Carb	Fib	Sug	Sod
Strawberry Fields w/Walnuts	130	8	1	0	0	15	3	12	75
Honey Minted Fruit Toss	140	6	4	0	0	20	3	15	80
Bombay Curry w/Almonds & Coconut	210	16	4	0	10	17	4	11	85
Watercress and Orange	90	4	1	0	0	12	2	6	90
Cherry Chipolte Spinach	220	15	2	0	0	20	2	10	90
Outrageous Orange w/Cashews	200	14	2	0	10	16	2	8	95
Mandarin Spinach w/Walnuts	170	11	1	0	0	14	3	11	150
Roma Tomato, Mozzarella & Basil	120	9	2	0	10	7	1	2	180
Barlett Pear & Caramelized Walnut	180	12	2	0	5	13	2	10	220
Won Ton Chicken Happiness	150	8	1	0	10	12	2	4	220
San Marino Spinach w/Pumpkin Seeds	200	15	4	0	15	11	6	5	220
Ensalada Azteca w/Turkey	130	9	3	0	15	7	4	3	230
Summer Lemon w/Spiced Pecans	220	15	3	0	10	18	2	13	250

SIGNATURE SALADS *(1/2 CUP UNLESS NOTED)*

Menu Item	Cal	Fat	Sat	TFat	Chol	Carb	Fib	Sug	Sod
Carrot Ginger w/Herb Vinaigrette	150	12	1	0	0	9	3	6	40
Dijon Potato w/Garlic Dill Vinaigrette	150	12	1	0	0	9	3	6	40
Carrot Raisin, LF	90	3	0	0	5	17	2	15	80
Oriental Ginger Slaw w/Krab, LF	70	3	0	0	2	8	4	3	80
Ambrosia w/Coconut	170	6	3	0	5	30	2	20	80
Poppyseed Coleslaw	120	9	1	0	10	9	3	5	130
Confetti Avocado Slaw	120	7	1	0	5	12	3	3	150
Baja Bean and Cilantro, LF	180	3	0	0	0	29	5	2	190
Pineapple Coconut Slaw	150	10	3	0	15	14	2	10	190
Marinated Summer Vegetables, FF	80	0	0	0	0	19	4	14	210
Southern Black-Eyed Pea	130	6	0	0	0	18	3	4	220
Tomato Cucumber Marinade	80	5	0	0	0	8	1	2	220
Citrus Noodles w/Snow Peas	140	6	1	0	0	19	2	5	240
Italian Garden Vegetable	110	8	1	0	0	9	2	2	240
Roasted Potato w/Chipotle Chile	140	6	1	0	0	18	4	3	250
Joan's Broccoli Madness	180	14	3	0	10	11	3	9	250

SALAD DRESSINGS

Menu Item	Cal	Fat	Sat	TFat	Chol	Carb	Fib	Sug	Sod
Sweet Maple	170	17	2	0	5	6	0	6	50
FF Honey Mustard	45	0	0	0	10	10	0	9	160
Basil Vinaigrette	160	17	1	0	0	1	0	0	160
FF Ranch	50	0	0	0	0	2	0	1	180
Ranch	130	13	2	0	10	1	0	1	180
Balsamic Vinaigrette	180	19	2	0	0	1	0	1	190
Thousand Island	110	11	2	0	5	3	0	2	190

SOUP PLANTATION / SWEET TOMATOES

Menu Item	Cal	Fat	Sat	TFat	Chol	Carb	Fib	Sug	Sod
TOPPINGS									
Tomato Basil Croutons, 5 pcs	45	3	1	-	0	3	0	0	90
Chow Mein Noodles	70	3	1	-	0	9	1	0	100
Plain Croutons	35	1	0	-	0	7	1	0	120
SOUPS (1 CUP UNLESS NOTED)									
Turkey Vegetable	180	8	3	-	30	15	2	4	140
Classical Shrimp Bisque	240	16	7	-	70	15	1	5	230
Country Corn & Red Potato Chowder	160	6	3	-	15	24	4	6	330
Cream of Chicken	250	15	6	-	40	21	2	3	350
Tomato Parmesan and Veg, LF	120	3	1	-	5	18	3	3	460
Big Chunk Chicken Noodle, LF	160	3	2	-	20	17	2	3	480
Chunky Potato Cheese w/Thyme	210	10	6	-	30	19	2	3	480
MUFFINS									
French Quarter Praline	290	15	2	-	20	38	2	21	100
Apple Cinnamon, Cranberry Orange, or Fruit Medley Bran Muffin (avg)	80	1	0	-	0	17	1	14	110
Cappuccino Chip	160	4	2	-	25	28	1	15	160
Spiced Pumpkin w/Cranberries	180	7	1	-	25	29	1	18	170
Wildly Blue Blueberry, small	140	5	1	-	10	22	1	9	180
Pauline's Apple Walnut Cake	180	7	3	-	25	28	1	21	180
Apple Raisin or Banana Nut	150	7	1	-	10	22	1	9	190
Cherry Nut or Zucchini Nut	150	7	1	-	10	22	1	9	190
Tangy Lemon	140	4	1	-	10	24	1	13	190
Choc Brownie or Choc Chip	170	8	2	-	10	22	1	10	190
Country Blackberry	170	6	2	-	15	27	1	13	190
Taffy Apple	160	6	1	-	10	25	1	18	190
Black Forest	230	9	2	-	10	36	1	19	190
DESSERTS (1/2 CUP UNLESS NOTED)									
Apple Medley or Banana Royale (avg)	75	0	0	0	0	19	1	12	5
Jello, Sugar Free	10	0	0	0	0	0	0	0	10
Jello, Regular	80	0	0	0	0	20	0	19	40
Rice Pudding	110	2	1	0	10	20	1	12	50
Vanilla Soft Serve, Reduced Fat	140	4	3	0	20	22	0	19	70
Choc Frozen Yogurt, FF	95	0	0	0	0	21	0	15	80
Nutty Waldorf Salad, LF	80	3	0	0	0	12	3	5	80
Choc Chip Cookie, 1 small	70	3	1	-	5	10	0	6	90
Choc Chip Cookie Bar, 1 pc	90	4	2	-	5	13	0	7	120
Butterscotch or Tapioca Pudding, LF (avg)	140	3	0	-	10	24	0	24	160
Vanilla Pudding	140	4	0	-	10	24	0	24	160

218

Menu Item	Cal	Fat	Sat	TFat	Chol	Carb	Fib	Sug	Sod
SOUP PLANTATION / SWEET TOMATOES (CONT'D)									
Apple Cobbler	350	10	2	-	0	64	1	10	160
Butterscotch Toasted Coconut Focaccia, 1pc	190	7	3	-	5	27	1	8	170
Cheery Cherry Cobbler	340	10	2	-	0	61	2	10	180

(STEAK ESCAPE)

7" SANDWICHES

Menu Item	Cal	Fat	Sat	TFat	Chol	Carb	Fib	Sug	Sod
Portabello Vegetarian	311	1	-	-	0	65	-	-	733
Philly Cheesesteak	420	6	-	-	50	60	-	-	1004

Other 7" sandwiches exceed 1100mg sodium.

12" SANDWICHES

Menu Item	Cal	Fat	Sat	TFat	Chol	Carb	Fib	Sug	Sod
Portabello Vegetarian	442	2	-	-	0	93	-	-	1047

NOTE: Eat half the 12" for 200mg less sodium than the 7".
Other 12" sandwiches exceed 1500mg sodium.

KID'S SANDWICHES

Menu Item	Cal	Fat	Sat	TFat	Chol	Carb	Fib	Sug	Sod
Steak	210	3	-	-	13	29	-	-	445
Chicken	205	7	-	-	32	29	-	-	470

SALADS *(W/O DRESSING)*

Menu Item	Cal	Fat	Sat	TFat	Chol	Carb	Fib	Sug	Sod
Side Salad	40	1	0	0	0	8	-	-	20
Grilled Salad w/Steak	187	6	-	-	103	11	-	-	292
Grilled Salad w/Chicken	177	5	-	-	108	11	-	-	652

SALAD DRESSINGS

Menu Item	Cal	Fat	Sat	TFat	Chol	Carb	Fib	Sug	Sod
Balsamic Vinaigrette	90	3	-	-	0	3	-	-	35
Ranch	83	9	-	-	5	0	-	-	137

SMASHED POTATOES

Menu Item	Cal	Fat	Sat	TFat	Chol	Carb	Fib	Sug	Sod
Smashed Potato, Plain	246	0	0	0	0	53	-	-	43
Smashed Potato w/Portabello	290	1	0	0	0	63	-	-	93
Smashed Potato w/Steak	393	5	-	-	103	55	-	-	313
Smashed Potato w/Chicken	383	4	-	-	108	56	-	-	475
Loaded Smashed Potato, Ranch & Bacon	692	34	-	-	29	87	-	-	501

SIDE ITEMS

Menu Item	Cal	Fat	Sat	TFat	Chol	Carb	Fib	Sug	Sod
Kids Meal Fries	249	13	-	-	0	34	-	-	205

Other sides exceed 400mg sodium.

(SUBWAY)

BREAKFAST

Menu Item	Cal	Fat	Sat	TFat	Chol	Carb	Fib	Sug	Sod
Cheese on Deli Round	270	9	4	0	15	35	3	2	670
Cheese on 6" Bread	310	9	4	0	15	43	3	5	740

Other breakfast items exceed 1000mg sodium.

SUBWAY

Menu Item	Cal	Fat	Sat	TFat	Chol	Carb	Fib	Sug	Sod
SUBWAY (CONT'D)									
6" SUBS *(ON ITALIAN OR WHEAT BREAD)*									
Vegie Delite® w/o cheese	230	3	1	0	0	44	4	7	520
Absolute Angus Steak	420	20	8	-	70	44	4	7	730
Barbecue Rib Patty	420	19	6	0	50	47	4	8	830

Other subs exceed 900mg sodium.

NOTE: Sub values include lettuce, tomato, onion, green pepper, olives, pickles, and cheese. Omit pickles to reduce sodium by 125mg.

DELI STYLE SANDWICHES *(ON DELI ROLL)*									
Roast Beef	220	5	2	0	15	35	3	4	660
Turkey Breast	210	4	2	0	15	36	3	4	730
Tuna	350	18	5	1	30	35	3	3	750
Ham	210	4	2	0	10	36	3	4	770

NOTE: Sandwich values include lettuce, tomato, onion, green pepper, olives, and pickles. Omit pickles to reduce sodium by 125mg.

WRAPS									
Turkey Breast	190	6	1	0	20	18	9	2	1290
Tuna w/Cheese	440	32	6	1	45	16	9	1	1310

SOUPS – *exceed 900mg sodium.*

SALADS *(W/O DRESSING)*									
Veggie Delite®	60	1	0	0	0	12	4	5	90
Grilled Chicken & Baby Spinach	140	3	1	0	50	11	4	4	450
Tuna w/Cheese	360	29	6	1	45	12	4	5	600
Carb Conscious	360	29	6	1	45	12	4	5	600

SALAD DRESSINGS – *exceed 500mg sodium.*

BREADS									
Deli Style Roll	170	3	1	0	0	32	3	2	280
6" Italian (White)	190	3	2	0	0	38	1	5	340
6" Hearty Italian	210	3	2	0	0	41	2	5	340
6" Wheat	200	3	1	0	0	40	3	5	360
6" Honey Oat	250	4	1	0	0	48	4	9	380
6" Monterey Cheddar	240	6	4	1	10	39	2	5	400

TOPPINGS AND CONDIMENTS									
Lettuce, Tomato, Onions, Green Peppers, or Cucumbers (avg)	5	0	0	0	0	1	0	0	0
Vinegar, 1 tsp	0	0	0	0	0	0	0	0	0
Olive Oil Blend, 1 tsp	45	5	0	0	0	0	0	0	0
Banana Peppers, 3 rings	0	0	0	0	0	0	0	0	20
Olives, 3 rings	5	0	0	0	0	0	0	0	25
Swiss Cheese, 2 triangles	50	5	3	0	15	0	0	0	30

Menu Item	Cal	Fat	Sat	TFat	Chol	Carb	Fib	Sug	Sod
SUBWAY (CONT'D)									
Jalapeño Peppers, 3 rings	0	0	0	0	0	0	0	0	70
Mayonnaise, 1 tbsp	110	12	2	0	10	0	0	0	80
Light Mayonnaise, 1 tbsp	50	5	1	0	5	1	0	0	100
Mustard, Yellow or Deli Brown, 2 tsp	5	0	0	0	0	1	0	0	115
Pickles, 3 chips	0	0	0	0	0	0	0	0	125
SAUCES									
Sweet Onion, FF	40	0	0	0	0	9	0	8	85
Honey Mustard, FF	30	0	0	0	0	7	0	6	115
COOKIES AND DESSERTS									
Fruit Roll Up, 1	50	1	0	0	0	12	0	7	55
Choc Chunk or M&M® Cookie (avg)	205	10	5	0	12	31	1	17	100
Sugar Cookie	220	12	6	0	15	28	1	14	140
White Macadamia Nut or Choc Chip (avg)	215	11	5	0	15	29	1	18	155
Double Choc Chip or Oatmeal Raisin (avg)	205	9	4	0	15	30	1	18	170
Peanut Butter	220	12	5	0	15	26	1	16	200

(TACO BELL)

Contact Taco Bell® or their website (www.tacobell.com) for nutritional info.

TACOS
350-400MG SODIUM
Taco Supreme® • Crunchy Taco • Crunchy Taco, "Fresco Style"
500-550MG SODIUM
Grilled Steak Soft Taco, "Fresco Style"
550-600MG SODIUM
Spicy Chicken Soft Taco
600-650MG SODIUM OR LESS
Beef Soft Taco • Beef Soft Taco, "Fresco Style" • Beef Soft Taco Supreme® •
Grilled Steak Soft Taco

GORDITAS
500-550MG SODIUM
Gordita Supreme®, Steak or Chicken
550-600MG SODIUM
Gordita Baja®, Steak or Chicken, "Fresca Style" • Gordita Supreme®, Beef

CHALUPAS
550-600MG SODIUM
Chalupa Supreme, Steak or Chicken
600-650MG SODIUM
Chalupa Supreme, Beef

TACO DEL MAR

Menu Item	Cal	Fat	Sat	TFat	Chol	Carb	Fib	Sug	Sod

TACO BELL (CONT'D)

BURRITOS

EXCEED 1000MG SODIUM, THE LOWEST:
   Chili Cheese Burrito • Fiesta Burrito, Steak or Chicken

SPECIALTIES

650-700MG SODIUM
   Tostada, "Fresco Style"
Other specialties exceed 700mg sodium.

SIDE ITEMS

500-550MG SODIUM OR LESS
   Nachos
Other sides exceed 700mg sodium.

DESSERTS

200-250MG SODIUM
   Cinnamon Twists
250-300MG SODIUM
   Caramel Apple Empanada

(TACO DEL MAR)

BREAKFAST

Menu Item	Cal	Fat	Sat	TFat	Chol	Carb	Fib	Sug	Sod
Eggs, 2 oz scoop	90	7	2	-	220	1	0	0	250
Egg & Cheese Taco, flour, refried	200	10	4	-	125	17	1	1	510
Breakfast Taco, flour, refried	130	15	5	-	135	18	1	1	640

BREAKFAST SIDES

Menu Item	Cal	Fat	Sat	TFat	Chol	Carb	Fib	Sug	Sod
Diced Potatoes, 1.75 oz	60	1	0	-	0	11	1	0	20
Hash Browns	110	6	1	-	0	13	2	0	140
Sausage	100	8	3	-	20	1	0	0	220

TACOS

Menu Item	Cal	Fat	Sat	TFat	Chol	Carb	Fib	Sug	Sod
Hard Taco, Chicken	260	13	5	-	45	16	1	1	360
Hard Taco, Fish	270	15	4	-	30	23	1	1	360
Hard Taco, Pork	260	14	5	-	45	17	1	1	370
Soft Taco, Chicken	260	9	4	-	45	27	3	1	430
Soft Taco, Fish	270	11	4	-	30	34	3	1	440
Soft Taco, Pork	260	10	4	-	45	28	3	1	450

BURRITOS AND OTHER ENTREES – *exceed 800mg sodium.*

KID'S MENU

Menu Item	Cal	Fat	Sat	TFat	Chol	Carb	Fib	Sug	Sod
Kids Taco, Chicken	250	13	5	-	45	15	1	0	300
Kids Taco, Pork	250	14	5	-	45	16	1	0	320
Kids Quesadilla	320	14	6	-	30	34	2	1	320
Kids Chips & Cheese	400	22	7	-	30	38	2	0	350

Menu Item	Cal	Fat	Sat	TFat	Chol	Carb	Fib	Sug	Sod
TACO DEL MAR (KIDS MENU CONT'D)									
Kids Taco, Beef	270	15	6	-	30	16	1	1	460
Kids Quesadilla & Chips	600	27	8	-	30	71	4	1	490
Other kid's menu items exceed 750mg sodium.									
SIDES									
Guacamole	40	4	1	0	0	2	1	1	170
Whole Pinto Beans	90	0	0	0	0	20	6	1	200
Other sides exceed 400mg sodium.									
CONDIMENTS AND SAUCES									
Red or Green Sauce	5	0	0	0	0	1	0	0	45
Sour Cream	70	6	4	0	15	2	0	1	60
Other condiments and sauces exceed 150mg sodium.									
TORTILLAS									
Taco Shell	110	5	1	0	0	14	0	0	5
Corn Tortillas, 2	120	2	0	0	0	24	3	0	85
Other tortillas exceed 200mg sodium.									
DESSERTS									
Peanut Butter Cookie	240	13	6	-	40	27	0	15	95
Choc Chip/Nut Cookie	240	13	7	-	30	30	2	20	125
White Ch Mac Cookie	270	16	8	-	30	30	0	12	135
Choc Chip Cookie	240	12	8	-	30	34	1	23	140

TACO JOHN'S

Contact Taco John's® or their website (www.tacojohns.com) for nutritional info.

BREAKFAST

700-750MG SODIUM
  Breakfast Taco, Bacon
750-800MG SODIUM
  Breakfast Taco, Sausage
Other breakfast items exceed 800mg sodium.

TACOS

250-300MG SODIUM
  Crispy Taco • Steak Softshell
450-500MG SODIUM
  Softshell Taco
600-650MG SODIUM
  Taco Burger • Taco Bravo®
Other tacos exceed 750mg sodium.

Menu Item	Cal	Fat	Sat	TFat	Chol	Carb	Fib	Sug	Sod

TACO JOHN'S (CONT'D)

BURRITOS

700-750MG SODIUM
Bean Burrito w/o cheese
800-850MG SODIUM
Bean Burrito • Combination Burrito
Other burritos exceed 850mg sodium.

SALADS

0-50MG SODIUM
Side Salad w/o dressing
200-250MG SODIUM
Steak Festiva Salad w/o dressing
600-650MG SODIUM
Steak Taco Salad w/o dressing
Other salads exceed 750mg sodium.

SALAD DRESSINGS

350-400MG SODIUM
House Dressing
Other salad dressings exceed 450mg sodium.

LOCAL FAVORITES - *not available at all locations*

500-550MG SODIUM
Mexi Rolls® w/o Nacho Cheese
Other local favorites exceed 850mg sodium.

SIDES

300-350MG SODIUM
Guacamole, 2 oz
Other sides exceed 850mg sodium.

CONDIMENTS

0-50MG SODIUM
Super Hot Sauce • Sour Cream
100-150MG SODIUM
Hot or Mild Sauce
150-200MG SODIUM
Pico de Gallo • Salsa
Other condiments exceed 350mg sodium.

DESSERTS

100-150MG SODIUM
Giant Goldfish® Grahams • Choco Taco • Churro
200-250MG SODIUM
Apple Grande

Menu Item	Cal	Fat	Sat	TFat	Chol	Carb	Fib	Sug	Sod

(TACO TIME)

Contact Taco Time® or their website (www.tacotime.com) for nutritional info.

TACOS

550-600MG SODIUM
  Super Soft Taco • Soft Taco
600-650MG SODIUM
  Crisp Taco
Other tacos exceed 900mg sodium.

BURRITOS

450-500MG SODIUM
  Crsip Bean Burrito
550-600MG SODIUM
  Chicken and Black Bean Burrito
600-650MG SODIUM
  Veggie Burrito
Other burritos exceed 700mg sodium.

SALADS *(W/O DRESSING)*

800-850MG SODIUM
  Chicken Fiesta Salad
850-900MG SODIUM
  Chicken Taco Salad • Taco Salad, regular
Other salads exceed 1000mg sodium.

SALAD DRESSINGS

100-150MG SODIUM
  Thousand Island Dressing

NACHOS, ETC.

200-250MG SODIUM
  Cheddar Melt

SIDE ITEMS – *exceed 500mg sodium.*

SAUCES

100-150MG SODIUM
  Green Sauce • Hot Sauce

DESSERTS

0-50MG SODIUM
  Fruit-Filled Empanada
50-100MG SODIUM
  Cinnamon Crustos

Menu Item	Cal	Fat	Sat	TFat	Chol	Carb	Fib	Sug	Sod

TCBY

SOFT SERVE FROZEN YOGURT AND SORBET *(1/2 cup)*

Menu Item	Cal	Fat	Sat	TFat	Chol	Carb	Fib	Sug	Sod
Frozen Yogurt, NF, No Sugar Added	90	0	0	0	5	20	0	7	35
Sorbet, NF & Nondairy	100	0	0	0	0	24	0	19	30
Frozen Yogurt, NF	110	0	0	0	5	23	0	20	60
Frozen Yogurt, 96% FF	140	3	2	0	15	23	0	20	60
Low Carb Frozen Yogurt	110	7	5	0	25	16	7	3	60

HAND-SCOOPED FROZEN YOGURT AND SORBET

Menu Item	Cal	Fat	Sat	TFat	Chol	Carb	Fib	Sug	Sod
Rocky Road	220	7	4	0	5	36	1	27	25
Psychedelic Sorbet	290	0	0	0	0	75	0	55	30
Choc Choc Swirl	120	4	2	0	15	19	1	16	50
Strawberries & Cream	120	3	2	0	10	21	0	18	50
Mint Choc Chunk or Vanilla Choc Chunk	140	5	4	0	10	22	0	18	55
Cotton Candy or Rainbow Cream	120	4	2	0	15	20	0	16	60
Vanilla Bean	120	4	2	0	15	19	0	16	60
Vanilla, No Sugar Added	80	1	0	0	0	19	5	6	60

SMOOTHIES

20 oz w/o Yogurt:

Menu Item	Cal	Fat	Sat	TFat	Chol	Carb	Fib	Sug	Sod
Raspberry Revitalizer	300	0	0	0	0	79	6	71	0
Peachy Lean	360	0	0	0	0	96	1	93	30

NOTE: Raspberry Revitalizer has the least sodium, Peachy Lean has the most; the other varieties fall in between.

20 oz w/Yogurt:

Menu Item	Cal	Fat	Sat	TFat	Chol	Carb	Fib	Sug	Sod
Berry Slim or Healthy Balance	410	3	2	-	10	95	2	91	50
Raspberry DeLITE	360	3	2	-	10	85	4	81	50
Tropical Replenisher	370	3	2	-	10	87	1	85	50
Raspberry Revitalizer	370	3	2	-	10	84	3	77	50

32 oz w/o Yogurt:

Menu Item	Cal	Fat	Sat	TFat	Chol	Carb	Fib	Sug	Sod
Raspberry DeLITE	300	0	0	0	0	74	4	67	25
A Lotta Coloda	620	15	13	0	10	122	3	113	75

NOTE: Raspberry DeLITE has the least sodium, A Lotta Coloda has the most; the other varieties fall in between.

32 oz w/Yogurt:

Menu Item	Cal	Fat	Sat	TFat	Chol	Carb	Fib	Sug	Sod
Raspberry Revitalizer	530	4	2	0	10	124	4	113	75
Peachy Lean	620	4	3	0	10	151	1	147	100

NOTE: Raspberry Revitalizer has the least sodium, Peachy Lean has the most; the other varieties fall in between.

Menu Item	Cal	Fat	Sat	TFat	Chol	Carb	Fib	Sug	Sod

(TIM HORTONS)

DONUTS

150-200MG SODIUM
Yeast: Choc Dip • Honey Dip • Maple Dip
200-250MG SODIUM
Yeast: Dutchie
Cake: Sour Cream Plain • Old Fashioned Plain • Old Fashioned Glazed
Filled: Blueberry • Strawberry • Angel Cream

TIMBITS

0-50MG SODIUM
Dutchie
50-100MG SODIUM
All other timbits

MUFFINS – *exceed 450mg sodium*

BAGELS

350-400MG SODIUM
Cinnamon Raisin
400-450MG SODIUM
Sesame Seed • Poppyseed • Plain
Other bagels exceed 450mg sodium.

SPECIALTY BAKED GOODS

150-200MG SODIUM
Maple Pecan Danish
200-250MG SODIUM
Choc Danish • Cherry Cheese Danish
Other baked goods exceed 350mg sodium.

SANDWICHES

750-800MG SODIUM
Egg Salad w/Lettuce
Other sandwiches exceed 800mg sodium.

SOUPS – *exceed 850mg sodium*

750-800MG SODIUM
Egg Salad w/Lettuce

COOKIES

100-150MG SODIUM
Triple Choc • M&M w/Choc Chip • Choc Chip • Oatmeal Raisin •
Peanut Butter Choc Chunk

WENDY'S

Menu Item	Cal	Fat	Sat	TFat	Chol	Carb	Fib	Sug	Sod

TIM HORTONS (CONT'D)

SPECIALTY DRINKS

50-100MG SODIUM
  Iced cappuccino
150-200MG SODIUM
  Cafe Mocha • Hot Smoothee
200-250MG SODIUM
  French Vanilla • English Toffee
Other drinks exceed 400mg sodium.

WENDY'S

BURGERS AND SANDWICHES

Menu Item	Cal	Fat	Sat	TFat	Chol	Carb	Fib	Sug	Sod
Jr. Hamburger	280	9	4	1	30	34	1	7	600
Jr. Bacon Cheeseburger	370	17	7	1	50	34	2	6	750
Jr. BBQ Cheeseburger	330	13	6	1	40	36	1	8	800
Crispy Chicken Sandwich	380	15	3	2	35	43	1	5	810
Jr. Cheeseburger	320	13	6	1	40	34	1	7	820

NOTE: Remove dill pickles and eliminate 150mg sodium; change American cheese to Swiss and save 135mg sodium.

CHICKEN STRIPS AND NUGGETS

Menu Item	Cal	Fat	Sat	TFat	Chol	Carb	Fib	Sug	Sod
4 Piece Nuggets, Kids' Meal	180	11	3	2	25	10	0	1	390
5 Piece Nuggets	220	14	3	2	35	13	0	1	490

DIPPINGS SAUCES

Menu Item	Cal	Fat	Sat	TFat	Chol	Carb	Fib	Sug	Sod
Sweet and Sour Sauce	50	0	0	0	0	13	0	11	120
Barbecue Sauce	45	0	0	0	0	10	0	8	170
Spicy Southwest Chipotle Sauce	150	15	3	0	25	5	0	1	180

SALADS *(W/O DRESSING)*

Menu Item	Cal	Fat	Sat	TFat	Chol	Carb	Fib	Sug	Sod
Side Salad	35	0	0	0	0	8	2	4	25
Caesar Side w/o croutons	70	5	2	0	15	3	2	1	135
Mandarin Chicken® w/o noodles & almonds	170	2	1	0	60	18	3	13	480
Caesar Chicken w/o croutons	180	5	3	0	70	9	4	4	550

SALAD DRESSINGS AND TOPPINGS

Menu Item	Cal	Fat	Sat	TFat	Chol	Carb	Fib	Sug	Sod
Roasted Almonds	130	11	1	0	0	4	2	1	70
Homestyle Garlic Croutons	70	3	0	0	0	9	0	0	125
FF French Dressing	80	0	0	0	0	19	0	16	210
Caesar Dressing	120	13	3	0	20	5	1	0	220

Other salad dressings exceed 300mg sodium.

BAKED POTATOES

Menu Item	Cal	Fat	Sat	TFat	Chol	Carb	Fib	Sug	Sod
Plain Potato	270	0	0	0	0	61	7	3	25
Sour Cream & Chives Potato	320	4	2	0	10	63	7	4	55

Menu Item	Cal	Fat	Sat	TFat	Chol	Carb	Fib	Sug	Sod
WENDYS (POTATOES CONT'D)									
Plain Potato w/Buttery Best Spread	320	6	1	0	0	61	7	3	115
SIDE ITEMS									
Baked Lay's	130	2	0	0	0	26	2	2	200
French Fries, Kids' Meal	280	14	3	4	0	37	3	0	270
Other sides exceed 400mg sodium.									
DESSERTS AND FROSTY™									
Mandarin Orange Cup	80	0	0	0	0	19	1	17	15
LF Strawberry Flavored Yogurt	140	2	1	0	5	27	0	11	85
Junior Frosty™	160	4	3	0	20	29	0	22	75
Fix 'N Mix Frosty - M&Ms®	310	10	6	0	25	49	1	40	95
Fix 'N Mix Frosty - Butterfinger®	300	9	5	0	20	49	1	36	145
Small Frosty™	330	8	5	0	35	56	0	42	150

(WHATABURGER)

Contact Whataburger® or their website (www.whataburger.com) for nutritional info.

BREAKFAST

SANDWICHES

600-650MG SODIUM

Egg Sandwich

650-700MG SODIUM

Taquito w/Sausage and Egg

Other sandwiches exceed 700mg sodium.

SIDES

300-350MG SODIUM

Cinnamon Roll

Other sides exceed 400mg sodium.

SANDWICHES

BURGERS

300-350MG SODIUM

Whataburger,® no bun

450-500MG SODIUM

Double Meat Whataburger,® no bun

600-650MG SODIUM

Grilled Chicken, no bun

650-700MG SODIUM

Whataburger, Jr.® • Justaburger®

Other burgers and sandwiches exceed 700mg sodium

CHICKEN ENTREES – *exceed 700mg sodium.*

WHITE CASTLE

Menu Item	Cal	Fat	Sat	TFat	Chol	Carb	Fib	Sug	Sod

WHATABURGER (CONT'D)

SALADS *(W/O DRESSING)*

0-50MG SODIUM

  Garden Salad w/o Cheese

250-300MG SODIUM

  Garden Salad w/Cheese

Other salads exceed 650mg sodium.

SALAD DRESSINGS

350-400MG SODIUM

  Reduced Fat Ranch

Other salad dressings exceed 450mg sodium.

SIDE ITEMS

200-250MG SODIUM

  French Fries, small

Other sides exceed 450mg sodium.

DESSERTS AND SHAKES

0-50MG SODIUM

  Choc Chunk Cookie • Oatmeal Raisin Cookie • Peanut Butter Cookie

50-100MG SODIUM

  White Choc Macadamia Nut Cookie

200-250MG SODIUM

  Choc, Strawberry, or Vanilla Shake (Kid's, 16 oz)

Other desserts and shakes exceed 250mg.

(WHITE CASTLE)

SANDWICHES

Menu Item	Cal	Fat	Sat	TFat	Chol	Carb	Fib	Sug	Sod
White Castle Burger, 1	140	7	3	1	15	13	1	1	240
Cheeseburger, 1	160	9	5	1	20	13	1	2	360
Double White Castle, 1	250	14	6	1	30	19	1	2	400
Jalapeño Cheeseburger, 1	170	10	5	1	25	13	1	2	410
Fish w/Cheese, 1	180	8	3	1	25	18	1	2	420
Chicken Ring Sandwich w/Cheese, 1	190	10	4	-	30	17	1	2	490

SIDE ITEMS

Menu Item	Cal	Fat	Sat	TFat	Chol	Carb	Fib	Sug	Sod
French Fries, small (avg)	310	15	3	4	0	39	4	1	250
Onion Rings, 4 rings	230	12	2	3	0	28	1	4	260

Other sides exceed 300mg sodium.

SHAKES

NOTE: A small shake has anywhere from 280mg to 550mg sodium depending on the region of the country.

Menu Item	Cal	Fat	Sat	TFat	Chol	Carb	Fib	Sug	Sod

RESTAURANT QUICK REFERENCE

Use this guide to find the fast food restaurants offering the lowest sodium items in each of the following categories.

BURGERS, HOT DOGS WITH FRIES OR ONION RINGS

KRYSTAL

Menu Item	Cal	Fat	Sat	TFat	Chol	Carb	Fib	Sug	Sod
Krystal Sandwich	160	7	3	-	20	17	1	1	260
Cheese Krystal	180	9	4	-	25	17	2	1	430
Bacon Cheese Krystal	190	10	5	-	25	16	2	2	430
Fries, regular	470	20	8	-	20	53	7	0	90

WHITE CASTLE

Menu Item	Cal	Fat	Sat	TFat	Chol	Carb	Fib	Sug	Sod
White Castle Burger, 1	140	7	3	1	15	13	1	1	240
Cheeseburger, 1	160	9	5	1	20	13	1	2	360
Double White Castle, 1	250	14	6	1	30	19	1	2	400
Jalapeño Cheeseburger, 1	170	10	5	1	25	13	1	2	410
French Fries, small (avg)	310	15	3	4	0	39	4	1	250

WHATABURGER

Menu Item	Cal	Fat	Sat	TFat	Chol	Carb	Fib	Sug	Sod
Whataburger,® no bun									300-350
Double Meat Whataburger,® no bun									450-500
French Fries, small									200-250

FLAMERS

Menu Item	Cal	Fat	Sat	TFat	Chol	Carb	Fib	Sug	Sod
Charbroiled Chicken w/o pickles									300-350
Lemon Pepper Chicken w/o pickles									300-350
Cajun Chicken w/o pickles									300-350
Hamburger, 4 oz or 6 oz w/o pickles									400-450
BBQ Chicken w/o pickles									400-450

CULVER'S

Menu Item	Cal	Fat	Sat	TFat	Chol	Carb	Fib	Sug	Sod
Corn Dog (kids' meal)									500-550
Fries, Junior or Seasoned Green Beans									0-50

IN-N-OUT BURGER

Menu Item	Cal	Fat	Sat	TFat	Chol	Carb	Fib	Sug	Sod
Hamburger, Protein Style *(bun replaced with lettuce)*	240	17	4	-	40	11	3	7	370
French Fries	400	18	5	-	0	54	2	0	245

FLAMERS

Menu Item	Cal	Fat	Sat	TFat	Chol	Carb	Fib	Sug	Sod
Charbroiled Chicken w/o pickles									300-350
Lemon Pepper Chicken w/o pickles									300-350
Cajun Chicken w/o pickles									300-350

Menu Item	Cal	Fat	Sat	TFat	Chol	Carb	Fib	Sug	Sod
BURGERS, HOT DOGS WITH FRIES/ONION RINGS (FLAMERS CONT'D)									
Hamburger, 4 oz or 6 oz w/o pickles									400-450
BBQ Chicken w/o pickles									400-450
CARL'S JR.									
Sourdough Bacon Cheeseburger									450-500
French Fries (kids or small)									150-200
BURGER KING									
Whopper Jr.® w/o pickles									450-500
Whopper Jr.® w/o mayo									450-500
The Angus Steak Burger, Low Carb									450-500
French Fries, small, unsalted									200-250
Onion Rings, small									250-300
MCDONALD'S									
Hamburger									500-550
French Fries (small)									100-150

(SANDWICHES)

Menu Item	Cal	Fat	Sat	TFat	Chol	Carb	Fib	Sug	Sod
AU BON PAIN									
Classic Grilled Cheese	560	22	14	-	64	68	3	3	374
Grilled Chicken	394	24	4	-	55	28	1	0	494
D'ANGELO									
Classic Veggie No Cheese Pokket									400-450
Hamburger or Steak Pokket									400-450
Salad or Turkey Pokket									450-500
SONIC DRIVE-IN									
Breaded Chicken Sandwich									400-450
BOJANGLES									
Cajun Filet w/o Mayo	337	11	5	-	45	41	3	-	401
w/Mayo	437	22	7	-	55	41	3	-	506
Grilled Filet w/o Mayo	235	5	3	-	51	25	2	-	540
STEAK ESCAPE									
Steak, kid's	210	3	-	-	13	29	-	-	445
Chicken, kid's	205	7	-	-	32	29	-	-	470
KFC									
Honey BBQ KFC® Snacker									450-500
SCHLOTZSKY'S DELI									
Classic Swiss & Tomato Panini									500-550

(SUBS)

Menu Item	Cal	Fat	Sat	TFat	Chol	Carb	Fib	Sug	Sod
COUSINS SUBS									
7 1/2" Lower Fat Garden Veggie									350-400

Menu Item	Cal	Fat	Sat	TFat	Chol	Carb	Fib	Sug	Sod
SUBS (COUSINS SUBS CONT'D)									
7 1/2" Lower Fat Roast Beef									450-500
4" Mini Seafood w/Crab or Tuna									500-550
D'ANGELO *(SMALL ON HONEY WHEAT)*									
Turkey D'Lite (Kidz Meal)									350-400
Steak or Cheeseburger Sub (Kidz Meal)									450-500
Hamburger, Salad, or Turkey									450-500
SUBWAY									
6" Vegie Delite® w/o cheese	230	3	1	0	0	44	4	7	520

(WRAPS)

Menu Item	Cal	Fat	Sat	TFat	Chol	Carb	Fib	Sug	Sod
D'ANGELO *(WHITE WRAP)*									
Steak, Salad, or Hamburger Wrap									300-350
Turkey Wrap									350-400
Roast Beef Wrap									500-550
AU BON PAIN									
Riviera Chopped Wrap	227	14	4	-	21	21	2	16	431
Riviera Tuna Wrap	244	16	4	-	16	11	2	8	562

(POULTRY OR FISH WITH SIDE DISHES)

Menu Item	Cal	Fat	Sat	TFat	Chol	Carb	Fib	Sug	Sod
KOO KOO ROO									
Fresh Roasted Turkey, Sliced Breast									50-200
Add a side:									
Sticky Rice or Butternut Squash									0-50
Tossed Salad w/o Dressing									0-50
Baked Yams or Celery Sticks, 6									0-50
Steamed Vegetables									0-50
Cantaloupe and Honeydew									0-50
Lahvash, 1 pc									50-100
Italian Vegetable									100-150
Cucumber Salad or Tangy Tomato Salad									150-200
Kernel Corn or Green Beans									150-200
SKIPPER'S									
Grilled Salmon or Halibut Fillet									50-100
Grilled Chicken Breast									50-100
Add a side:									
Green Salad w/o dressing, lrg or sm									0-50
Plain Baked Potato or Grilled Veggies									0-50
Coleslaw, small									150-200

Menu Item	Cal	Fat	Sat	TFat	Chol	Carb	Fib	Sug	Sod

POULTRY OR FISH WITH SIDE DISHES (CONT'D)

LONG JOHN SILVER'S

Menu Item	Cal	Fat	Sat	TFat	Chol	Carb	Fib	Sug	Sod
Battered Shrimp									150-200
Baked Cod									200-250
Add a side:									
Corn Cobbette									0-50
Hushpuppie									200-250
Cocktail Sauce • Tartar Sauce									200-250
Cheesestick, Cole Slaw, or Fries (reg)									300-350

EL POLLO LOCO

Menu Item	Cal	Fat	Sat	TFat	Chol	Carb	Fib	Sug	Sod
Leg or Thigh									200-250
Kid's Meal Drumstick Chicken									200-250
Wing									300-350
Add a side:									
3" Corn Cobbette									0-50
Fresh Vegetables									50-100
3 Corn Tortillas									100-150

CHURCH'S CHICKEN

Menu Item	Cal	Fat	Sat	TFat	Chol	Carb	Fib	Sug	Sod
Original Leg									250-300
Add a side:									
Corn on the Cob									0-50
Cole Slaw or Collard Greens									150-200

POPEYES

Menu Item	Cal	Fat	Sat	TFat	Chol	Carb	Fib	Sug	Sod
Leg, Spicy (skin & breading removed)									250-300
Wing, Spicy (skin & breading removed)									300-350
Chicken Sausage Jambalaya									350-400
Chicken Étouffée									400-450
Add a side:									
Corn on the Cob									0-50

BOSTON MARKET

Menu Item	Cal	Fat	Sat	TFat	Chol	Carb	Fib	Sug	Sod
Roasted Sirloin (5 oz) or 1/4 Dark Original Rotisserie Chicken, no skin (5 oz)									250-300
Add a side:									
Cranberry Walnut Relish									0-50
Fresh Steamed Vegetables									0-50
Fresh Fruit Salad or Cinnamon Apples									0-50
Sweet Corn or Garlic Dill New Potatoes									100-150
Garden Fresh Coleslaw									150-200
Chicken Noodle Soup (6 oz)									150-200
Sweet Potato Casserole or Cornbread									200-250

Menu Item	Cal	Fat	Sat	TFat	Chol	Carb	Fib	Sug	Sod

POULTRY OR FISH WITH SIDE DISHES (CONT'D)

KFC

Menu Item	Cal
Whole Wing, Original or Extra Crispy	350-400
Add a side:	
Corn on the Cob, 3" or 5.5"	0-50
Baked! Cheetos®	200-250
Cole Slaw	300-350
Mashed Potatoes w/o Gravy	300-350

(TACOS, BURRITOS AND OTHER MEXICAN)

RUBIOS FRESH MEXICAN GRILL

Menu Item	Cal
Origingal Fish Taco (Kid's Meal)	100-150
HealthMex MahiMahi Taco	150-200
MahiMahi or Chicken Street Taco	200-250
Original Fish Taco	200-250
2 Taquitos (Kid's Meal)	200-250
Carnitas Street Taco or 3 Chicken Taquitos	250-300
Fish Taco Especial	300-350
Carne Asada Street	350-400
HealthMex Chicken Taco	350-400

DEL TACO

Menu Item	Cal
Taco	150-200
Soft Taco	300-350
Carne Asada Taco or Crispy Fish Taco	450-500

BAJA FRESH MEXICAN GRILL

Menu Item	Cal
Baja Style, Charbroiled Steak	200-250
Baja Style, Chicken	200-250
Baja Style, Charbroiled Shrimp	250-300
Baja Style, Savory Pork Carnitas	250-300
Grilled MahiMahi or Baja Fish Taco	400-450

EL POLLO LOCO

Menu Item	Cal
Taco Al Carbon	200-250
Chicken Soft Taco	500-550

LA SALSA FRESH MEXICAN GRILL

Menu Item	Cal
Taco La Salsa® w/Chicken (w/o chips)	250-300
Taco La Salsa® w/Steak (w/o chips)	300-350
Baja Fish Taco (w/o chips)	350-400
Taco La Salsa® w/Carnitas (w/o chips)	350-400
Baja Style Shrimp (w/o chips)	450-500

Menu Item	Cal	Fat	Sat	TFat	Chol	Carb	Fib	Sug	Sod
TACOS, BURRITOS AND OTHER MEXICAN (CONT'D)									
TACO JOHN'S									
Crispy Taco or Steak Softshell									250-300
Softshell Taco									450-500
JACK IN THE BOX									
Regular Beef Taco	160	8	3	1	15	15	2	4	270
Beef Monster Taco®	240	14	5	2	20	20	3	4	390
TACO DEL MAR									
Hard Taco, Chicken	260	13	5	-	45	16	1	1	360
Hard Taco, Fish	270	15	4	-	30	23	1	1	360
Hard Taco, Pork	260	14	5	-	45	17	1	1	370
Soft Taco, Chicken	260	9	4	-	45	27	3	1	430
Soft Taco, Fish	270	11	4	-	30	34	3	1	440
Soft Taco, Pork	260	10	4	-	45	28	3	1	450
Kids Taco, Beef	270	15	6	-	30	16	1	1	460
Kids Quesadilla & Chips	600	27	8	-	30	71	4	1	490
TACO BELL									
Taco, Regular or Taco Supreme®									350-400
Crunchy Taco, "Fresco Style"									350-400
TACO TIME									
Crsip Bean Burrito									450-500

(**PIZZA**)

DOMINO'S PIZZA
Build a Pizza *(1/8 SLICE UNLESS NOTED)*:

Menu Item	Cal	Fat	Sat	TFat	Chol	Carb	Fib	Sug	Sod
Crusts									
Crunchy Thin, 12"	80	4	1	0	0	12	1	1	15
Crunchy Thin, 14"	110	5	1	0	0	16	1	1	20
Ultimate Deep Dish, 12"	160	3	1	0	0	28	1	3	110
Ultimate Deep Dish, 14"	220	4	1	0	0	38	2	3	150
Toppings									
Pineapple, Mushrooms, Bell Peppers, Tomatoes									
Onions, Chili Peppers, & Garlic (avg)	3	0	0	0	0	3	0	1	1
Anchovies	0	0	0	0	0	0	0	0	35
Cheddar Cheese (avg)	32	3	2	0	7	0	0	0	50
Crunchy Thin Crust *(1 SLICE)*:									
Vegi Feast®, 12"	160	10	4	0	15	16	2	2	355
Barbecue Feast, 12"	210	12	5	0	20	20	1	5	375
Philly Cheese Steak, 12"	180	11	6	0	20	13	1	1	375
Deluxe Feast®, 12"	180	12	4	0	15	16	2	2	395

Menu Item	Cal	Fat	Sat	TFat	Chol	Carb	Fib	Sug	Sod

PIZZA (CONT'D)

LITTLE CAESAR'S

Cheese, thin crust, 12", 1/8 slice									150-200
Cheese, 14" thin crust, 1/10 slice									200-250
Cheese, 12", 1/8 slice									250-300
Pepperoni, 14" thin crust									250-300
Cheese, 14", 1/10 slice									300-350
Cheese, 16", 1/12 or 18", 1/14 slice									300-350
Cheese, deep dish, medium, 1/8 slice									300-350

ADD TOPPINGS *(PER SLICE)*

Mushrooms, Pineapple, Onions, Tomato									0-50
Green Peppers & Black Olives									0-50
Sausage, Ham, Beef, or Hot Peppers									50-100

GODFATHER'S PIZZA

Mini, Original Crust, 1/4

Cheese									200-250
Hawaiian or Super Hawaiian									250-300
Pepperoni or Veggie									250-300

Medium, Thin Crust, 1/8

Pepperoni									200-250
Cheese									250-300
Veggie, Hawaiian, or Super Hawaiian									300-350

Large, Thin Crust, 1/10

Cheese									300-350

HUNGRY HOWIES PIZZA

Thin Crust

Cheese, medium, 1/8 slice									250-300
Cheese, large, 1/10 slice									300-350

PAPA MURPHY'S

Thin Crust:, 1/10 slice

	Cal	Fat	Sat	TFat	Chol	Carb	Fib	Sug	Sod
Cheese deLITE	140	7	4	0	20	13	1	2	270
Veggie deLITE	150	8	4	0	20	13	1	1	275
Gourmet Vegetarian	160	9	4	0	21	13	1	1	290
Veggie Mediterranean	165	9	4	0	20	15	2	3	325
Hawaiian deLITE	150	7	4	0	22	15	1	4	335

(POTATOES)

WENDY'S

	Cal	Fat	Sat	TFat	Chol	Carb	Fib	Sug	Sod
Sour Cream & Chives Potato	320	4	2	0	10	63	7	4	55
Plain Potato w/Buttery Best Spread	320	6	1	0	0	61	7	3	115

Menu Item	Cal	Fat	Sat	TFat	Chol	Carb	Fib	Sug	Sod

POTATOES (CONT'D)

ARBY'S

Menu Item	Cal	Fat	Sat	TFat	Chol	Carb	Fib	Sug	Sod
Sour Cream Baked Potato									0-50
Baked Potato w/Butter and Sour Cream									150-200
Deluxe Baked Potato									300-350

STEAK ESCAPE

Menu Item	Cal	Fat	Sat	TFat	Chol	Carb	Fib	Sug	Sod
Smashed Potato w/Portabello	290	1	0	0	0	63	-	-	93
Smashed Potato w/Steak	393	5	-	-	103	55	-	-	313
Smashed Potato w/Chicken	383	4	-	-	108	56	-	-	475
Loaded Smashed Potato, Ranch & Bacon	692	34	-	-	29	87	-	-	501

SCHLOTZSKY'S DELI

Menu Item	Cal	Fat	Sat	TFat	Chol	Carb	Fib	Sug	Sod
Bacon & Cheddar									250-300

(SALADS)

SOUP PLANTATION / SWEET TOMATOES

TOSSED SALADS

Menu Item	Cal	Fat	Sat	TFat	Chol	Carb	Fib	Sug	Sod
Strawberry Fields w/Walnuts	130	8	1	0	0	15	3	12	75
Honey Minted Fruit Toss	140	6	4	0	0	20	3	15	80
Bombay Curry w/Almonds & Coconut	210	16	4	0	10	17	4	11	85
Watercress and Orange	90	4	1	0	0	12	2	6	90
Cherry Chipolte Spinach	220	15	2	0	0	20	2	10	90
Outrageous Orange w/Cashews	200	14	2	0	10	16	2	8	95
Mandarin Spinach w/Walnuts	170	11	1	0	0	14	3	11	150
Roma Tomato, Mozzarella & Basil	120	9	2	0	10	7	1	2	180
Barlett Pear & Caramelized Walnut	180	12	2	0	5	13	2	10	220
Won Ton Chicken Happiness	150	8	1	0	10	12	2	4	220
San Marino Spinach w/Pumpkin Seeds	200	15	4	0	15	11	6	5	220
Ensalada Azteca w/Turkey	130	9	3	0	15	7	4	3	230
Summer Lemon w/Spiced Pecans	220	15	3	0	10	18	2	13	250

SIGNATURE SALADS *(1/2 CUP UNLESS NOTED)*

Menu Item	Cal	Fat	Sat	TFat	Chol	Carb	Fib	Sug	Sod
Carrot Ginger w/Herb Vinaigrette	150	12	1	0	0	9	3	6	40
Dijon Potato w/Garlic Dill Vinaigrette	150	12	1	0	0	9	3	6	40
Carrot Raisin, LF	90	3	0	0	5	17	2	15	80
Oriental Ginger Slaw w/Krab, LF	70	3	0	0	2	8	4	3	80
Ambrosia w/Coconut	170	6	3	0	5	30	2	20	80
Poppyseed Coleslaw	120	9	1	0	10	9	3	5	130
Confetti Avocado Slaw	120	7	1	0	5	12	3	3	150
Baja Bean and Cilantro, LF	180	3	0	0	0	29	5	2	190
Pineapple Coconut Slaw	150	10	3	0	15	14	2	10	190
Marinated Summer Vegetables, FF	80	0	0	0	0	19	4	14	210
Southern Black-Eyed Pea	130	6	0	0	0	18	3	4	220

Menu Item	Cal	Fat	Sat	TFat	Chol	Carb	Fib	Sug	Sod
SALADS (SOUP PLANTATION / SWEET TOMATOES CONT'D)									
Tomato Cucumber Marinade	80	5	0	0	0	8	1	2	220
Citrus Noodles w/Snow Peas	140	6	1	0	0	19	2	5	240
Italian Garden Vegetable	110	8	1	0	0	9	2	2	240
Roasted Potato w/Chipotle Chile	140	6	1	0	0	18	4	3	250
Joan's Broccoli Madness	180	14	3	0	10	11	3	9	250
SALAD DRESSINGS									
Sweet Maple	170	17	2	0	5	6	0	6	50
FF Honey Mustard	45	0	0	0	10	10	0	9	160
Basil Vinaigrette	160	17	1	0	0	1	0	0	160
AU BON PAIN *(W/O DRESSING)*									
Garden, small	50	1	0	0	0	10	3	2	10
Fresh Fruit & Yogurt	115	0	0	0	3	26	2	20	83
Garden, large	110	2	0	0	0	19	5	3	300
Caesar	240	11	6	0	25	23	4	4	310
Steak w/Cranberries & Mandarin Oranges	290	7	4	0	40	46	7	27	400
SALAD DRESSINGS *(2 TBSP)*									
Orange Citrus Vinaigrette	120	10	2	0	0	7	0	7	90
FF Raspberry	80	0	0	0	0	18	0	16	190
HUNGRY HOWIE'S									
Large or Small Garden									0-50
Large Chef, 1/4									300-350
Small Chef, 1/2									350-400
SALAD DRESSINGS									
Greek									50-100
French Style									150-200
D'ANGELO *(W/O DRESSING)*									
Tossed									0-50
Turkey									50-100
Roast Beef									200-250
SALAD DRESSINGS									
Honey Mustard									200-250
MCDONALD'S *(W/O DRESSING)*									
Side Salad or Asian Salad w/o chicken									0-50
Fruit & Walnut Salad									50-100
Caesar Salad w/o Chicken									150-200
Bacon Ranch w/o Chicken									250-300
CULVER'S									
Side Salad									100-150
Side Caesar									150-200
Garden Fresco									350-400

Menu Item	Cal	Fat	Sat	TFat	Chol	Carb	Fib	Sug	Sod
SALADS (CULVERS CONT'D)									
SALAD DRESSINGS									
Raspberry Vinaigrette									150-200
Ranch, Reduced Calorie									150-200
WHATABURGER									
Garden Salad w/o Cheese									0-50
Garden Salad w/Cheese									250-300
WENDY'S *(W/O DRESSING)*									
Caesar Side w/o croutons	70	5	2	0	15	3	2	1	135
Mandarin Chicken® w/o noodles & almonds	170	2	1	0	60	18	3	13	480
SALAD DRESSINGS AND TOPPINGS									
Roasted Almonds	130	11	1	0	0	4	2	1	70
Homestyle Garlic Croutons	70	3	0	0	0	9	0	0	125
ROUND TABLE PIZZA									
Garden Salad									200-250
Caesar Salad									350-400
KOO-KOO-ROO *(W/O DRESSING)*									
House Salad									200-250
Other salads exceed 850mg sodium.									
SALAD DRESSINGS									
Ranch or Caesar									200-250
PAPA MURPHY'S									
Caesar Salad	85	4	3	0	10	6	4	3	240
Garden Salad	160	11	6	0	23	10	5	3	380
EL POLLO LOCO *(W/O DRESSING)*									
Garden Salad									250-300
SALAD DRESSINGS									
Creamy Cilantro Dressing									250-300
STEAK ESCAPE									
Grilled Salad w/Steak	187	6	-	-	103	11	-	-	292
SALAD DRESSINGS									
Balsamic Vinaigrette	90	3	-	-	0	3	-	-	35
Ranch	83	9	-	-	5	0	-	-	137
SCHLOTZSKY'S DELI *(W/O DRESSING)*									
Caesar									300-350
Garden									450-500
DEL TACO									
Taco Salad									350-400
TACO JOHN'S									
Steak Festiva Salad w/o dressing									200-250

Menu Item	Cal	Fat	Sat	TFat	Chol	Carb	Fib	Sug	Sod
SALADS (TACO JOHN'S CONT'D)									
SALAD DRESSINGS									
House Dressing									350-400

SOUPS

Menu Item	Cal	Fat	Sat	TFat	Chol	Carb	Fib	Sug	Sod
SOUPLANTATION / SWEET TOMATOES									
Turkey Vegetable	180	8	3	-	30	15	2	4	140
Classical Shrimp Bisque	240	16	7	-	70	15	1	5	230
Country Corn & Red Potato Chowder	160	6	3	-	15	24	4	6	330
Cream of Chicken	250	15	6	-	40	21	2	3	350
AU BON PAIN									
Old Fashioned Tomato Rice, LS	80	1	0	0	0	16	2	4	230
Southwest Vegetable, LS	70	2	0	0	0	11	2	2	250
Jamaican Black Bean, LS	112	1	0	0	0	30	17	3	310
Tomato Basil Bisque, LS	140	5	4	0	20	20	4	12	330
D'ANGELO'S									
Hearty Vegetable, small									250-300
BRUEGGER'S									
Moroccan Stew									300-350

BREAKFAST – EGGS, FRENCH TOAST AND SANDWICHES

Menu Item	Cal	Fat	Sat	TFat	Chol	Carb	Fib	Sug	Sod
AU BON PAIN									
Arugula and Tomato Frittata	290	13	7	0	260	27	2	3	210
MCDONALDS									
Scrambled Eggs, 2									200-250
Hash Browns or English Muffin									250-300
TACO DEL MAR									
Eggs, 2 oz scoop	90	7	2	-	220	1	0	0	250
Egg & Cheese Taco, flour, refried	200	10	4	-	125	17	1	1	510
BREAKFAST SIDES									
Diced Potatoes, 1.75 oz	60	1	0	-	0	11	1	0	20
Hash Browns	110	6	1	-	0	13	2	0	140
Sausage	100	8	3	-	20	1	0	0	220
BURGER KING									
French Toast Sticks, 5 sticks									400-450
KRYSTAL									
Krystal Sunriser	240	14	5	-	255	14	2	1	460
DEL TACO									
Breakfast Burrito									500-550

QUICK REFERENCE
Bagels, Muffins, Pastries and Other Baked Goods

Menu Item	Cal	Fat	Sat	TFat	Chol	Carb	Fib	Sug	Sod

(BAGELS, MUFFINS, PASTRIES AND OTHER BAKED GOODS)

KRISPY KREME DOUGHNUTS

Menu Item	Cal	Fat	Sat	TFat	Chol	Carb	Fib	Sug	Sod
Cinnamon Twist	230	9	3	0	5	33	1	19	85
Sugar	200	12	3	4	5	21	0	10	95
Original Glazed	200	12	3	4	5	33	1	21	95
Original Glazed Doughnut Holes	200	11	3	4	5	24	1	13	95
Choc Iced Glazed	250	12	3	4	5	33	1	21	100
Choc Iced w/Sprinkles	260	12	3	4	5	38	1	24	100
Glazed Cinnamon	210	12	3	4	5	24	1	12	100
Maple Iced Glazed	240	12	3	4	5	32	1	20	100
Glazed Raspberry Filled	300	16	4	5	5	38	1	22	130
Cinnamon Bun	260	16	4	5	5	28	1	13	125
Glazed Lemon Filled	290	16	4	5	5	35	1	18	135
Powdered Strawberry Filled	290	16	4	5	5	33	1	13	135
Choc Iced Kreme Filled	350	20	5	6	5	38	1	23	140
Choc Iced Custard Filled	300	17	4	5	5	35	1	19	140
Glazed Kreme Filled	340	20	5	6	5	38	1	23	140
Powdered Blueberry Filled	290	16	4	5	5	33	1	14	140
Cinnamon Apple Filled	290	16	4	5	5	32	1	14	150
Key Lime Pie	320	17	5	5	5	40	1	24	150
Dulce De Leche	290	18	5	5	5	30	1	12	160
Caramel Kreme Crunch	350	19	5	5	5	43	1	25	170
New York Cheesecake	320	19	5	6	10	35	1	17	190

AU BON PAIN

MUFFINS, PASTRIES AND OTHER BAKED GOODS *(1 BAKED GOOD)*

Menu Item	Cal	Fat	Sat	TFat	Chol	Carb	Fib	Sug	Sod
Danish Pretzel	603	24	12	-	53	92	1	63	104
Cherry Strudel	390	19	0	0	0	49	1	5	135
Apple Strudel	410	18	0	0	0	56	1	19	140
Almond Artisan Pastry	464	30	14	-	123	41	2	12	143
Strawberry Puff Pastry	242	13	6	-	42	30	1	20	143
Hurricanes	622	12	3	-	2	130	4	80	146
Blueberry Sweet Cheese Artisan Pastry	408	23	13	-	105	44	1	14	151
Dutch Apple Nuns	307	12	3	-	24	49	3	19	162
Cinnamon Roll	300	13	7	0	30	39	2	8	250

CROISSANTS *(1 CROISSANT)*

Menu Item	Cal	Fat	Sat	TFat	Chol	Carb	Fib	Sug	Sod
Choc	340	17	10	0	30	42	3	17	190
Plain	270	15	8	0	40	28	1	4	200
Apple	230	10	6	0	25	31	2	11	230
Raspberry	340	18	10	1	55	39	1	16	270
Sweet Cheese	350	20	12	1	70	36	1	11	290

Menu Item	Cal	Fat	Sat	TFat	Chol	Carb	Fib	Sug	Sod

BAGELS, MUFFINS, PASTRIES AND OTHER BAKED GOODS (CONT'D)

DUNKIN' DONUTS

Menu Item	Cal	Fat	Sat	TFat	Chol	Carb	Fib	Sug	Sod
French Cruller									100-150
Glazed Lemon or Frosted Lemon Cake									150-200
Lemon Filled Munchkins									150-200
Glazed Cake Munchkins									150-200
Glazed Munchkin									200-250
Plain or Powdered Munchkin									200-250
Cinnamon Cake Munchkin									200-250
Jelly Filled Munchkin									200-250
Glazed Choc Cake Munchkin									200-250

SOUP PLANTATION / SWEET TOMATOES

Muffins:

Menu Item	Cal	Fat	Sat	TFat	Chol	Carb	Fib	Sug	Sod
French Quarter Praline	290	15	2	-	20	38	2	21	100
Apple Cinnamon, Cranberry Orange, or Fruit Medley Bran Muffin (avg)	80	1	0	-	0	17	1	14	110
Cappuccino Chip	160	4	2	-	25	28	1	15	160
Spiced Pumpkin w/Cranberries	180	7	1	-	25	29	1	18	170
Wildly Blue Blueberry, small	140	5	1	-	10	22	1	9	180
Pauline's Apple Walnut Cake	180	7	3	-	25	28	1	21	180
Apple Raisin or Banana Nut	150	7	1	-	10	22	1	9	190
Cherry Nut or Zucchini Nut	150	7	1	-	10	22	1	9	190
Tangy Lemon	140	4	1	-	10	24	1	13	190
Choc Brownie or Choc Chip	170	8	2	-	10	22	1	10	190
Country Blackberry	170	6	2	-	15	27	1	13	190
Taffy Apple	160	6	1	-	10	25	1	18	190
Black Forest	230	9	2	-	10	36	1	19	190

MY FAVORITE MUFFIN

Menu Item	Cal	Fat	Sat	TFat	Chol	Carb	Fib	Sug	Sod
All reg muffins except Lemon Poppyseed									100-150
Lemon Poppyseed or FF Cinnamon Bun									150-200
FF Raspberry Amaretto Muffin									150-200
FF Blueberry or FF Cherry Pie Muffin									150-200
Honey Grain Bagel									300-350

TIM HORTONS

Menu Item	Cal	Fat	Sat	TFat	Chol	Carb	Fib	Sug	Sod
Maple Pecan Danish									150-200
Choc Danish									200-250
Cherry Cheese Danish									200-250
Cinnamon Raisin Bagel									350-400
Sesame Seed									400-450
Poppyseed									400-450
Plain									400-450

Bagels, Muffins, Pastries and Other Baked Goods

Menu Item	Cal	Fat	Sat	TFat	Chol	Carb	Fib	Sug	Sod
BAGELS, MUFFINS, PASTRIES AND OTHER BAKED GOODS (CONT'D)									
BIG APPLE BAGELS									
Quiche Lorraine Bagel									250-300
Spinach Bagel									250-300
CHICK-FIL-A									
Cinnamon Cluster	370	12	5	2	35	60	1	30	260
Sunflower Multigrain Bagel	220	3	0	0	0	41	2	6	350

RESOURCES

DASH DIET

NHLBI Health Information Center (Publication #01-4082)
P.O. Box 30105
Bethesda, MD 20824-0105
301.592.8573 or 240.629.3255 (TTD)
www.nhlbi.nih.gov

ONLINE PRODUCTS AVAILABLE FROM MANUFACTURERS

Allen Canning Company
P.O. Box 250
Siloam Springs, AK 72761
www.allencanning.com

Alvarado Street Bakery
500 Martin Ave.
Rohnert Park, CA 94928
707.585.3293
www.alvaradostreetbakery.com

American Spoon
P.O. Box 566
Petoskey, MI 49770
888.735.6700 or 800.222.5886
www.spoon.com

Aunt Candice Foods
P.O. Box 93
Oak Grove, MI 48863
866.670.5968
www.auntcandicefoods.com

Authentic Foods
1850 W. 169th St., Suite B
Gardena, CA 90247
800.806.4737 or 310.366.7612
www.glutenfree-supermarket.com

Awrey Bakeries
12301 Farmington Road
Livonia, MI 48150
866.743.7525
www.awrey.com

Blazing Blends
908-507-4339
www.blazingblends.com

Canterbury Naturals
15500 Woodinville-Redmond Rd, C-400
Woodinville, WA 98072
800.588.9160 or 425.486.3334
www.conifer-inc.com

'Cause You're Special
P.O. Box 316
Phillips, WI 54555
866.669.4328 or 715.339.6959
www.causeyourespecial.com

Dixie Diners'
P.O. Box 1969
Tomball, TX 77377
800.233.3668
www.dixiediner.com

Dr. Praegers
www.drpraegers.com

ONLINE PRODUCTS AVAILABLE FROM MANUFACTURERS (CONT'D)

Eden Foods, Inc.
701 Tecumseh Rd.
Clinton, MI 49236
888.424.EDEN
www.edenfoods.com

Ener-G Foods
5960 First Ave. So.
Seattle, WA 98001
800.331.5222 or 206.870.4740
www.ener-g.com

French Meadow Bakery
2610 Lyndale Ave. So.
Minneapolis, MN 55408
877.NO.YEAST or 612.870.4740
www.frenchmeadow.com

Garden of Eatin'
800.434.4246
www.gardenofeatin.com

Gloria's Gourmet Foods
800.782.5881 or 802.388.6581
www.gloriasgourmet.com

Hodgson Mill
www.hodgsonmill.com

HolGrain (Conrad Rice Mill Inc.)
P.O. Box 10640
New Iberia, LA 70562
800.551.3245 or 337.364.7242
www.holgrain.com

The Lollipop Tree, Inc.
www.lollipoptree.com

Med-Diet Labs, Inc.
800.MED.DIET
www.med-diet.com

Melissa's
P.O. Box 21127
Los Angeles, CA 90021
800.588.0151
www.melissas.com

Montana Mills Bread Co.
2171 Monroe Ave., #205A
Rochester, NY 14618
877.MMBREAD
www.montanamills.com

Mozzarella Company
800.798.2954 or 214.741.4072
www.mozzco.com

Mr. Spice (Lang Naturals)
850 Aquidneck Ave.
Newport, RI 02842
800.SAUCE.IT or 401.848.7700
www.mrspice.com

Natural Ovens Bakery
P.O. Box 730
Manitowoc, Wi 54221-0730
800.772.0730
www.naturalovens.com

Nu-World Foods
630.369.6851
www.nuworldfoods.com

Pacific Bakery
P.O. Box 950
Oceanside, CA 92049
760.757.6020
www.pacificbakery.com

Papa Cheese Country Store
715.669.7620
www.papacheese.com

Private Harvest
www.privateharvest.com

ONLINE PRODUCTS AVAILABLE FROM MANUFACTURERS (CONT'D)

Rising Sun Farms
5126 So. Pacific Hwy.
Phoenix, OR 97535-6606
800.888.0795 X-211
www.risingsunfarms.com

Roberts American Gourmet
800.626.7557
www.robscape.com

Seneca Foods
3736 S. Main St.
Marion, NY 14505
315.926.8100
www.senecafoods.com

Tasty Baking Co. (Tastykake)
2801 Hunting Park Ave.
Philadelphia, PA 19129
800.33-TASTY
www.tastykake.com

Tillen Farms
866.972.6879
www.tillenfarms.com

Uncle Dave's Kitchen
www.vermontfinest.com

Vogue Cuisine, Inc.
3710 Grand View Blvd.
Los Angeles, CA 90066
888.236.4144
www.voguecuisine.com

Wax Orchards Inc.
22744 Wax Orchards Rd. SW
Vashon Island, WA 98070
800. 634.6132
www.waxorchards.com

Wolferman's
PO Box 15913
Shawnee Mission, KS 66285-5913
800.999.0169
www.wolfermans.com

Zadie's Low Sodium Seasonings
816.525.7004
www.zadies.com

ONLINE WEBSITES WITH LOW-SODIUM PRODUCTS

Amazon.com
www.amazon.com
Carries many low-sodium products

The Better Health Store
305 N. Clippert
Lansing, MI 48912
877.876.8247
www.thebetterhealthstore.com
Carries Amy's, Annie's Homegrown, Arrowhead Mills, Atkins, Barbara's Bakery, Bearitos, Bob's Red Mill, Breadshop, Cascadian Farm, Clif, Eat Well Be Well, Eden Foods, Ener-G, Enrico's, Erewhon, Flax Z Snax, Garden of Eatin, Guiltless Gourmet, Hain, Health Valley, Muir Glen, Nature's Path, Terra Chips, Tree of Life, Westbrae Natural, and more

CarbSmart, Inc.
18685-101 Main St., #101
Huntington Beach, CA 92648
www.carbsmart.com
Carries Arrowhead Mills, Atkins, Baja Bob's, Bob's Red Mill, Carborite, Dixie Diner, Eat Well Be Well, Fran Gare's, Gringo Billy, Heavenly Desserts, Jok 'n Al, La Nouba, Flax Z Snax, Mt. Olive, Steel's, Walden Farms, and more

The Dietary Shoppe, Inc.
4436 Ridge Ave.
Philadelphia, PA 19129
215.242.5302
www.DietaryShoppe.com
Carries Amy's, Annie's Naturals, Authentic Foods, Carmel, 'Cause You're Special, The Cravings Place, Ener-G, Erewhon, Glutano, Gluten Free Pantry, Health Valley, Jennie's, Mr. Spice, Nature's Path, Orgran, Steel's, Wax Orchards, and more

eDiet Shop
P.O. Box 1037
Evanston, IL 60204-1397
800.325.5409 or 847.679.5409
www.edietshop.com
Carries Baja Bob, Bernard, Calorie Control, Longhorn Grill, San Sucre, Steel's, Sweet N' Low, Walden Farms

eFood Pantry
2520 S. Grand Ave. East
Springfield, IL 62703
800.238.8090
www.efoodpantry.com
Carries Fifty/50, Frank Sinatra, Orgran, Pritikin, Sweet'N Low

Fresh Direct
www.freshdirect.com
Online regional grocer carrying many low-sodium products

GlutenFreeMall.com
www.glutenfreemall.com
Carries Authentic Foods, 'Cause You're Special, Creme De La Creme, Glutano, Mr. Spice, Nu-World Foods, Tartex and more

The Gluten-Free Pantry
P.O. Box 840
Glastonbury, CT 06033
800.291.8386
www.glutenfree.com
Carries Bumble Bar, Ener-G, Glenny's, Glutano, Gluten-Free Pantry, Omega Smart, Orgran

Healthy Heart Market
800.753.0310
www.healthyheartmarket.com
Carries 4C, Albertos, Arrowhead Mills, Ass Kickin', B&G, Bearitos, Bernard, Bob's Red Mill, Breadshop, Campbell's, Cannon, Chef Paul Prudhommes, Consorzio, Deboles, Diana's, Eden, Ener-G, Enrico's, Featherweight, Fisher & Wieser, Fortners, Frog Ranch, Frontier, Fry Krisp, Garden of Eatin, Garlic Survival, Gloria's, Gorgio, Hail Caesar, Health Valley, Mr. Spice, Muir Glen, Nantucket Off-Shore, Neera's, New Traditions, RW Knudsen, Robert's American Gourmet, Sadaf, Sgt. Pepper's, Slow Cooker Gourmet, Sweet 'N Low, and more

Kosher.com
866.567.4379
www.kosher.com
Carries Gefen, Goodman's, Kineret, Miko, Osem, Ratner's, Rokeach, Season, Streit, Tabatchnick and more

MyKosherMarket.com
www.mykoshermarket.com
Carries Empire Kosher, Gefen, Goodman's, Hain, J&J, Kineret, Osem, Ratner's, Rokeach, Season, Streit, Tabatchnick, and more

ONLINE WEBSITES WITH LOW-SODIUM FOODS (CONT'D)

MotherNature.com
www.mothernature.com
Carries Atkins, Eden, Genisoy, Spice Hunter, Rapunzel, and more

Netgrocer.com
www.netgrocer.com
Online grocer carrying many low-sodium products

Peaceworks
www.peaceworks.com
Carries Be Natural, Kind, Meditalia, Moshe & Ali

Peapod.com
www.peapod.com
Online regional market carrying many low-sodium foods

The Rice Diet Store
1644 Cole Mill Road
Durham, NC 27705
919.383.7276 x-226
www.ricedietstore.com
Carries Annie's Naturals, Bean Cuisine, Bearitos, Bionaturae, Cherchie's, Consorzio, Crown Prince, Desert Pepper, Eden, Enrico's, Frontier, Health Valley, Mr. Spice, Muir Glen, Nature's Path, Season, and more

Rokeach Kosher Food
80 Avenue K
Newark, NJ 07105
973.589.6145
www.rokeach.com
Carries Carmel, Mrs. Adler's, Rokeach

Salt Watcher, Inc.
2002 Covert St.
Pittsburgh, PA 15210
412.882.0243
www.saltwatcher.com
Carries 4C, Abeles & Heymann, Albertos, Barbara's Bakery, Bean Cuisine, Bearitos, Belgioioso, Bells, Blue Crab Bay, Blue Diamond, Cannon, Chef Paul Prudhommes, Consorzio, Crown Prince, Desert Pepper, Eden, Edward & Son, Enrico's, Ezekiel, Fifty/50, Fischer & Wieser, Frontier, Garden of Eatin', Garlic Survival, Gunthers, Haddon House, Hail Caesar, Health Valley, Heluva, Hillandale Farms, Jaclyns, KaMe, Kuner's, LaCostena, Lum Taylors, Manischewitz, Merry Goat, Muir Glen, Oetker, Osem, OTC, Paula's, Pearl Valley, Pitaland, RC, Reko, Season, San Sucre, Spice Hunter, Steels, Streits, Sweet 'N Low, Terra Chips, Tom Douglas, Venus, Zatarain, and more

www.ShopNatural.com
Carries Amy's, Annie's Homegrown, Annie's Naturals, Arrowhead Mills, Barbara's Bakery, Bionaturae, Bob's Red Mill, Breadshop, Cascadian Farm, Clif, Crown Prince, Deb-El, Deboles, Eden, Ener-G, Erewhon, Frontier, Garden of Eatin, Genisoy, Hain, Health Valley, Lundberg, Muir Glen, Natural Value, Nature's Path, Oetker, Orgran, Pamela's, RW Knudsen, Westbrae, and more

SimonDelivers.com
www.simondelivers.com
Online regional market carrying many low-sodium foods

RESOURCES

WellnessGrocer.com
888.272.8775
www.wellnessgrocer.com
Carries Alvarado Street Bakery, Amy's, Annie Chun's, Annie's Naturals, Arrowhead Mills, Barbara's Bakery, Bionaturae, Bob's Red Mill, Breadshop, Colavita, Consorzio, Crown Prince, Debole's, Eden, Ener-G, Enrico's, Food for Life, Frontier, Garden of Eatin', Gluten Free Pantry, Hain, Health is Wealth, Health Valley, Ian's, Jaclyn's, Maranatha, Moosewood, Muir Glen, Nature's Path, No Pudge, Rapunzel, Robert's American Gourmet, RW Knudsen, Season, Terra Chips, Tofurky, Westbrae, and more

WorldPantry.com, Inc.
1024 Illinois St.
San Francisco, CA 94107
866.972.6879 or 415.581.0067
www.worldpantry.com
Carries Annie Chun's, Bette's Diner, Heaven & Earth, Prairie Thyme, Tillen Farms

INDEX

InData Group, Inc.
P.O. Box 11908
Olympia, WA 98508-1908
360.432.7844 (tel)
800.897.8440 (toll free)
360.432.7838 (fax)

Pocket Guide to Low Sodium Foods is available from your local bookstore and online book retailers. To order autographed books directly from the publisher:

Internet orders: www.lowsaltfoods.com

Fax orders: 360.432.7838 (send this form)

Telephone orders: 800.897.8440 (credit card orders)

Mail orders: InData Group, Inc.
 P.O. Box 11908
 Olympia, WA 98508-1908, USA
 (send this form)

Please send me:

_____autographed copies of *Pocket Guide to Low Sodium Foods* at $8.95 each.   _____

Sales tax: Washington residents, please add 8.3%   _____

Shipping: U.S.(Priority) - $4.00 for first book and $2.00 for each additional book. International - $9.00 for first book and $5.00 for each additional book.   _____

TOTAL   _____

Credit Card ___VISA ___MasterCard   Exp. Date   _____

Credit Card #   _____

Name   _____

Address   _____

City _____State_____ Zip   _____